Wakefield Press

TRUSTED

Karen Starko is a physician, epidemiologist, and clinical trialist who trained in internal medicine at Boston City Hospital and in infectious diseases at Brown Affiliated Hospitals and Harvard University. She was an Epidemic Intelligence Service officer in the Field Services Division of the Center for Disease, United States Public Health Service, stationed at the Arizona Department of Health Services from 1978 to 1980.

TRUSTED

Children and Aspirin

A Deadly Dance of Science, Business, and Politics

Karen M. Starko

**Wakefield
Press**

Wakefield Press
16 Rose Street
Mile End
South Australia 5031
www.wakefieldpress.com.au

First published 2023

Cover designed by Stacey Zass
Edited by Julia Beaven, Wakefield Press
Typeset by Michael Deves, Wakefield Press
Printed in Australia by Pegasus Media & Logistics

ISBN 978 1 74305 957 9

A catalogue record for this
book is available from the
National Library of Australia

NATIONAL
LIBRARY
OF AUSTRALIA

CORIOLE
McLAREN VALE

Wakefield Press thanks
Coriole Vineyards for
continued support

For Oli, Steve, Alex, Caitlyn, Sarah, and Caroline

Paris savant says Aspirin revives withering flowers.

Special cable to the *New York Times*, 3 September 1923.

Contents

Author's Note

In 2001 the Centers for Disease Control (CDC) invited me to Atlanta to speak at the 50th Anniversary of the Epidemiology Intelligence Service (EIS). I had been an EIS officer from 1978–1980 when I investigated seven children with Reye's syndrome, a mysterious illness that had already killed thousands of perfectly healthy children. The investigation had been a breakthrough. I was honored by the invitation yet realized that my investigation was only a small part of a long history. Telling the story of this decades-long medical mystery, the keen, early observations, the forgotten clues, the blind alleys, and the role of opinion, marketing, and public health laws and regulations seemed essential.

In *Trusted*, I rely heavily on academic publications, government reports, news reports, and the perspectives of parents and professionals touched and motivated by the tragic deaths. A list of those interviewed can be found at the end of the book. Quotes from interviews are verbatim (lightly edited); conversations with me from the investigation period are reconstructed from my memory. During research for this book, records of the foundations were in storage and not available. I include historical details and perspectives learned after I began research for this book. These include the history of marketing practices, the possible role of aspirin in the 1918 influenza pandemic deaths, the crisis of accidental aspirin ingestion by toddlers from the 1950s to 70s, details of the growing pharmacology knowledge, and the history of public health law.

Two numbers should be kept in mind. Over the years, dose instructions for children appeared in many different forms: grains, milligrams (mg), milligrams per day, milligrams per kilogram of weight, etc. This undoubtedly led to some confusion. In 1965, F.T. Shannon, referring to aspirin, noted that "Standard reference works are often vague as to dosage and do not always relate dosage to weight."[1] In this book, I have converted all reported dosages to a standard mg/kg/day for a 16-kg four-year-old and, if not otherwise stated, I assumed a dose frequency of every four hours. The number you should keep in mind is that the recommended dose for children primarily ranged from 60–90 mg/kg/day. (See Appendix 1) A second important number is the level of salicylate in the blood. It was generally believed that levels above 25 mg/dL were necessary to treat those with serious rheumatic diseases[2] and that these patients should be carefully monitored for toxicity.

Finally, this book concerns classical Reye's syndrome, the illness that occurred in large numbers from 1950 through the mid-1980s and likely in smaller numbers for many years prior and after. Other similar illnesses, sometimes called Reye's-like illnesses, are uncommon and occur because of genetic errors in metabolism or ingestion of drugs such as valproic acid and others.[3] Cases of "Reye's syndrome" occurring now likely represent one of these conditions.

Karen M. Starko, July 2022

Glossary and Abbreviations

Glossary

Aspirin	Acetylsalicylate, a member of the salicylate family of drugs
Adenosine triphosphate (ATP)	Molecule that powers all body functions, including the critical function of preventing swelling of cells
Cerebral edema	Swelling of the brain
Dinitrophenol (DNP)	A drug formerly used for weight loss, chemical cousin to salicylate
Hepatocyte:	The main cell in the liver
Liver enzymes:	Proteins (most often SGOT and SGPT) spilled into the blood when the liver cell membrane is disrupted
Metabolism:	Life-sustaining chemical processes that: 1. Convert energy in food to a form that can be used by the body, 2. Convert food to the building blocks of the body (proteins, lipids, etc.), 3. Eliminate waste, e.g. drugs, chemicals, etc.
Mitochondria:	An organelle or small structure within cells. Mitochondria carry out the critical role of burning (oxidizing) food molecules (carbohydrates, fats, and proteins) and capturing the released energy in the chemical bonds of a molecule called ATP (adenosine triphosphate)
Poisoning	A condition of being markedly diminished by a substance; intoxication; toxicity (these terms are used interchangeably herein)
Salicylate	A drug that is converted to salicylate in the body such as salicylate, aspirin, sodium salicylate, methyl salicylate, and salicylate itself.
Salicylate levels	Studies show that blood levels above about 25 mg/dL were required to suppress severe inflammation in adults. However, at this level toxicity was common.

Abbreviations

AAP	American Academy of Pediatrics
CCC	Committee on the Care of Children
CDC	Center(s) for Disease Control
DHHS	Department of Health and Human Services
EIS	Epidemic Intelligence Service
FDA	Food and Drug Administration
FTC	Federal Trade Commission
HRG	(Public Citizen) Health Research Group
NIH	National Institutes of Health
NRSF [Colorado]	National [American] Reye's Syndrome Foundation (Colorado)
NRSF [Michigan]	National Reye's Syndrome Foundation (Michigan)
NRSF [Ohio]	National Reye's Syndrome Foundation (Ohio)
OTC	Over-the-counter, a term for drugs that can be purchased without a prescription
PHS	Public Health Service

Tables and Figures

Illustrations by Chapter

Preface

Quietly, through much of the mid-20th century, heartbroken parents on every continent buried their child just days after what seemed to be a simple cold or flu. Doctors found little evidence that the infection itself was the cause, but they did observe a striking pattern—symptoms of sudden, severe brain swelling and, in the very young, hypoglycemia. For decades the illness went largely unnoticed amid the major childhood infectious diseases slowly being dramatically reduced with antitoxins, antibiotics, or vaccination: smallpox and diphtheria first, pertussis during the 1930s, rheumatic fever and meningitis during the 1940s, polio during the 1950s, and measles during the 1960s. In 1963, meticulous Australian pathologist R.D.K. Reye and colleagues published their observation that the clinical pattern was accompanied by autopsy findings of an extremely wet brain and an unusual type of fat in cells known as fatty degeneration. The illness became known as Reye's syndrome. The adjective "rare" was soon applied. The truth is that in developed countries most child deaths after infancy are rare. Nevertheless, the term seemed to stall research interest as Reye's syndrome quietly took its place among the common causes of death in children.[1] For every death, many more children were hospitalized.[2] To raise awareness and promote research, devastated parents created foundations.

By 1978, there seemed to be no way to get a firm handle on causes or treatments. After attending a crash course in epidemiology as a rookie Center for Disease Control medical officer, I studied seven children hospitalized with the illness and their classmates and found a statistical link with taking recommended doses of aspirin, the popular, go-to medication upon which almost all parents relied to treat the minor illnesses of their children.

The link implied that either aspirin was responsible or that I had erred in my study methods. The former seemed preposterous and I, fresh out of training, possessed little experience-honed confidence. Whether driven by curiosity, a desire to protect my own child, or a compulsion to put the messy finding to rest, the link compelled me to devote time each day to the matter. I began with the *Index Medicus*, a truly huge, thin-papered tome containing a listing of every medical article ever written. There I found a long history explaining features of the mysterious illness and a parallel story of decades-long concerns regarding therapy with aspirin, also known as salicylate (aspirin belongs to the salicylate drug family). Complicating matters, however, was a sense that even when a fact seemed indisputable, a counter narrative of interpretations, beliefs, and assumptions seemed to stand by its side.

This is the story of the mysterious brain swelling illness, my journey of discovery, and the work of researchers, parents, public health professionals, and media that led to a warning on the product label for all. The arguments I will advance are that facts key to the solution of Reye's syndrome were known before Reye first described the syndrome, that these facts were scattered in libraries of paper-bound books and narrowly focused specialty silos, that discordant safety assessments influenced the market for aspirin, and that public health laws (and lack thereof) were instrumental in both the unfortunate duration of the tragedy and its spectacular solution.

The illness was generally not reportable to health authorities, but the number of children affected was likely staggering. From 1950 to 1985 in the United States as many as 100,000 children may have been affected including over 10,000 (and possibly up to 28,000) who died. (See Appendices 2 and 3) By comparison, as of 30 December 2021, 735 children died of COVID-19 in the United States.[3] Though the illness was reported in many countries including Australia, Canada, Czechoslovakia, England, Scotland, South Africa, and Thailand, the total number affected worldwide is still unknown.

Part I describes my early 1979 case-control study linking Reye's syndrome with aspirin use, the skepticism I encountered, parents' struggles, and a pivotal meeting arranged by a grieving father. Part II reveals the eye-opening saga of aspirin and children—from invention to convention, from prescription to over-the-counter marketing, from therapy to a difficult-to-diagnose poisoning, and from the idea of parental overuse to a possible issue with the drug regimen itself. In Part III, you will learn that Reye and colleagues (concurrently with rampant postwar marketing of aspirin during the 1950s) meticulously studied 21 children linking the devastating, mysterious illness with a unique pathology finding and that researchers found reasons to ignore aspirin. I uncover critical information in a government freezer and a draft FDA document in Part IV, as more case-control studies demonstrate the link and CDC publishes the link in 1980. Part V shows the responses of those who do not believe the studies, academics who recommend a warning to the public, industry's experts who believe the studies are grossly flawed, and FDA's 1982 decision to require a warning on the product label. Finally, Part VI chronicles successful efforts to delay a warning label requirement, and the four additional years waiting for results of even more studies while, despite efforts to alert the public, over a thousand more children die. The warning label was required in 1986.

The link is now accepted, and, where warnings are required on aspirin (and salicylate) packaging, Reye's syndrome is rare. Its demise in the United States was hailed as a public health triumph and the American Academy of Pediatrics recognized my work as a Milestone at the Millennium.[4,5] Yet, the story of how the oft-fatal illness arose and sustained itself behind obscure descriptions over many decades has not been revealed. Even today a mist of inuendo questioning the aspirin link remains. Read this book and you will be convinced that the previously recommended and untested dose schedules of aspirin for children were responsible for the unnecessary demise of thousands of children—and that science saved the day.

PART I

THE ODDS
1978–1979

Chapter 1

A Call

A Lethal Children's Disease. Cause and Cure: Unknown

National Reye's Syndrome Foundation, Brochures,
Bryan, Ohio, 1977 and 1979

Silver Bell is a remote village adjacent to the massive open pits of the American Smelting and Refining Company's copper operation in the southern Arizona desert. It was there in the summer of 1978 that eight-year-old Rodney Ray Hime came down with a cold and died.

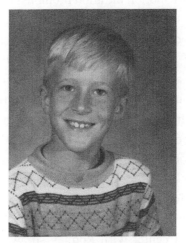

Rodney Ray Hime, Silver Bell, Arizona
1970–1978
Courtesy of Betty Hime

Rodney, his sister Teresa, and his parents, Ray, a bulldozer operator, and Betty, a housewife, had returned early from their vacation in the White Mountains of eastern Arizona for Rodney's Little League championship game when he became ill. Ray, assistant coach of the

Silver Bell Steelers, thought his son should rest, but it was only a cold and Rodney had begged to play. Bill Shaw later wrote in *The Arizona Daily Star*: "First base chores were handled by third grader Rodney Hime, a great-looking kid with lively brown eyes, a mop of blond hair and a broad easy smile. He was only 8 but already carried himself like a winner, a kid destined to experience victory many times in life." On Monday, 17 July, with the temperature hovering around 100 degrees, Rodney hit the winning run and secured the championship.[1]

Over the next several days, Rodney watched TV and rested quietly at home. By the week's end, he felt better. Nevertheless, Betty kept the appointment she had made with his doctor. "Must have had the flu," the doctor pronounced. On the way home, though, Rodney vomited. The vomiting was abrupt, unusually violent, and worse, it continued. Unsettled, Betty called the doctor. He prescribed a suppository.

When Rodney began blankly staring into space, Betty once again dialed the doctor. Her spot-on intuition prompted the doctor to instruct the Himes to take Rodney to St Mary's, the local hospital. Upon a glance, the emergency staff knew that something was very wrong with the boy. Results of a blood test revealed that a liver enzyme called SGOT (serum glutamic-oxaloacetic transaminase) was abnormally high. Suspecting some sort of acute liver damage, the physician asked Ray and Betty whether Rodney could have taken any drugs or poisons. No, they said, he had only taken baby aspirin and the suppository that his doctor had recommended. Perplexed, the physician told them to take Rodney to the Tucson Medical Center, a larger facility that would be better equipped to deal with Rodney's situation.

On Sunday 23 July 1978, with growing apprehension, the Himes sped to the medical center with Rodney sprawled across the back seat. He sat up abruptly, looked around without focusing his eyes, and vomited again. He began thrashing about. His brain was swelling.

The doctors at the medical center quickly prepared to perform a spinal tap to see if Rodney had bacterial meningitis. If so and if treated early, it was curable. The staff asked Betty and Ray to hold Rodney for the procedure, but Rodney fought them, and nurses took over.

Afterwards, Rodney was taken to the ICU. No longer combative, he had descended into an irreversible coma.

At midnight, Rodney's doctor wearily lowered himself onto a chair next to the Himes. Rodney did not have bacterial meningitis. The doctor was convinced the boy had Reye's syndrome.

Reye's syndrome, he explained, was named after R.D.K. Reye, an Australian pathologist, who had described 21 children with an illness that had, for a decade, perplexed doctors at his hospital. His report entitled "Encephalopathy and fatty degeneration of the viscera [organs]. A disease entity in childhood" had been published in the respected medical journal *The Lancet* in 1963.

Encephalopathy is a general term for dysfunction of the brain. Fatty degeneration is the accumulation of many tiny fat drops called vesicles within most cells in an organ. Pathologists often focus on the liver because of the ease with which a biopsy can be obtained. Fatty degeneration is rare and distinct from common fatty liver. Reye noted that only a few conditions were known to cause fatty degeneration. The children he studied seemed to have none of these.

The tiny fat droplets would disappear quickly if Rodney got better, but the brain swelling was serious. The doctor explained that because the bony skull cannot expand, swelling compresses the brain and can destroy brain cells. Yet, like the liver, the brain could recover. Questions swirled. It started with a cold but was not contagious. How did this happen? Was it something from the copper mine or the desert, or something Rodney had caught on vacation in the mountains? The doctor then told them the illness was often fatal. The rest was a blur.

Specialists were called in—a gastroenterologist for the liver and a neurologist for the brain. There was talk of removing a portion of Rodney's skull to relieve the pressure, but the doctors decided against it. Rodney received intravenous medications and was placed on a ventilator. His temperature skyrocketed, and the nurses placed him on cooling blankets. Nothing worked. Ray and Betty watched and waited. Ten days later, the doctors told them that an EEG confirmed that Rodney's brain would not recover.

On 6 August 1978, Rodney Ray Hime, the dearly loved and perfectly healthy eight-year-old only son of Ray and Betty Hime, died.

Ray Hime, obsessed with finding out why his son had died, learned that John and Terri Freudenberger of Bryan, Ohio, had established the National Reye's Syndrome Foundation (NRSF Ohio) in 1974 after their five-year-old daughter Tifinni died of Reye's syndrome. The foundation's brochure entitled "Reye's Syndrome. A Children's Lethal Disease. Cause and Cure: Unknown" reflected the Freudenbergers' frustration.[2] Here's what was known. Reye's syndrome mainly struck children. It often occurred during outbreaks of influenza or chickenpox. Some families had more than one child with it, but it was clearly not contagious. And when it began, it was frightening and fast, occurring over only hours or a few days. Curiously and inexplicably, the age of the stricken had changed over the past three decades. The average age at onset had gotten older. It seemed infants had mainly been reported during the 1950s; now older children and teenagers made up most cases. Parent groups in Ohio and Michigan were uncovering numerous cases and were demanding a system to count cases as the illness was not generally reportable to health authorities. The Freudenbergers traveled to Arizona and met with the Himes. Hime donated $1000, his life savings, to the foundation and started Chapter 34.

From that time on, Hime worked to raise awareness of the illness. He forced himself to speak in public. On 12 December 1978, he made his first speech to the Pima [County] Pediatric Society meeting in Tucson. The doctors there promised to help.[3] Later, Hime found my name in a newspaper article and kept it in case he needed to talk with someone at the Arizona state health department.

Seven Children

A moment of opportunity is often recognized only in retrospect. The moment came on the day after Christmas, December 1978 as a phone call about seven children with a mysterious illness.

The offices of the Arizona Department of Health Services near downtown Phoenix were almost empty that day. I was reviewing disease reports and looking forward to spending a few days at home with my husband and baby when the phone rang. The caller was John Sullivan-Bolyai, a pediatrician-in-training at the Indian Health Service hospital. When we established that I was the medical officer from the Center for Disease Control (CDC) recently stationed at the health department, he quickly got to the point.

He explained that seven children, each gravely ill with Reye's syndrome, were hospitalized nearby. Seven children gravely ill? Reye's syndrome? I searched my memory and vaguely recalled memorizing a list of serious, post-viral illnesses in children, Reye's syndrome among them. As we talked, I pulled Nelson's 1975 *Textbook of Pediatrics* from the bookshelf above my desk and read: "This disorder is emerging as one of the more common causes of death in childhood ... mortality ... 40–80%."[4] Sullivan-Bolyai had my attention.

The path to that moment had been unusual. Eight years earlier, at the age of 22, I had been teaching third grade in Pennsylvania and in the evenings travelling the road past the Three Mile Island nuclear plant to attend classes for a doctorate in school psychology at Millersville State Teachers College, when I met Winifred Kost, MD, the mother of one of my third graders. Her caring nature and problem-solving skills inspired me. Then during spring break in Daytona Beach, I picked up a magazine laying on a lounge and saw an article about Mary Calderone, the founder of sex education in the United States who had attended medical school at age 30. On the spot, her story seemed to open a door and I decided to apply to medical school. It was a crazy idea. Women comprised only a tiny fraction of physicians, yet the idea set me on fire. In 1971, after a year of pre-med classes, a stint as a blood-draw technician, and a medical school interview at an unnamed school where I was asked what I would do if I had children, I accepted a place where clinical excellence and community service were priorities, Temple University School of Medicine in Philadelphia. I received a stellar humanistic education there. About 13% of my class, a high percentage at the time, were women. Now, eight years later, I had completed medical school, a residency in internal medicine at Boston

City Hospital, and a fellowship in infectious diseases in Boston and Rhode Island and was married and the mother of a 10-month-old son.

I had planned to provide hands-on care for the ill but during my training, my husband-to-be, physician Donald P. Francis, a career CDC medical officer, convinced me that preventing an illness was as important as treating one. So I joined the CDC's Epidemic Intelligence Service (EIS), a two-year on-the-job training program in epidemiology and disease control. The CDC had been created after WW II to prevent malaria from spreading across the United States. In 1947, CDC paid Emory University $10 for 15 acres on Clifton Road in Atlanta and established its headquarters there. The EIS was created in 1951 as an early warning system against biologic warfare and man-made epidemics. Over the years, its scope expanded from infectious diseases to include among others chronic diseases and environmental health.

In July 1978 I had packed our belongings in Rhode Island, taken our four-month-old to New Jersey to my parents' home, and flown to Atlanta for CDC's annual three-week "crash" training course in epidemiology required for my new job. My husband had gone ahead to our new home in Phoenix. Staying at the slightly shabby Emory Pines Motel next to the center, with my baby in New Jersey, my husband in Phoenix beginning his new assignment at CDC's Hepatitis Laboratory, and our belongings, mostly items my husband had collected from his work in Africa and India, in a moving van on its way to Arizona, I wondered if I had made the right choice. The cramped dark motel room did nothing to lift my spirits. Sweating, tired, and homesick, I lay on the bed and wrestled with my uncertainty and the misery at leaving my baby, even though my mother was to bring him to Atlanta in a few days.

While I felt incredibly fortunate to have the opportunity of learning epidemiology at the CDC, I also felt the burden of taking "a man's position," and guilt for everything I was not—not being a full-time mom and not being a physician with a single priority. Maternity leave had not been available after the birth of my son. Being one of the few women accepted into the EIS program as a commissioned officer, postponing was not an option.

Every July about 50 new officers, most having just finished their medical training, headed to headquarters in Atlanta for the EIS course that would make them instant experts, or at least persons with a nodding acquaintance with the tools of epidemiology, the study of diseases in populations, and disease control. According to Professors Philip E. Sartwell and John M. Last, of the University of Ottawa and the Johns Hopkins University School of Hygiene and Public Heath respectively, modern epidemiology, which developed during the 19th century, embraced the ideas of careful clinical observation, precise counting of well-defined cases, and determination of risk.[5] The contributions of one British statistician William Farr were enormous. Farr defined and clarified the concepts of vital statistics, personal and environmental causes of disease, rates and probability, dose response relationships, herd immunity, incidence and prevalence, and the concepts of retrospective and prospective studies. Little did I know how great a role in my life these concepts would play.

The EIS course was exciting. There was talk of smallpox eradication, the 1976 swine flu episode, the new and mysterious Legionnaires' disease, and potential solutions to chronic and environmental diseases. My classmates and I ate grits and curries and talked of world travel. The instructors charged us with nothing less than protecting the health of the nation and instructed us to seek preventable illnesses and stamp them out. Young and idealistic, we learned the tools of epidemiology, specific techniques to identify risk factors or causes of illnesses and to develop methods of prevention. The world of disease prevention opened before my eyes. After the first day, I begged my mother to bring my baby to Atlanta and she booked the next flight.

Upon completion of the course, each of the new officers reported to their assignments. Mine was in Arizona. Approximately half of us were assigned to CDC headquarters and would become expert in one or two disease areas. The other half, like me, were assigned to state health departments to become involved in whatever was going on locally. The rules were clear. At all times, on order of the Surgeon General, officers were to be available for epidemic duty, domestic and foreign, and of utmost importance, a request for aid from a state or local government was to be considered the highest priority. My duties, laid out in a letter from CDC to the Arizona Director of Health, included events I was required to attend, such as courses on workplace hazards, surveillance, and immunizations and the annual EIS Conference in April in Atlanta.

I gathered my baby, my mother, and a thin pile of course handouts and flew to Phoenix. My husband had gone to a small town on the East Coast to investigate an epidemic of fatal hepatitis related to MDMA ingestion in young people. When we arrived in Phoenix, our air-conditioning and kitchen sink were not functioning, boxes from our move from Rhode Island were still unpacked, and my internal medicine board examination and new assignment were imminent. I spent the next few weeks of afternoons studying in the library. My mother was a godsend. She wrote to my father back in New Jersey, "It's been a long hot summer and this place is a disaster … It's been three weeks and still no kitchen sink, we eat out or take out mostly. It's like pioneering." I was certain she was wondering if medical school had been worth it. Yet by October, I had passed my board exam, my mother had flown home, we had hired a nice babysitter, and I had begun my new job as a public health expert, my qualifications being the three-week crash course.

Then came the call. *Seven children. Reye's syndrome? A mini epidemic?* Sullivan-Bolyai knew a lot. Prior to his current position, he explained, he had studied the illness as an EIS officer in the Viral Disease Division at CDC headquarters. I listened carefully as Sullivan-Bolyai brought me up to date on what was known. Its cause was a mystery. The syndrome consisted of two phases—an initial mild viral illness (the prodrome or antecedent illness) followed by the main illness which came on suddenly and progressed at a terrifying speed: hyperventilation, severe vomiting, and the neurologic symptoms of confusion or combativeness followed by seizures and/or coma sometimes with low blood sugar and the presence of ketones (in the blood or urine) that showed the body was becoming more acidic than normal. Ketones represent accelerated fat metabolism when sugar is low. CDC had become involved in the 1960s and had detected a trend. Chickenpox or type B influenza were common prodromes. Sullivan-Bolyai knew that influenza type A had recently hit Phoenix and encouraged me to study influenza A in the hospitalized children.

As a field officer, I was free to choose specific projects. My supervisor, J. Lyle Conrad, a seasoned career public health physician, watched over the 40 or so field officers from his desk in Atlanta and I liked the independence this arrangement afforded. I knew I could investigate the children's illness, or simply choose another project. Yet I wondered why Reye's syndrome had remained a mystery for so long, especially as the textbook had called it a common cause of death in childhood. I recalled that, in contrast, two years earlier, after 11 Legionnaires had died of a mysterious illness, headlines filled the nation's papers and CDC had urgently sent teams of researchers to Philadelphia to investigate. I was in training then and we braced for cases. Now here was a fatal illness involving children that seemed to have been stamped "cold case." I thanked Sullivan-Bolyai and drove home. That evening however, as I cared for our baby, I could not shake thoughts of the call, the children, and the unsolved mystery.

Chapter 2

The Arizona Study—A Suspect

It is a truth very certain that, when it is not in our power to determine
what is true, we ought to follow what is most probable.

René Descartes, *Discourse on Method*, 1637

Shoe leather epidemiology

I awoke early. Coffee. I talked to our baby as I dressed. He crawled around happily playing with his toys. *What should I do about the seven children?* Dress like a physician. I looked younger than my 31 years. No jewelry. No makeup. I slipped on my black slacks and white shirt, rolled my long hair into a bun, and looked for my shoes. The EIS symbol is a shoe with a hole in the sole, denoting "shoe leather epidemiology." Its message: "Get out of the office. Wear down that shoe. Find out what is really going on." Should I go to the hospitals to see the children?

My husband donned his helmet and strode towards his bicycle to pedal to work. Seven children hospitalized at once? Could our baby get this? My heart fluttered; my thoughts focused. This illness was a taker. I put my notebook in my shoulder bag and looked for my car keys as my baby looked up at me with trusting eyes. I would do anything to protect him. I gave him a hug and tickled him. I couldn't protect the seven children. Could I learn something that could protect him?

My sitter, an elderly woman with the dubious skill of clucking like a chicken, rang the bell. I gave her instructions for the day and chugged off to Good Samaritan Hospital in the old tan diesel Mercedes my husband had driven from Europe to India, leaving a trail of stink in the clear Arizona air.

The woman at the Good Samaritan reception desk greeted me and looked me up and down. "I'm from the state health department and would like to talk with the physician treating the children with Reye's syndrome."

She paged Dr Allen Kaplan. I waited. Kaplan, the hospital's pediatric neurologist, soon came to reception. He looked kind and spoke rapidly.

"I never expected to be treating so many ICU patients," he told me as we walked toward the ICU. "Brain swelling. That's the problem. We had to put bolts through their skulls."

"Bolts?" I asked.

"Yes. Intra-cranial devices to monitor the pressure inside. You see, when the brain swells inside the bony skull, it has no place to expand so it compresses itself destroying brain cells. We choose treatments based on the severity of the pressure. We must do everything we can to lower it. Some physicians will even cut a large hole in the skull." With horror, I pictured the gelatinous brain protruding from the opening.

He continued, "We are treating the children with hyperventilation to lower carbon dioxide in the blood. That reduces brain swelling."

As we walked past gurneys and men in white coats to the pediatric intensive care unit, he explained, "Yes, the children here have Reye's syndrome. The others are at St Joes and in Scottsdale."

I listened carefully, my adrenaline-fueled focus increasing. I pelted him with questions. "How did it start? What happened next? What tests had been done to rule out other conditions—say a worsening infection or a poisoning? Could the children have something else?"

I could see Kaplan was very busy and trying to be patient. He explained, "Each of the children had the flu. It's going around you know. And about four days later, often when the child seemed to be recovering, the abrupt and severe vomiting characteristic of Reye's syndrome started. When the delirium set in, parents brought them to the hospital. It all happens very quickly." He rattled off a list of tests that had been done: "Blood counts, blood chemistry, tests for infection." Then he paused to be sure I was listening, "They have abnormal tests of liver function, the hallmark of Reye's syndrome."

When we reached the pediatric intensive care unit, Kaplan introduced me to an ICU nurse and left. "See for yourself," he told me.

The ICU was surprisingly quiet. Twinkling Christmas lights blinked in the periphery as nurses talked in hushed tones. Small, pale bodies, surrounded by plastic tubing and the soft humming of life-support machines, seemed to be floating on the clean white sheets, like in a scene from a Michael Crichton novel. Was this real? I'd spent several years working at inner-city hospitals where I'd cared for the sickest of the sick, heart failure patients, and young adults with terminal cancer. I was proud of the way I could handle tough situations. But I was not prepared for this. On a visceral level I felt the possible, imminent death of a child and immediately recalled why I'd had specialized in adult medicine rather than pediatrics.

I first looked over the children's charts. A nurse stopped to talk. She explained, "The delirium phase is quite frightening. The children are wild, hallucinating, and pushing away loved ones. Some yell that they can't see. I was afraid. One girl reminded me of the child Regan in *The Exorcist*." The charts indicated the children had been in the delirious or combative stage or had progressed into a coma as they entered the hospital. Tests had been done to rule out other mimicking conditions such as meningitis, poisoning, or drug overdose. These children appeared to have textbook cases of Reye's syndrome.

I walked toward the beds. The children lay on cooling blankets to slow the metabolism of the brain, making it less vulnerable to damage. The bolt monitor was being held in place in their heads with gauze and tape. Nurses were monitoring the pressure levels. Ventilators were cranked up to overdrive in hopes of blowing out enough CO_2 to reduce the brain swelling. Some of the children were medically paralyzed and, therefore, totally dependent on the unwavering attention of those caring for them. I observed all of it. Speechless, I quietly left the unit.

After taking a moment to steel myself, I then approached the waiting room to talk with the parents. I could see from outside the door that the room was darkened and quiet. I knocked then entered. All eyes turned toward me. I took a breath and introduced myself. "I'm from the state health department," I told the parents as I sat down and leaned forward, my elbows on my knees. "I'm trying to learn why your children have become so ill." I waited. "There are others with the same illness," I said, confirming what they already knew. "Sometimes by talking with parents and doing tests we can learn new things that may help your child or others."

They stared at me. I asked the names of their children. They softly answered.

"Since the illness seems to start with a virus, we would like to see what virus it was. I would like to take some swab samples from your child's throat and rectum. I also would like to take some blood and urine." I held my breath ready for the possibility of eliciting anger or fear. "May I do that?"

After obtaining permission for these procedures, I asked if we could talk. The parents, as anxious as I was for answers, were eager to tell me everything they knew. One mother described her foster daughter's behavior to me and later to newspaper journalist.

> [She] was screaming and crying, but it wasn't like she was in pain. She was hallucinating. I thought maybe she had taken some drugs. I know she wouldn't do it on purpose, but I thought maybe someone had given her some candy with something in it. She was violent and it was like she was fighting off someone who wasn't there. She was acting like someone on LSD.[1]

Having told their stories, the frightened parents timidly began to ask me questions. One by one, I answered as best I could until there was silence.

Most remarkably, the parents' stories were almost identical. Perfectly healthy children. Came down with the flu and seemed to be getting better when, about four days after onset, intractable vomiting began. Four days from health to illness. Only four days. What had happened during those four days?

A case-control study

Within the CDC, the Viral Diseases Division was tracking Reye's because the syndrome usually started with a virus. Yet the illness of the seven children didn't seem like any complication of a virus that I'd ever seen. In my limited experience, there was rarely a period of seeming recovery before the child's state deteriorated. In any case, there was no incriminating evidence—such as tissue inflammation—either in the textbook description of Reye's or in these children, to suggest a progressive infection. Nelson's textbook indicated that Reye's syndrome looked like the work of a toxin or poison and admonished against giving aspirin or phenothiazine which could worsen both liver and brain function.[2] But what could the toxin be?

Although I had no suspects, I did have a tool to study these children. During the summer at CDC, I had been given a simple five-page booklet called "Choosing Controls." It described a key concept of epidemiology—the comparison of ill cases with a control group, those free from the illness, in a case-control study.

Case-control studies have successfully linked or associated many diseases to their cause. Well-known links include those between scurvy and vitamin C deficiency, lung cancer and smoking, and diethylstilbestrol (DES) exposure in pregnant women and vaginal cancer in their daughters. Case-control studies, however, have a key limitation: they show *associations* and, as epidemiologists are fond of saying, association does not always represent causation.

However, case-control studies are by far the most efficient way to identify possible causes for uncommon illnesses. When properly done, they provide a statistic, the *probability* that the presence of the characteristic (such as vitamin C intake, smoking, or DES) in the two groups differs by chance alone. If the probability of chance is low and the study is properly done, the characteristic may be important. I had already tried it once that autumn during an investigation of an outbreak of serious gastrointestinal illness in northern Arizona.[3] It made sense to pursue a case-control approach for the children with Reye's syndrome.

On 29 December, the chief of the State Laboratory Jon Counts handed me a few pages copied from W. Lawrence Drew's 1976 book, *Viral Infections. A Clinical Approach*. It read:

The pathogenesis of Reye's syndrome is not understood. The close association with an acute viral illness suggests that viruses play a role ... There is often a history of ingestion of medication such as salicylates or antiemetics [drugs used to treat vomiting]; occasionally, various toxic substances such as isopropyl alcohol have also been implicated in this syndrome ... [And] speculation about a synergistic role between a virus and a toxic agent should "give pause for some thought, particularly when treating infants and young children symptomatically with drugs for otherwise uncomplicated viral infections." [4]

The chapter was written by C. George Ray, a man I would meet quite by chance the following May, a man who would change the pace of my investigation.

I decided to focus on viruses, toxins, and medications. I found it curious that influenza and chickenpox (varicella) viruses were the most common prodromal illnesses associated with Reye's. These extremely common viruses are quite different from one another. What could they possibly have in common with Reye's, or, for that matter, with the many other types of viral infections (for example, dengue, Epstein-Barr) that sometimes immediately preceded Reye's? I found an equally long list of suspected drugs and toxins, including aflatoxins (naturally occurring in several varieties of mold), endotoxins (from bacteria), hypoglycin (naturally occurring in certain fruit), insecticides, isopropyl alcohol, antiemetics, pteridines (in the excreta of insects), salicylates (including aspirin, known to chemists as acetylsalicylate), valproic acid (to prevent seizures), and warfarin (an anticoagulant). A 1976 FDA report said there was "insufficient evidence to show that anti-emetics, aspirin, and acetaminophen are clearly causally related to Reye's syndrome, although this possibility cannot be eliminated." [5]

With these possibilities in mind, and because of the parents' descriptions, I divided the children's illnesses into two distinct parts: the prodrome and the severe phase, which began with unusually violent vomiting. It seemed that whatever caused Reye's syndrome happened between the onset of the flu and this very remarkable vomiting—an average period of only four days.

The next task was to choose the cases and controls. There are two ways to select cases: all cases, an approach that is theoretically ideal but often impractical, or a random sampling of cases. If we studied a sample and the cases were not like "all" cases, our "selection" could result in a *selection bias* and bias our results. In the end, I decided to look at all the children in Arizona over the age of one year who had been hospitalized with Reye's in December of 1978. The smallest patients were excluded because Reye's could be confused with genetic metabolic diseases that often show up during the first year of life.

For assistance, I went to Lee Dominguez, a seasoned state public health investigator. Dominguez was trained to interview and perform contact tracing for those with transmissible diseases. He was experienced in eliciting detailed and sensitive information. We canvassed all the hospitals in the state and, in the end, came up with only the seven original cases.

Next came choosing a comparison group. The controls were chosen to be just like the children with Reye's, except they did not have Reye's syndrome. As the cases were school-aged, I decided to select controls from the classrooms of the afflicted children. Dominguez and I called each of the principals and asked for class lists to choose control children for the study. Each agreed to help. With class lists in hand, we randomly chose three male classmates for each boy with Reye's and three female classmates for each girl. In other words, the controls were matched for age and gender.

At the same time, I wrote (with a pen) a questionnaire and copied (mimeographed) 28 copies. The questionnaire was short, only three pages, and focused on the age and gender of all the people in the household, illnesses of each family member in December, medications and vitamins taken, history of childhood illnesses, recent immunizations, the presence of tonsils, whether there were pets in the home (and, if so, what type), and the type of heat used in the home. We also completed CDC's Reye's Syndrome Case Investigation Form, which asked for general information.

Beyond the questionnaires, we assembled the blood and biological samples from the throat, rectum, and urine of the Reye's children and had them shipped to the State Laboratory for virus culture and serology (antibody tests), where state experts Dora Woodall and Warren Stromberg processed them.

Two of the seven children died. The autopsy reports showed fatty livers and brain swelling described as "widespread" or "advanced."

We needed answers quickly before memories faded. It was already too late to collect biologic samples from the control children. We called all the case and the control families. Each agreed to participate and answered our questions seriously and thoughtfully. Then the tedious task of hand-tabulating the information began.

The results

After drawing the curtains in the evening in our small English-style cottage and our baby falling asleep, I worked on the questionnaires. My husband had just finished a doctoral program in virology at Harvard and encouraged me: "Look at the viral illness. There must be something going on there." Under the tiny desk light in the bedroom, I laid out the pages, three for each child. I wished my desk was larger as the papers spilled over the edges.

All seven of the children with Reye's syndrome had a flu-like illness before the profuse vomiting set in.[6] Of the 21 control children, 16 had been ill with a similar flu-like illness and had recovered. I decided to compare those 16 with the seven who had developed Reye's syndrome. With detailed information on the symptoms of the parents, brothers, and sisters of each case and control child, I constructed elaborate charts to check ideas about the influenza phase, particularly the four days between onset and vomiting. I asked many questions of the data by making lists and looking for patterns. Did the illness in the children with Reye's differ in some way? Could the virus have mutated as it passed from one family member to another? Did it matter whether the victim was the first or last person in the family to get the virus? Did the victim's symptoms differ from those of other family members? Did birth order make a difference? One by one I crumpled my charts and threw them on the bedroom floor. On those nights, tired and annoyed by the tedium, I dropped into bed.

Finally, frustrated by dead-end ideas, I turned my attention to the medications. Right off the bat I could see that the children with Reye's syndrome were different. They had taken more medications during the influenza phase. While the control children, on average, had taken two medications, the Reye's children had taken three, even though their illnesses up to the point of vomiting were shorter.

Bingo, a difference between the two groups. A wedge into the problem. The explanation for this, though, dangled out of reach. What did it mean? Were the Reye's children sicker in the beginning? Were the parents more concerned? And how could I know? It seemed questions only begot more questions. No real catch, but the finding compelled me to go on.

I listed the medications. None seemed extraordinary. Most were the usual over-the-counter (OTC) medications commonly given to children. A few had also been given the antibiotics erythromycin and tetracycline.

I stared at the list. What could I do with this? Many of the parents had provided only brand names. To do any kind of analysis I needed ingredients—that is, the specific chemical or so-called generic name of each component. Neither my medical textbooks nor the *Physician's Desk Reference (PDR)* contained this information. Surely someone before had needed to know this. I located a book about non-prescription drugs and ordered it. Impatient, I stopped at drug stores, found the exact medications the parents had named, and extracted the information identifying the ingredients from the tiny printing on the labels. A list of ingredients was required by public health law.

Finally, I listed the ingredients separately for the two groups as shown in Table 2.1. The lists were similar except for one ingredient. All seven of the Reye's children had taken a drug in the salicylate family— for most it was aspirin itself—while only half of the ill control children had done so. A similar per cent of the case and control children had used the other medications, including acetaminophen (commonly known as Tylenol).

Working list of medications
taken by children with Reye's Syndrome and ill
Control Children Arizona, early 1979[7]

I banged the salicylate numbers into my hand-held calculator. A probability of less than 0.05 popped up on the screen. This meant that the difference in aspirin use between cases and controls would happen *by chance less than five times in 100 studies.* The finding in scientific terms was "statistically significant." Seeing a probability of chance at 0.05 or less is always exciting to an epidemiologist. Although statisticians today might add context to describing p values this way,[8] I felt I had latched onto something.

Table 2.1 Medications Taken by Patients with Reye's Syndrome and Control Subjects Arizona, December 1978[9]
Summarized with permission from *Pediatrics*, Vol. 66, p. 861.
Copyright © 1980 by the American Academy of Pediatrics

Medication	Reye's Syndrome	Controls
Salicylate-containing medication*	100%	50%
Acetaminophen	0%	25%
Decongestant and acetaminophen	14%	0%
Decongestant, anti-tussive and acetaminophen	0%	6%
Antitussive (for cough)	14%	19%
Decongestant	29%	31%
Antitussive and decongestant	29%	6%
Bronchodilator	14%	19%
Antibiotic	14%	25%
Hexylresorcinol lozenge	0%	6%

*Salicylate-containing medications included adult aspirin, children's aspirin, decongestant aspirin combination, aspirin-containing gum, bismuth subsalicylate (Pepto-Bismol), and aspirin/acetaminophen combinations.

Then, reality set in. Good grief, the finding was laughable. Aspirin was the drug of choice for children with any viral infection and the standard recommendation of physicians.

But there was more. The Reye's children had taken larger amounts of salicylate than had the controls—about 5 grams (the equivalent of about 16 adult aspirin tablets) in the days before being hospitalized (the average time before hospitalization was 5.9 days) versus 3 grams taken by the control children during the entire illness. My pediatric textbook recommended a dose of not more than 3.6 grams in 24 hours.[10] Recommended doses at the time were about 60–90 mg/kg/day for children over one year of age. (Appendix 1) I had not recorded the children's weights but the amounts taken did not seem to be in the realm of potentially fatal poisoning.

Further, all five of the Reye's children with a fever had taken aspirin, but none of the four febrile controls had done so. I next found that the more severe the neurologic impairment the more salicylate the child had taken.

Only one child had been tested for salicylate poisoning. The blood level was 27.1 mg/dL, a level considered potentially toxic. For serious rheumatic diseases, levels of 25–35 mg/dL were often recommended—with careful monitoring.[11] Curiously, the child hadn't taken a dose during the 72 hours prior to admission suggesting that, earlier, the level had been even higher.[12]

There were only three explanations for these findings. First, the results might be within the 5% chance of being a fluke. Second, perhaps some bias had flawed the study. And finally, dare I think, salicylate did play a role in Reye's syndrome.

Even with the figures before me, I found it utterly impossible to believe that the most popular medication ever created—not to mention one that came in tablets specifically for children—was involved in this deadly illness. Surely, some bias must have had crept into my work.

The tension of the unexplained

The state epidemiologist retired, and I was appointed Acting Arizona State Epidemiologist. My workdays became filled with phone calls and investigations. I wished I could just forget the questionnaires—and the aspirin finding. I still had my medical school pharmacology book, the 1970 edition of Goodman and Gilman, as it was known to every medical student. There on page 328 it read, "Salicylate does not influence the course of the common cold or upper respiratory infection ... If symptomatic improvement tempts the individual to be ambulatory and active ... the drug may do more harm than good."[13] Hmmm, the drug was only for symptomatic relief.

On the way home from work one day, after a few quiet minutes of driving, I found myself turning the old diesel, like the pad on a Ouija board, from McDowell Avenue onto Central toward the Maricopa County Medical Society Library a few blocks away.

The library was cool, dark, and empty. The librarian directed me to the *Index Medicus*, a series of huge bound books with miniscule printing that contained a comprehensive index of every medical journal article written since 1879. Impressive. Start here, she told me, leaving me alone. My babysitter did not know where I was. I quickly scanned the pages for "aspirin" and "Reye's syndrome," and, on a form the librarian had given me, placed orders for articles that seemed relevant. This was taking forever. My baby was at home. I left but every day after work returned for a few minutes. Some articles were in the volumes in the basement; others slowly arrived. Each article became a hit, like an addiction. Eye-opening information revealed. Never the whole story but each piece asking for more.

I quickly learned that the symptoms of aspirin (salicylate) poisoning and those of Reye's syndrome were identical. In 1906, in a report entitled, "Salicylate Poisoning in Children," Frederick Langmead of the Hospital for Sick Children on Great Ormond Street in London had written one of the most complete clinical descriptions of what he called the "much feared symptoms of salicylate poisoning" ever written:

> drowsiness, deepening into coma, and, if untreated, ending in death, and air hunger of the Kussmaul type increasing with the drowsiness. The child is flushed, the eyes are bright, and there is usually great thirst. Vomiting usually, but not always, precedes these symptoms. The drowsiness may be replaced or be associated with delirium ... I found acetone [a ketone] in large amounts in all the cases in which it was looked for.[14]

The air hunger that Langmead described is often a response to blood that has become too acidic; however, it is often subtle and not obvious to the untrained eye. Its presence is an important clue to the diagnosis of diabetes or salicylate intoxication (the name used for poisoning with aspirin or any of the members of the salicylate family), both of which are characterized by production of acidic ketones. The clinical illness that Langmead described was exactly like the one Reye described almost 60 years later. From the major symptoms of air hunger (aka hyperventilation or hyperpnea), vomiting and coma, to the more subtle ones, Reye's syndrome and aspirin poisoning were clinically the same. Similar too were laboratory findings including ketones and amino acids (possible evidence of disturbed metabolism) in the urine, low levels of the clotting factor prothrombin, and, in the very young, low blood sugar. In fact, some doctors had suspected aspirin had a role in the illness. Importantly, though, Reye's syndrome was distinguished by a rare pattern of fat in cells called fatty degeneration.

On 5 February, I placed aspirin on top of the list of suspect toxins in a memo to my Arizona supervisor,[15] and again three weeks later in a press release I had drafted for the Arizona Department of Health Services.[16] In early March, when a *Phoenix Gazette* reporter called concerned about pesticides, I conceded the money was probably with a viral infection but remarked, "there is a much stronger case against aspirin."[17]

You see, the articles I had ordered had begun to arrive in quantity. They came in no particular order and the information was chronologically fragmented. I had little time to organize it. "By far the two most common manifestations of salicylism in infants and children are hyperpnea and vomiting," Vanderbilt University pediatrician Harris D. Riley had written in 1956.[18] I read that during the 10-year period from 1945 to 1955, poisoning during therapy was more common than accidental ingestion.[19] Yet even before I could truly understand it all, I felt a growing apprehension, because just by skimming, I could see the reports contained some damning evidence about aspirin use in children.

I began a mental list of "reasons" that doctors had used to eliminate aspirin as a cause of Reye's syndrome. I thought of these as the "pillars" supporting their conclusion:

1. The syndrome had mysteriously emerged in the 1960s when Reye described it, whereas aspirin had been used for many decades.

2. Aspirin (salicylate) poisoning could be easily diagnosed with a blood test.

3. The recommended dose schedule (dose, frequency, duration) was safe for children.

4. Not all children with Reye's syndrome had taken aspirin.

5. The pathology lesion fatty degeneration defining Reye's syndrome was not found in salicylate poisoning.

6. The government was monitoring safety.

I would return to these six pillars, one by one, as the tangled history of Reye's syndrome and aspirin poisoning unfolded in the documents I was gathering.

Chapter 3

It Can't Be

Statistician Richard Royall of Johns Hopkins Bloomberg School of Public Health in Baltimore, Maryland, said that there are three questions a scientist might want to ask after a study: 'What is the evidence?' 'What should I believe?' and 'What should I do?'
Regina Nuzzo, *Nature*, 2014

Over the next few months, each report I read strengthened the idea that aspirin might be involved in the genesis of Reye's syndrome. While my study was the first comparative study to implicate aspirin in Reye's syndrome, it consisted of only seven cases—hardly a smoking gun.

When did Reye's syndrome begin?

A widely quoted assumption about Reye's syndrome was that it had arisen mysteriously in the mid-20th century. This was easy to debunk. A careful tracing backwards through medical writings revealed that, although Reye's syndrome had gotten its name during the early 1960s when Reye described a series of cases, a similar brain swelling illness had been around since at least the early 1920s.

Humans are drawn to the new and unexplained. Thus, when Arthur F. Anderson learned that five young children had died in children's hospitals in Boston with a strikingly similar, very unusual, and profound brain disorder during ten hot days in July 1923, he immediately reported them in the *Boston Medical and Surgical Journal*.[1] Though some recognize Brain, Hunter, and Turnbull's 1929 report[2] as the first report of the illness later called Reye's syndrome,[3] most credit Anderson.[4, 5, 6, 7, 8] The explosive brain swelling illness began with intractable vomiting lasting four to seven days, followed shortly thereafter by stupor, and convulsions. Two children were noted to be breathing deeply and rapidly. Curiously, their breath smelled of acetone and ketones were found in their urine. For the four who came to autopsy, marked cerebral edema (brain swelling) was the most notable finding. Anderson's report was descriptive. Description, the first step in scientific inquiry, serves to identify features of an illness. Analytic (comparative) studies, however, are needed to test ideas about cause, risk factors, and treatments. Without an analytic study in which two groups are compared and probability tests applied, all ideas are simply just that—ideas.

Two years after Anderson's report, five more rapidly fatal similar illnesses in New York were reported.[9] According to the physicians, the illnesses in Boston and New York had not previously been "recognized and described."[10] Frighteningly, even with powerful drugs, the seizures could often not be controlled. None of the children had evidence of inflammation, a characteristic common in encephalitis. The extent of the swelling shocked the physicians who wrote, "the brain is so soft as to give one the sensation of flowing." An infectious agent did not appear to be involved, so physicians deemed the illness "toxic" in origin.

Pathologists further defined patterns. Besides brain swelling, some looked for and found fat in the liver and other organs. Some also found cloudy swelling. In the 1955 edition of *Human Pathology*, Howard T. Karsner, formerly of Western Reserve University and Medical Research Advisor to the United States Navy, pointed out that cloudy swelling commonly precedes fatty degeneration.[11]

Brain swelling is dangerous. A healthy brain is the consistency of firm Jell-O and has thick snakelike convolutions (the gyri) and slit-like fissures (the sulci). It fits snuggly into the hard cranium or skull and is bathed in a thin layer of clear liquid called cerebrospinal fluid, which also moistens the contiguous spinal cord. When the brain swells, however, the skull, which normally protects it from injury, becomes it captor. Pressure builds. As swelling increases, the enlarged swollen brain may be forced dangerously downward onto the brain stem where vital structures regulate breathing and heart function. With extreme swelling the brain can liquefy.

At first, the new illness was called either encephalitis or encephalopathy and, because of limited patient data, early writers struggled to distinguish them. *Encephalitis*, which is often due to a viral infection, is characterized by inflammation, the presence of white blood cells within the brain itself. *Encephalopathy* on the other hand, does not involve inflammation. Encephalopathy is usually caused by a toxin or derangement in metabolism. For example, in 1929, after studying 40 cases of "encephalitis" in children, physician Bert Beverly of the Children's Memorial Hospital in Chicago wrote "encephalitis" had become more common during the previous 10 years mainly due to "toxic encephalitis." He detailed three fatal cases and found that each had swelling of the brain, two had fatty changes of the liver, and all had cloudy swelling of the kidneys.[12] The same year, assistant physicians Russell Brain and Donald Hunter with Hubert M. Turnbull, Director of the Bernhard Baron Institute of Pathology of the London Hospital and Professor of Morbid Anatomy, described six children with an acute illness unlike any with which they were familiar. An autopsy of one three-year-old revealed ring hemorrhages in a congested and swollen brain, fat in the kidneys and "extreme ... degeneration of the liver." They concluded that the changes were likely "caused by a single agent."[13]

In 1930, A.S. Low recognized that Anderson had been the first to describe the brain swelling illness which "seemed to constitute a heretofore not observed type of encephalitis" in children after a cold, fever, or diarrhea with fever.[14] The mysterious brain swelling illness came to be called, "toxic encephalopathy," but a toxin was never identified. By 1961, Boston neurologist Gilles Lyon and associates at the Massachusetts General Hospital and Harvard Medical School uncovered 40 reports published before 1960 and deemed "toxic encephalopathy" a major problem accounting for *"6% of all infant and childhood deaths coming to autopsy at Massachusetts General Hospital in the previous decade* [emphasis added]."[15] After assessing 16 cases, most from records of the hospital, they too concluded that the condition was a discrete disorder characterized in most by brain swelling. The state of the liver and other organs was not mentioned. The neurologists did not consider salicylate poisoning and reported aspirin use in only one case. In fact, aspirin was so far from the neurologists' minds that they recommended it for fever reduction in the patients, even though brain swelling had been observed in children with salicylate toxicity during the 1940s.[16, 17]

Despite the many prior descriptions of a brain swelling illness, it was the report by pathologist R.D.K. Reye and colleagues entitled "Encephalopathy and fatty degeneration of the viscera [organs]. A disease entity in childhood" that rang bells around the world. Although some previous reports had noted fatty degeneration, most had simply noted fat or cloudy swelling likely because under a microscope, especially early in the course, the microvesicles of fat are barely perceptible, as shown in the diagram in Figure 3.1.[18] When a fat stain is applied, however, the amount of fat is striking. Reye had applied a fat stain and carefully documented fatty degeneration.[19]

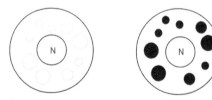

Figure 3.1 Diagram of Liver Cells with Fatty Degeneration (N=nucleus)
Fat microvesicles may be barely perceptible with routine stains. (left).
With a fat stain (right), multitudes of small fat drops (black dots) are confirmed.

After Reye's report, any child with a mild childhood infection followed within days by hyperventilation, vomiting, and coma, with laboratory tests showing abnormal liver function, low blood sugar (particularly in infants), and ketones had Reye's syndrome. Reye was struck by the severity of the brain swelling and the grossly yellow, fatty liver but because the microscopic fatty degeneration pattern is extremely rare, its presence became the syndrome's *sine qua non* marker.

As physicians slowly realized that the toxic brain swelling

illness—known as Reye's syndrome—was a leading cause of child death, the long history had been forgotten and many believed the illness had mysteriously appeared during the 1960s when Reye had described it. I had uncovered the first misconception about the illness.

To headquarters

I decided to bring the Arizona study findings to headquarters, where they could be further investigated. Mostly I worried about the liver pathology. If aspirin did cause Reye's syndrome, aspirin must cause fatty degeneration, and there seemed no information about that.

In April 1979, I flew to Atlanta for the annual EIS Conference. My feelings about flying had changed since becoming a mother. Once a woman who would go anywhere anytime, I now dreaded flying and being away from my baby. Love. Hormones. Anxiety. Nevertheless, attending the conference was a requirement for EIS officers and I was to present a summary of the *Salmonella* investigation I had completed in northern Arizona. I had practiced my speech over and over as it was strictly limited to 10 minutes. The entire CDC would be there. Female field officer. Mother. I wanted to do a good job. I also scheduled a meeting with Larry Schonberger in the Viral Diseases Division to discuss the Reye's syndrome data. Schonberger was the Chief of the Enteric [gut] and Neurotropic [nerves] Viral Diseases Branch of the Viral Disease Division, the branch overseeing Reye's syndrome activities.

I stayed at the home of Bill Foege, the CDC Director. Foege had been a mentor to my husband during his work in the smallpox program in India. Foege's wife Paula graciously hosted me. In the morning I drove the winding two-lane roads lined by thick greenery and blossoming dogwoods past Emory University to the Clifton Road campus. CDC comprised a series of large non-descript rectangular structures which reminded me of the electronics factory where my mother had worked. I informed the woman at the front desk of my appointment with Schonberger. She gave me a pass. I stopped at the cafeteria. A hair-netted worker asked me if I wanted streak-o-lean with my biscuits and sweet tea. Excuse me? Bacon, she clarified. I nodded. After eating, I walked the long dimly lit corridors to Schonberger's office. My thoughts swirled. I wasn't experienced at this. As a physician I could easily rattle off symptoms, signs, tests, and diagnoses, but this was different. I was going to talk about concepts I had just learned: cases, controls, study design, statistics. I knocked. Schonberger, a few years my senior, opened the door and greeted me collegially, his expression open and friendly. I relaxed a bit.

Schonberger had a medical degree from Case Western Reserve and had been working in the Viral Disease Division since 1976. In the winter of 1971, as an EIS officer, he had been assigned to one of CDC's first Epi-Aids concerning Reye's syndrome. Epi-Aid is the term used to denote an investigation resulting from a request from a state. Schonberger had studied 10 afflicted children in North Carolina hospitals and had concluded there was no common viral etiology (three different viruses, none being influenza or chickenpox were implicated) or common medication.

The first CDC officer to investigate the illness, however, had been 26-year-old George Magnus Johnson, an EIS field officer stationed in North Carolina in 1962. In 1980, Johnson would tell the tale of his harrowing investigation to the attendees at the Scientific Session of the Sixth Annual National Reye's Syndrome Foundation Conference.[20] He had become involved after Gertrude Jones of the North Carolina State Board of Health noticed for the 10th time in two weeks a physician report marked "death, encephalitis, unknown cause." For the next three months Johnson followed a trail of 16 cases from the mountains to the piedmont to the lowlands of North Carolina. None had survived long enough to be transferred to the major medical centers of North Carolina: Duke, the University of North Carolina, or Bowman Gray. Dr Lee Large at the Charlotte Presbyterian Hospital had noted the pathology findings suggested an "exogeneous poison." In April 1963, Johnson traveled on the Peach Blossom Special to Atlanta to present the cases at CDC. There, Johnson recalled, Alexander Langmuir, the brilliant and blunt creator of the EIS, had stood up and in his slow, booming voice announced, "Gentleman, this may be of great significance. Any time we can find more about sudden brain death in children we must do so. I commend the author of this paper."

The *North Carolina Medical Journal* published Johnson's report in October 1963, the same month as Reye's report.[21] Johnson wrote that "marked cerebral edema seemed to be the only consistent finding." Four cases had "marked fatty metamorphosis" of the liver, including one with fatty degeneration. A virus had been isolated in four cases. One six-year-old had been treated with aspirin for a cold and an 18-month-old had been found in her crib with a bottle of APCs (a pill combining aspirin, phenacetin, and caffeine).

Over the ensuing years, in addition to Johnson and Schonberger, other EIS officers had conducted formal investigations including ones in New England, North Carolina, Chicago suburbs, St Louis, Ohio, Colorado, Michigan, and seven southern states. Physician Michael B. Gregg, Director of the Viral Diseases Division, had signed off on most of them through 1980. In addition to supervising the Division, Gregg was editor of the *MMWR* (*Morbidity and Mortality Weekly Report*), CDC's premier weekly report of disease statistics and breaking news. Philip Brachman, MD, an anthrax expert presided over the entire Bureau of Epidemiology and was also the main conduit to the Director's Office until Walter Dowdle took over the new Center for Infectious Diseases in the early 1980s.

Between 1973 and 1976, Schonberger obtained a Master of Public Health degree from Johns Hopkins and worked at the Maryland state health department. He returned to CDC in 1976, joined the Viral Diseases Division, and recruited his first EIS officer, John Sullivan-Bolyai, the physician who had called me about the Arizona children. Later Schonberger explained his goal was to determine the incidence of Reye's syndrome in the United States, a number as mysterious as the illness itself. He explained that it is hard to get resources when the number of cases is unknown. Schonberger was now overseeing officers who worked on diseases assigned to his branch, such as polio and infectious encephalitis. He had recently completed a seminal investigation which linked a sudden surge of a rare illness called Guillain-Barré syndrome to the swine flu vaccine. Because of Guillain-Barré, the national vaccine program endorsed by the president of the United States with great fanfare had been a debacle, and heads, including that of the CDC Director, had rolled. Tensions remained high.

Schonberger explained that Reye's syndrome was not a defined program at CDC. EIS officers worked on it as time allowed. (That was about to change.) For now, however, he was the standard skeptical scientist. Schonberger told me about a tiny infant with Reye's syndrome he had encountered during his first investigation. He had been excited and had figured that because she was so young, he could learn everything she had ever been exposed to and crack the case. But nothing had turned up, at least back then.

I began by describing the Arizona study. "Well, I studied ... 7 cases and 16 controls." The study suddenly seemed very small. Aspirin. I focused on the probability, "less than 5% chance of being a fluke."

I sensed I was losing him. The room was feeling smaller. Our time was passing quickly. I switched to a discussion of some of the things I had learned about aspirin. He stopped me.

"It's not aspirin," he said bluntly.

I felt my face burning. Then, more gently, he explained, "CDC has looked at aspirin. It's not involved. There are lots of studies." I knew CDC had published a report in 1970 categorically stating that medications were not involved. I was ready for that. I had studied the report.

"But," I said, "they were using hospital records. They didn't interview the parents. We know hospital records can be incomplete." Surprised by my own assertiveness, I pressed on.

"Other investigators have found 100% aspirin use in children with Reye's syndrome. Look, I've done a lot of reading and have not come across any proof that aspirin is not involved in Reye's syndrome."

I waited. Then, despite a clear sense I was overstepping my rank, I pressed the point, "If you have proof, may I see it?"

Schonberger stared at me. He paused and seemed to soften. A good scientist, he took the challenge and promised to find the data showing aspirin did not cause Reye's syndrome and send it to me. He then told me that CDC and the state of Ohio were conducting a case-control study that had begun in December 1978. Ohio had been particularly interested in the possible role of medications. He promised to see if the study questions were detailed enough to get at the role of aspirin. I thanked him and left.

The meeting ended cordially but had not gone the way I had expected. I had envisioned that Schonberger had resources to push this ahead and would tell me I had done a great job and take it off my hands. Instead, I had volleyed it to him, and it seemed he had tapped it right back. Disappointed, I left for Phoenix feeling I had hit a wall.

Silver Bell, Ray Hime, and C. George Ray

The first day back in the office I remembered an invitation I had received from Ray Hime whose son had died of Reye's syndrome the previous summer (Chapter 1) asking me to speak about Reye's syndrome to parents in Silver Bell. I had said yes. Where on earth was Silver Bell?

Late in the afternoon of 10 May 1979 I checked the map. Silver Bell was near Tucson. I marked the fastest route, a short cut, and jumped in the state car. Unfortunately, the short cut was an unpaved road through the desert. Once committed, I had to keep going. No other vehicle appeared for miles. I was sweating and afraid I would miss the event entirely. Worse, there was no way to check my bearings other than the setting sun. Finally, the giant copper pits came into view. I arrived at the last minute. Hime was waiting outside the community center and about 100 people were seated inside. Hime warmly greeted me and introduced me to C. George Ray, Professor of Pediatrics at the University of Arizona. Hime had also convinced him to make the trip to Silver Bell.

George Ray was a soft-spoken man, a quintessential pediatrician. He was also an academic and an expert on viruses. To my surprise, he had been an EIS officer in 1964 and had written about Reye's syndrome in 1976. I liked him immediately. Once in the community room, Hime spoke briefly, Ray described the clinical illness, and I discussed observations learned by epidemiology methods mostly the characteristics of time, place, and person. Afterwards, Dr Ray and I sat in the back of the room enjoying the lovely, warm desert evening. I told him about the case-control study and some of the things I had learned at the Maricopa County Medical Society Library. He listened intently. I braced for another smack down. Finally, he took a breath and in his quiet, scholarly way, with words I will never forget, said, "I think you are on to something—you should pursue this." He sat back in the folding metal chair. The door was open to the outside and the softly glowing desert evening light poured in accompanied by distant sounds of children playing and dogs barking.

"You know," he said, "Ted Mortimer thinks aspirin has something to do with Reye's syndrome. He has been quite stuck on this for many years." I had heard of Mortimer, an old-timer from Ohio and a nationally respected pediatrician who sat on many national committees.

The reasons that aspirin had been dismissed as a cause of Reye's syndrome came to mind. Ray's enthusiasm provided the impetus to question them. One seemed to stand out—fatty degeneration of the liver. It defined Reye's syndrome. It seemed, therefore, if aspirin produced it, weren't the illnesses one and the same?

Chapter 4

The Parents

In the English language there are orphans and widows,
but there is no word for the parents who lose a child.
Jodi Picoult, *My Sister's Keeper*, 2004

After the meeting in Silver Bell, Schonberger called. He had looked for the "disconfirming evidence" and could not find any. He now agreed that existing studies showing low rates of aspirin use in Reye's children were far from definitive because many of the histories had been recorded from hospital records rather than real-time interviews with the parents. Later, he told me that he had located the record of the infant he had studied as a young officer and had carefully scanned its contents. He now saw a compulsively complete note by a medical student. The student had written that the infant had been given aspirin.

At the time, two foundations were intensively devoting time and resources to Reye's syndrome. Ray Hime's organization, the National Reye's Syndrome Foundation [Ohio], had been founded by John and Terri Freudenberger in 1974. Devastated by the sudden death of their daughter Tifinni, the Freudenbergers, owners of a manufacturing business in the rural village of Bryan, Ohio, were now extending their management skills to the entire country with the goal of spreading the word about Reye's syndrome. Theirs was one of the first grassroots parent organizations rallying around a childhood illness. Tifinni had become feverish one Sunday evening in April 1973 and woke the next morning with chickenpox. On Thursday she started to vomit, prompting her mother to take her to the doctor, who prescribed medicine. The vomiting continued into Friday. More medicine was prescribed. Then, when the little girl had to be carried and started to thrash and cry out, the Freudenbergers asked to see the doctor a third time. This time he suspected Reye's syndrome. By Friday evening Tifinni, now in a coma, was in an ambulance speeding to the Children's Hospital in Columbus. She was placed in isolation in the intensive care unit. The following Sunday, Palm Sunday, she died.

According to the Freudenbergers, eleven months later in the same small Ohio village, the parents of six-year-old Stephanie Huffman called the same doctor when their daughter developed similar signs. He quickly diagnosed Reye's syndrome. Stephanie survived. The physician had said vomiting had been the clue because vomiting is not a symptom of chickenpox.

The Freudenbergers met the Huffmans and incorporated a foundation to raise money for the study, treatment, cure, and prevention of Reye's syndrome in 1974. They asked the Bryan Jaycees for support. Soon plans were in full swing to make Reye's syndrome a national program of the Jaycees, to raise money with Christmas cards, to publish a pamphlet, and to develop a speaker's bureau. The Freudenbergers wanted to make Reye's syndrome a household word. Ohio was among the top states reporting cases to the CDC.

The Freudenbergers filed for non-profit status and looked for someone to accept their donation of approximately $600 in memorial funds. When they heard about a meeting that Ohio State researcher J. Dennis Pollack was organizing at an old hotel in downtown Columbus, they arranged to talk with him.

Pollack's Reye's Syndrome Conference was the first ever dedicated solely to Reye's syndrome. Pollack had no funding and did it through goodwill, tenacity, and charm. (Later, he did get sponsors including the Children's Hospital Research Foundation, the NIH, the FDA, the John W. Champion Center, and Ross Laboratories, a division of Abbott Laboratories.) Pollack had become interested in Reye's after earning a PhD and taking a position at Ohio State where he began studying influenza and fatty acids. He found high levels of fatty acids in children with Reye's syndrome and knew that mitochondria, where fatty acids are processed, might be involved.

In 2006, Pollack told me, "It was something that had to be done. No one had really investigated the disease in what I thought would be a technical and appropriate manner. Being a laboratory guy, not a clinical guy, I thought there were a lot of loose research ends." He involved Ohio State colleagues and worked with Milo Hilty, a clinician at the Children's Hospital. He called each doctor and scientist who had ever written anything on Reye's. "And one guy led to another guy and led to another woman … And some were obviously more interested, more excited, and more supportive than others … those are the people you're interested in."

Pollack edited the proceedings of the conference and had them published in 1975 in the first book solely dedicated to Reye's syndrome.[1] The content was impressive, both for what had been learned and what was still unknown. The *Proceedings* included 38 papers by 71 contributors on topics ranging from diagnostic pathology to etiologic and metabolic aspects to treatment. For example, Jerome Haller of Tufts reviewed the experience of doctors at three hospitals—one each in New Jersey, Georgia, and Massachusetts—who had been studying four treatment regimens and had randomized 21 children. Unfortunately, they had not enrolled enough children to make a definitive statement about the relative merits of the treatments (supportive therapy alone or with peritoneal dialysis, exchange transfusion—in which the blood is removed and exchanged, or glucose and insulin—to drive glucose into cells). In the conference summary, Ohio State physician Milo Hilty of the Children's Hospital in Columbus speculated on interactions between viruses, toxins, and genetics and suggested that, of the implicated drugs, aspirin was "a likely candidate to either be involved in the pathogenesis or to contribute to the severity of the illness."[2]

Pollack encouraged the Freudenbergers to create a scientific advisory board. He chaired it himself until the mid-1980s when Thomas Glick, a former EIS officer, took over. The focus of the foundation was not to fund research (there was too little money for that), but to share information. Pollack suggested the foundation support a medical journal to advertise the disease and generate interest among the scientific community. "A lot of scientists," he explained, "will do something just because they are curious even though it's not earth-shattering and won't change the spin of the earth."

By 1979, because of the tireless efforts of the Freudenbergers, the National Reye's Syndrome Foundation [Ohio] had 48 chapters throughout 21 states and Canada.[3]

At the same time another foundation, the National Reye's Syndrome Foundation of Michigan, was focusing on organizing a major study on Reye's syndrome. Three couples—the Dieckmans and the Crawfords of Michigan, and the Pettines of Massachusetts—had formed the National Reye's Syndrome Foundation [Michigan] after their sons had died of Reye's syndrome shortly after Thanksgiving 1975.

Eleven-year-old John Dieckman, the youngest child of John (Sr) and Doris Dieckman of Benzonia, Michigan, had missed several days of school the week before Thanksgiving.[4] The freezing northern Michigan winter had arrived, and John had a sore throat. By Saturday, though, he was well enough to play basketball at Benzie County Central High School. He came home noticeably tired and on Sunday started to vomit. The family doctor prescribed something for vomiting. By Monday the vomiting had abated, but the boy was worse, disoriented with episodes of bizarre, frightening behavior. "There was no way to communicate with him, no way to get through to him," his father said later. "He would become violent, then quiet … then violent, and then quiet again … He would double up his fist and slam it just as hard as he could against anything. … Doris and I were with him almost constantly." Around 8 pm, after two contacts with their physician, the Dieckmans drove their son 35 miles to a medical center in Traverse City. Twelve hours later, doctors told them that John had Reye's syndrome.

John was flown by air ambulance to the University of Michigan in Ann Arbor and admitted to Mott Children's Hospital. By evening, he had sunk into a coma. In the intensive care unit, he was intubated and hooked up to a ventilator. Medications were used to control the pressure building in his brain. Researchers had recently shown that on average the brains of children with Reye's syndrome *were 28% heavier [swollen] than normal.*[5] Unbelievably, there was another child in the ICU with the same "rare" Reye's coma. His name was Jimmy Crawford, the son of Judith and James Crawford of Ann Arbor.

John emerged from the coma and was transferred to the pediatric ward. On 10 December, in the elevator, as the Dieckmans were leaving the hospital with John, they met the Crawfords on their way to see Jimmy. The next day the Dieckmans drove home to Benzonia. John spent the evening playing with his two sisters and went to bed in his parents' bedroom around 11 pm. At 1 am, he awoke, got out of bed, and, as his father recalled, "took four steps and said, 'Dad, I can't breathe' … and that was the end. Boom—just like that." The official cause of death was listed as acute pulmonary edema, but the real cause, according to John's father, was Reye's syndrome. The case was unusual in that death had occurred suddenly in the wake of an apparent recovery.

The report of John's death never reached the CDC. Michigan doctors were not required to report Reye's syndrome. According to Dieckman, the CDC had received no case reports of Reye's syndrome in Michigan in 1975, yet he knew of more than 40 cases. For the first five months of 1976, the CDC again had received no Michigan reports; Dieckman knew of 17, including that of Jimmy Crawford. Dieckman came to believe that Reye's syndrome was not the rare disease it was made out to be. And he was right. The reality was that soon surveys by CDC and others would find that Reye's syndrome was a top killer of children and for each fatal case there were many non-fatal ones.

After Jimmy Crawford died, his parents decided to support Reye's syndrome research. Crawford recalled, "My wife and I traveled to the Boston area … We had some memorial funds, and we wanted to give the money to a hospital research center that was conducting basic-science work. But we were amazed to find out that nothing was going on. I mean, this was Boston … supposedly the top medical research centers in the world. And absolutely nothing was happening."[6] While they were in Boston, they met with Boston Floating Hospital pediatric neurologist Jerome Haller, whose assessment of the research situation was discouraging. He suggested they talk with Louis Pettine of Fall River.

Four-year-old Michael Pettine, the eldest son of Louis and Susan Pettine, was admitted to the Boston Floating Hospital for Infants and Children on 18 November 1975.[7] Michael had had the flu and was ready to go back to school when he started to vomit. Pettine, a buyer for clothing chain Anderson Little was away on business when his son was hospitalized. He flew back to Boston and learned the diagnosis. Pettine thought, "My son was in one of the finest hospitals in the country … they perform miracles in that place. So, they were going to straighten out the problem."[8] The next day the Pettines asked a young resident about their son's recovery. When he told them he had seen 16 cases and 14 had died, they were stunned by the gravity of the situation and cried. On Friday 21 November 1975, Michael Pettine was pronounced dead.

Pettine told me that gifts in Michael's memory had poured in but after they visited Haller, they realized the amount would buy little in terms of research.

In early February 1976, the Crawfords contacted the Pettines.[9] They met for dinner in Braintree, Massachusetts, talked for six hours, and agreed to work on stimulating public awareness of Reye's syndrome. The Crawfords told the Pettines about the Dieckmans. The three couples got together in April and founded the National Reye's Syndrome Foundation [Michigan]. John Dieckman became president, Jim Crawford vice-president, and Lou Pettine treasurer.

Pettine later recalled that the three men had flown to the CDC and talked with a "nice guy" who in their estimation provided little information. Frustrated by having so many questions and so few answers, they decided to make as many contacts in the field as they could and put together a conference of smart people. They had about $15,000. The rest they charged or paid for out of their pockets.

Over the next five years they worked tirelessly, especially John Dieckman, whose voice was persistent and effective. He was the person everyone got behind. Crawford recalled, "You can't imagine somebody so highly motivated on a cause and effect as that man was. And frankly, it almost engulfed him … When he'd go to a meeting in DC … he'd take out a picture of his son. He was almost in a trance ... I can't even explain to you how highly motivated he was to get something done with this thing."

Many details stuck with Crawford when I spoke to him in 2011. He told me that his son had not taken aspirin. "We started doing publicities and ads and parents started calling us up. And whenever we got a few parents together, we'd fly into that city ... meet a few parents and they would regroup and come back with 10, 12, 15, 20 parents ... they just didn't have anywhere to turn ... It's hard to say you took emotions out of it, but we kind of did ...We had a goal." The men typically travelled two or three weekends a month putting in 25 to 35 hours a week: "lots of travelling, lots of trips to DC, lots of trips with parents." While traveling, speaking, lobbying, writing letters, and reading the latest medical literature, Dieckman served on the local school board and worked as assistant manager at a frozen foods plant. The budget of the Michigan chapter was now about $30,000. It had no employees or consultants and paid no rent. The officers were volunteers. The mailing address was Dieckman's home.[10]

Their outreach was particularly effective in Michigan. Chris Lumsden, a young mother from Grand Rapids who thought one of her children had had a mild form of Reye's syndrome, arranged for Dieckman to address more than 300 people gathered at her local elementary school. Three journalists and a television reporter interviewed Dieckman. The interview was carried on media across the state. Presentations were also made at manufacturing facilities and local unions. Bake sales were held. Information pamphlets were distributed to PTA groups. Lumsden even persuaded a major grocery-general merchandise chain, Meijer's, to publish information on Reye's syndrome in its weekly ad, which had a circulation of one million readers.[11]

The numbers had become "pretty significant," Crawford recalled. "We had a few hundred people that had been afflicted, either grandparents or parents that had lost children or had children stricken with Reye's syndrome that were now damaged or had brain damage."

Their March 1979 brochure summarized the void of knowledge and research on Reye's syndrome: "Unfortunately, it is impossible to know how many cases of Reye's syndrome are occurring ... in only a handful of states is the disease reportable." It noted that research "is limited and uncoordinated." The foundation sent out a reprint of the 1976 FDA bulletin warning parents to "avoid anti-emetics" and recommending against the use of aspirin and acetaminophen because of the unproven possibility that they might make the illness worse.[12]

The NRSF [Michigan] also worked to make Reye's syndrome a reportable disease in all states, to establish a dedicated position at CDC, and to educate doctors. Dieckman's dream, however, was to unlock the mystery of Reye's syndrome. He planned to secure funds for a definitive study and wanted it up-and-running by the fall of 1981. Thus, the foundation sought to raise $25,000 for a series of information-pooling meetings that would serve as the basis for an NIH grant application.[13] In March 1979, three months after the seven Arizona children had become ill, researchers from 15 medical centers around the country attended the first meeting in Chicago.[14] The meeting focused on forming a study group to assess the areas of treatment, surveillance and epidemiology, and basic science related to etiology (cause) and mechanisms. The foundation would underwrite up to $30,000 for the application, while a physician in Denver, who had received a substantial private grant, planned to develop a research footing with a pilot study.[15]

Meanwhile, Dieckman and Crawford were "team[ing] up like a couple of high-pressure pitchmen, delivering the hard sell for research grants."[16] Their long hours were paying off. On 9 July 1979, Michigan Congressman Guy Vander Jagt addressed the United States House of Representatives and asked for support of the multicenter, three- to five-year study. About five to 10 million dollars would be needed.[17] The Senate Appropriations Committee asked the NIH to report on its Reye's syndrome work.[18]

Wallace Berman, the young Chief of Pediatric Gastroenterology at the Medical College of Virginia, was now Chairman of the NRSF [Michigan's] Multi-Center Study Research Group. He and Dieckman presented the Reye's situation at the American Legion's National Convention in Houston, Texas. The American Legion, an organization of veterans composed of 30,000 posts and auxiliaries, agreed to "enter the battle" against Reye's syndrome and became the first national organization to mandate an educational program on Reye's syndrome emphasizing awareness.[19]

In June 1979, two months after my visit to Schonberger at CDC, representatives of the NRSFs of Ohio and Michigan attended an NIH-sponsored workshop on influenza B in Bethesda, Maryland, which included a session on Reye's syndrome. Schonberger, Eugene Hurwitz, the EIS officer managing the study in Ohio, and other CDC personnel also attended, as did Michigan and Ohio researchers, and more than 50 other doctors, researchers, and interested parties.[20] The attendees learned that influenza B affected primarily children and young adults and was *not* generally fatal. Researchers reported that Reye's syndrome cases increased during influenza B years (for example, 1969, 1974, and 1977), and that data from the winter of 1978–1979 also found an association with influenza A.

I later learned about the NIH meeting when I saw the conference report, which concluded that Reye's syndrome might be preventable with an influenza B vaccine.[21] I did notice that aspirin was not mentioned at all.

PART II

POISONING, MARKETING, AND REGULATION 1800s–1970s

Chapter 5

Trusted—The Most Popular Medicine in the World and Early Alerts

Like Phenacetin and Heroin [other Bayer drugs] before, it [Aspirin]
quickly appeared in pharmacies from Siberia to San Francisco,
and physicians prescribed it for every malady under the sun …
Aspirin was on the way to becoming a resounding commercial triumph.

Charles C. Mann and Mark L. Plummer,
describing Bayer's early marketing campaigns in *The Aspirin Wars:*
Money, Medicine, and 100 Years of Rampant Competition, 1991

Aspirin was not only everyone's favorite remedy for everyday aches, pains, and fevers but it was also trusted. Aspirin was a staple in my parents' medicine cabinet and the go-to treatment for just about everything. Advertisements describing its safety and doctors' endorsements were common on TV and in the magazines my mother bought, like *Good Housekeeping* and *Ladies Home Journal*. I was using Tylenol for our infant simply because our pediatrician had recommended it. At the time I was unaware of the ongoing competition among aspirin companies, the new marketing threat of Johnson & Johnson's acetaminophen brand Tylenol,[1] or industry's earlier struggles with the FDA over safety caps and warning labels. I include this important history in Part II as I describe what I did learn about doctors' longstanding concerns about aspirin use in children. By late 1979, I was able to list most of these concerns in the manuscript I submitted for publication.

Confidence, loyalty, and trust

Trust is born, in part, from familiarity. Humans have extracted salicylates from plants since ancient times. In 1763 in Oxfordshire, England, Reverend Edward Stone proved salicylate could reduce fever.

A century later, in 1876, Scottish physician Thomas John Maclagan demonstrated its ability to decrease inflammation in rheumatic fever. Rheumatic fever, an acute febrile arthritis of several joints often with involvement of the heart, was common and potentially deadly. While salicylate had no effect on the inflammation in the heart, it had a dramatic effect on fever and arthritis and became a cornerstone of treatment.

During the 1800s advances in chemistry powered a fast-growing pharmaceutical industry which produced new medicines with major impacts on human health—and eye-opening profits. New laws protected entrepreneurs with patents and trademarks and the collective psyche had not yet fully embraced the concept of protecting the consumer. Germany "emerged as the world's leader in medicine."[2]

The German company Farben (Farbenfabriken vormals Friedrich Bayer and Company), also known as Bayer, began looking for a "blockbuster." Under the direction of Friedrich Carl Duisberg, Jr, head of Bayer's research and patent program, Bayer's first drug, Phenacetin, hit the market in 1887 with patent protection in the US.[3] Phenacetin's success launched Bayer as one of the world's first major pharmaceutical companies. Phenacetin was used to treat fever and pain in such popular formulations as headache powders and APC (aspirin, phenacetin, and caffeine) tablets for almost a century before evidence emerged that it caused serious kidney damage and had carcinogenic properties. It was withdrawn from the US market in 1983.[4] (Other countries including Australia had banned it years earlier.[5]) Phenacetin became one of the first modern drugs used by perhaps millions for many years before serious side effects were noticed.

In 1897, Bayer chemist Felix Hoffmann documented a process for making acetylsalicylic acid (later Arthur Eichengrün claimed Hoffmann did so under his direction).[6] However, the section chief, Professor Heinrich Dreser, rejected it on grounds that large doses caused panting (hyperventilation) and heart racing in dogs. Undeterred Duisberg enlisted an outside pharmacologist who provided "glowing" assessments.[7] In January 1899, Bayer named acetylsalicylic acid "Aspirin."* Dreser wrote a brief paper for distribution to the medical profession entitled, "Pharmacological Facts about Aspirin (acetylsalicylic acid)."[8]

Late that summer, Bayer sent free samples to a few hundred doctors, hospitals, and pharmacists across Germany and Europe explaining that Aspirin was an effective remedy for acute rheumatic fever and inflammation without the gastric side effects associated with other salicylates, and that it "showed some promise as an analgesic."[9] (According to K.D. Rainsford of the Biomedical Research Centre, Sheffield Hallam University, aspirin is "much more irritant to the stomach than either salicylic acid or sodium salicylate. ... Thus, the whole origin of aspirin appears to have been built on the early successful promotion of a completely false premise ..."[10])

The recipients of the free samples were asked to try it and publish their findings. One reported that he himself had taken 75 grains [a single dose of 4500 mg total or 75 mg/kg for a 60 kg person] "without toxic effects, except violent headache and tinnitus" and that a lower dose produced "flashes of light." Notwithstanding these symptoms, he recommended a dose (apparently for acute and chronic rheumatism) of 15 grains [900 mg] three times a day [45 mg/kg/day for a 60 kg adult].[11] Doctors' acceptance created general confidence. The beneficial effects were immediate and obvious, and doctors said so. Soon, Aspirin replaced sodium salicylate for the treatment of rheumatic diseases. Its most common use, however, would soon become the relief of pain, particularly muscle pain and headache. Amazingly, according to business historians Charles Mann and Mark Plummer, by November 1899, Aspirin was in widespread use around the world and, by 1902, more than 150 "almost universally favorable" scientific studies had been written.[12]

Securing patent protection, however, was difficult. Hoffman's

---

* Its root was derived from the fact that salicylate could be extracted from the meadowsweet plant, whose Latin genus is Spiraea, the "A" prefix was added to indicate acetylation (the addition of an acetyl group to the molecule), and the "in" made it easier to say.

procedure was simply an improvement on previous methods. Acetylsalicylic acid had first been created (and shelved) in 1853 in France, and again later in Germany. As a result, only two countries granted Bayer a patent—the United Kingdom and the United States. Nevertheless, Bayer marketed Aspirin elsewhere—in fact, almost everywhere from Latin America to Africa to China. In 1903, Bayer set in motion the development of a 75-acre Aspirin factory in Rensselaer, New York.[13]

Bayer marketed Aspirin as an "ethical" medicine, one usually referred to by a Latin name and sold only with a doctor's prescription (as compared with patent or proprietary medicines). Cognizant of the AMA's wary view of marketing, Bayer "promoted only to the medical profession ... and advertis[ed] in the *Journal of the American Medical Association* [*JAMA*]."[14] Its ads were simple—"Aspirin for headaches, Somotose for insomnia, Heroin for coughs."

Wiley shows salicylate increases metabolism

Harvey Wiley's suggestion that relatively small amounts of salicylate might be harmful did nothing to affect the public's love affair with Aspirin. Wiley was one of a new school of experimental pharmacologists learning about drugs through experiments rather than simply accepting the "*materia medica*," the plants and minerals used to remediate illnesses over the past centuries.[15] Wiley, Chief of the US Bureau of Chemistry (the forerunner of the FDA), was concerned with the increasing use of food preservatives such as boric acid and salicylate. He experimented by giving salicylate in increasing quantities from 0.2 to 10 grams per day to healthy young men and observing them for physical changes. (For a man weighing 60 kg, the amounts would be equivalent to 3 to 167 mg/kg/day.)

In 1906, Wiley wrote the "general effect [of salicylate] on the system is depressing in that the tissues are broken down more rapidly than they are built up." Wiley had observed salicylate's ability to increase metabolism. "Thus, the normal metabolic processes are interfered with in a harmful way," Wiley continued.[16] Wiley's view was that a substance "does not lose its power of injury to health because it is diluted or given in small quantities." Small quantities, he thought, only "masked the injurious effects." He continued with zeal: "If the use of small quantities is permitted, then there can never be any agreement among experts or others respecting the magnitude of the 'small quantity,' and continued litigation and disagreement must follow."[17] Wiley's predictions about litigation and disagreement were correct. Even today experts argue over acceptable benefit-to-risk ratios. After all, most substances, even water, can be harmful—in some amount. Prior to his experiments, Wiley had been relying on the testimony of experts, many from industry, but now he was convinced by his own data.[18] Industry attacked him claiming that it alone, not the government, should define what was harmful. Simply, industry wanted government off its back.

An enlightened public, however, was clamoring for something to be done about food adulteration. In 1906, Congress—bolstered by Wiley's work, Upton Sinclair's novel *The Jungle* exposing disgusting manipulations of foods by the Chicago meatpacking industry, and the backing of President Theodore Roosevelt—passed the Pure Food and Drug Act (the Wiley Act).[19] The legislation prevented "the manufacture, sale, or transportation of adulterated or misbranded or poisonous or deleterious foods, drugs, medicines, and liquors" and regulated "traffic therein, and for other purposes."[20] Specifically, the information on the *label* was to be true (that is, not misbranded) and the contents of the package not adulterated. Great ideas, but the devil would be in the details.

The Act also required manufacturers to list the presence of 10 compounds, including potentially addictive ones like alcohol, cocaine, heroin, and cannabis. However, substances for which quantity (dose) was the key difference between safety and harm were not specifically addressed. Wiley was not the first to offer an opinion on the importance of quantity. Sixteenth century physician Paracelsus had famously suggested, "All things are poison, and nothing is without poison: the *Dosis* alone makes a thing not poison."[21]

By 1911, salicylate as a preservative was replaced by benzoic acid.[22]

Half a century later, in 1958, Congress finally passed a law defining "food additive." Unless a substance was on the "generally recognized as safe" list, the FDA would have to approve it. Salicylate is not on the list.[23] Meanwhile, to comply with the Wiley Act, the manufacturer's *label* simply had to avoid false statements. It must have seemed that the less said the better. Besides, advertisements were not considered part of the label; there manufacturers could be more creative.

Wiley's experiments seemed to have no practical effect on the new and growing Aspirin market as Aspirin became a model for self-medication. An over-the-counter version allowed consumers to medicate themselves. This dual marketplace spawned heated debate. The AMA, for example, believed self-medication with "brand names and patents did nothing but drive up costs and mislead patients."[24] Others thought the AMA's ideas were self-serving. Helping oneself or one's family had strong appeal and pills from a local store were cheap. Initially, most consumers had never heard of Bayer, which sold Aspirin almost exclusively to wholesalers like the United Drug Company (UDC) of Boston, which repackaged it under its name.[25,26] Then, in a flash of commercial brilliance, Bayer decided to emphasize its trademark, the easy to recognize quasi-religious Bayer cross, and easily obtained trademarks for "Aspirin" throughout the world. Trademarks were protected indefinitely by an international agreement in 1883. According to Mann and Plummer: "Bayer would try to make consumers so thoroughly identify relief with 'Bayer Aspirin' that its rivals would have no chance … [Beginning in 1914] Each tablet was stamped with the Bayer Cross … which for the first time let customers see the name of the company that cured their headaches."[27] Bayer Aspirin became perhaps the most widely recognized brand in the world.

Kidneys and danger at the beginning of treatment

On 12 October 1901, a five-year-old boy was admitted to London's Hospital for Sick Children on Great Ormond Street with signs of acute rheumatic fever—arthritis in several joints, fever, and heart involvement—and died. It was not the disease that killed him. His doctor, 27-year-old Frederick Langmead, whose "diagnostic skill, especially with small children was later deemed exceptional"[28] identified the culprit: salicylate poisoning. Doctors had frequently encountered salicylate intoxication when treating rheumatic fever. However, Langmead was surprised. He had treated the child with relatively small doses of sodium salicylate—about 75 mg/kg/day divided into four doses.*

Langmead reported his observations in *The Lancet* where he captured both the enthusiastic endorsement and dire warnings of salicylate by Harveian Lecturer and senior physician D.B. Lees in 1903.[29] Sodium salicylate, Lees had said, was among "the most valuable of recently introduced medicines." Yet Lees was no Pollyanna. He recognized its toxicity and recommended, as a prophylactic measure, the administration of sodium bicarbonate (common baking soda) at twice the salicylate dose. (Later doctors learned that bicarbonate increases the kidney's ability to remove salicylate from the body.) Lees had taught that "*by gradually increasing an initial small dose he can administer the drug in such large doses as these without producing any of the much-feared symptoms of salicylate poisoning.*" [Emphasis added] Lees had also warned doctors to watch for early symptoms. Deepening respiration, he said, necessitates immediate discontinuation.[30] In 1909, Lees' warning took on a more urgent tone, "As soon as any unpleasant symptom due to salicylate occurs in an adult, or vomiting in a child, the drug should be suspended."[31]

Langmead described the illnesses of eight children. The five-year-old boy at first had improved. Then, after several weeks, he vomited and developed fever and marked air hunger. His breath smelled of acetone and he quickly deteriorated. A postmortem examination revealed no specific cause for the death. Seven other patients followed similar courses but survived. The final patient was noteworthy in that his symptoms *continued to worsen even after the drug was discontinued.*

---

* He was treated with 5 grains [300 mg] every six hours without bicarbonate. If he weighed 16 kilograms (36 pounds), his dose would have been 75 mg/kg/day.

Langmead was perplexed about the great variation in the dose that produced toxicity as well as his observation that some of the toxic children received "quite small doses." He surmised that constipation and deficient elimination of urine seemed to allow "a concentration of the poisonous products."[32] Indeed, in 1879, French physician Blanchier had already observed that if the kidneys were impaired, slow elimination of "accumulated salicyl will give rise to trouble."[33] Inadequate flow of urine was identified as the first factor contributing to salicylate toxicity.

Langmead now suggested a second factor—a danger at the beginning of treatment. He did not know what it was but offered a recommendation that, if followed, might have saved many lives. The "time to use the drug most cautiously is, therefore at the beginning of its administration so that the personal factor may be estimated." His idea, however, would be ignored, resurrected in mid-century—and ignored again.

Individual differences; toxic and fatal dose elusive

The AMA became "a major broker of American pharmaceutical policy" via its Council on Pharmacy and Therapeutics, which advised the government and physicians through its publication, the *Journal of the American Medical Association* (*JAMA*).[34] It called upon physician Paul J. Hanzlik of Cleveland's prestigious Western Reserve University to "clear up" physician thinking about the idea that some of the many salicylates being marketed were less toxic than others. Hanzlik reviewed the records of 400 hospitalized adults (three-fourths with rheumatic fever) who had been given a salicylate, including Aspirin, sodium salicylate, and others, and published his data in 1913.[35] Each had received the equivalent of about two to four (adult) 325-mg tablets every hour. No tests were available to use as indicators of toxicity, so he used patient symptoms to estimate the *median toxic dose*, that is, the dose at which half developed signs of toxicity such as ringing of the ears, deafness, or vomiting for which the physician had typically stopped treatment.

Hanzlik estimated that under this regimen the median cumulative toxic dose for Aspirin was about 11,000 mg and 8000 mg for an adult male and female, respectively. Importantly, salicylate had usually been given with bicarbonate, which meant the true toxic amount was lower. Half of the patients had become toxic during the first day. The toxic dose differed widely among individuals, as shown in Figure 5.1 for synthetic salicylate, even differing at times for the same person.

All drugs show individual differences in whether they work (efficacy) and in toxicity (safety). The only way to determine the reasons for these differences is by formal clinical experiment. At least for now, individual differences were identified as another factor in determining salicylate toxicity.

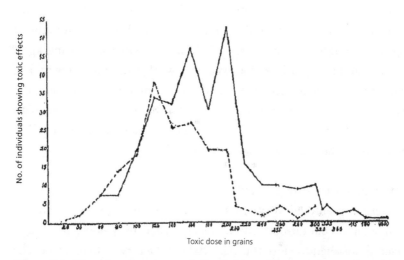

Figure 5.1 Chart showing range and distribution of the toxic doses of synthetic salicylate. The continuous line represents males; the broken line, females.[36]

Hanzlik remained interested in salicylates. In 1917, he found that salicylate causes swelling of the body. About 20 hours after beginning treatment, body weight increased and persisted until the salicylate was excreted from the body in about three-and-a-half days. Hanzlik called this phenomenon "salicyl edema."[37] Salicyl edema was seemingly of no practical use until the early 1920s when French florists recognized that aspirin could be used to revive wilted flowers by making them swell back to their original state.[38] What Hanzlik had observed was the ability of salicylate to affect a process basic to human life—the maintenance of just the right amount of water inside cells.

Unable to find a single toxic amount, Hanzlik must have been frustrated. So, later, after moving to Stanford University, he attempted to answer an even more basic question. What is the lethal amount? In 1927, after reviewing the medical literature of the previous 50 years, he settled upon the disturbing conclusion that the lethal dose also "varied."[39] Nevertheless he made an estimate.* If his estimate is applied to a four-year-old child weighing about 16 kg, the fatal single dose would be about 3,200 mg or 200 mg/kg. Researchers had previously concluded that 5000 mg of sodium salicylate caused potentially lethal symptoms in dogs.[40,41] Doctors would later agree that Hanzlik was about right. In 1966, manufacturers agreed to limit the amount of aspirin in children's containers to 2916 mg (36 tablets) (182 mg/kg, if taken all at once, by a 16 kg four-year-old) so that the amount would be under the estimated "fatal if taken all at once" amount.[42] Curiously, the average amount *taken over several days* by the Arizona children with Reye's syndrome, 5165 mg, exceeded the estimate of the fatal "all at once" dose. These amounts seemed quite close.

Bayer loses patent protection

As Germany entered WWI in 1914, Britain commandeered most of its phenol, a coal-tar-derived chemical needed to make Aspirin, and Bayer almost had to close the giant Aspirin factory in Rensselaer. The English Board of Trade cancelled the Aspirin trademark (Britain had already negated Bayer's patent in 1905[43]) and ordered Bayer to "wind up its British affairs."[44] Worse yet, other companies were producing fake Aspirin.[45] The government of Australia also suspended the German patents and trademarks and, in 1915, granted a license to manufacture

---

* For sodium salicylate based on his work on adults, he estimated the fatal dose was between 1000 and 1500 milligrams per kilogram for all animals studied, and for methyl salicylate and aspirin 50 to 80% less. Using his most conservative estimate (80% of 1000 milligrams per kilogram), an estimate of the fatal dose for aspirin would be 200 mg/kg.

and sell the product in the Commonwealth to H.W. Shmith and G.R.R. Nicholas[46] who, two years later, registered the drug under the trade name Aspro.[47] Their company hired New Zealander George Davies, who devised a brilliant sales strategy including gift packs, defined market areas, and hard-sell advertising.[48] Slogans were his specialty: "Aspro is the tablet that has made Australia famous."[49] Aspro was even marketed for a new illness "one degree under" with which almost everyone could identify.[50]

That was not all. The impending loss of the lucrative US patent in 1917 put Bayer in another predicament. Companies like Dow Chemical of Midland, Michigan, were preparing to make acetylsalicylic acid.[51] The United Drug Company (UDC), which had been repackaging Aspirin for Bayer, began buying acetylsalicylic acid from a company in St Louis, Missouri, called Monsanto Chemical Works, labeling tablets 5 grains Aspirin UDC.[52] Facing this competition, Bayer abandoned its conservative marketing and began advertising to the public. "In the fall of 1916, Aspirin ads appeared in newspapers across the United States, headlined with 'Bayer' above a picture of an Aspirin box."[53] The early ads focused on purity and genuineness.[54]

In 1917, US federal Judge Learned Hand approved generic use of the word "aspirin."[55] Immediately, the AMA advised physicians to avoid the term "Aspirin" when prescribing acetylsalicylic acid and reprimanded the company for "attempting to impress on the lay mind that there is no satisfactory Aspirin, except Aspirin-Bayer."[56] "Aspirin" simply became aspirin, an iconic medicine for relief of common ailments. Nevertheless, Bayer had two valuable assets: a trademarked name and a widely recognized symbol, the Bayer cross.

The great influenza deals aspirin a lucrative hand

Now fortune visited aspirin in the form of the worst recorded influenza pandemic in history. All told the Great Influenza claimed millions around the world and over 500,000 victims in the United States alone. On 13 September 1918, as a deadly second wave of influenza hit, the *New York Times* summarized United States Surgeon General Rupert

Blue's recommendations of bed rest, abundant food, fresh air, and Dover's powder (a combination of opium and ipecac) as well as his statement that salts of quinine and aspirin had been used "apparently with much success in the relief of symptoms."[57] A US Navy circular recommended a cathartic and aspirin and warned not to take large doses of aspirin. While "large doses" was not defined, the Navy's own *materia medica* advised a dose of aspirin up to 1300 mg (about four adult tablets).[58] The British War Office recommended a similar dose.[59] A London physician advised a dose schedule of 20 grains [1200 mg] per hour for 12 hours non-stop and every two hours thereafter.[60] Monsanto Chemical Works of St Louis advertised acetyl salicylic acid for shipment in the periodical *Drug and Chemical Markets*.[61] And Bayer ads emphasized its American staff and control of the Alien Property Custodian, which had seized the assets.[62]

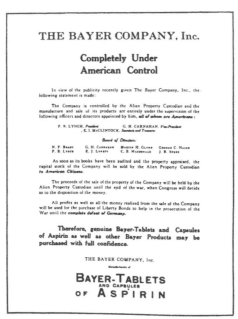

Advertisement
Drug and Chemical Markets, 18 September 1918

Homeopaths, generally shocked at the harsh compounds used by physicians of the day, thought that aspirin was a poison and boasted that under their care, few flu victims died.[63,64] Today, salicylates are known to cause pulmonary edema (swelling of the lungs) in some adults.[65] Could aspirin-induced lung swelling have exacerbated the effects of an influenza infection in some individuals?[66] More than 60 years would pass before doctors tested aspirin for the treatment of influenza. (See Chapter 25) Meanwhile, beginning in 1918 and for the next 50 years—absent valid testing—influenza and aspirin were firmly linked in the minds of physicians and consumers alike.

In December 1918, as the Great War ended, the United States government auctioned Bayer's assets to the highest bidder. Sterling Products, Inc. of Wheeling, West Virginia, founded by childhood friends William E. Weiss and Albert H. Diebold, paid $5,310,000 for the facility in Rensselaer and Bayer's drugs and dyestuffs.[67] Sterling was known mainly for its patent medicines with secret (proprietary) ingredients, such as Neuralgine for pain and Sterling Remedy for nicotine addiction.[68] The scorn of the AMA did not stop Sterling and others from advertising. Aspirin production and sales doubled between 1918 and 1920.[69] But Sterling needed Bayer's manufacturing expertise. In April 1923, Sterling and Bayer reached several agreements distributing work and profits. Regarding marketing, one contract granted Sterling exclusive rights to sell aspirin in the "Weiss countries," the United States, Canada, Great Britain, Australia, and South Africa. Farben would control the Bayer Cross in the rest of the world. Sterling would continue to sell aspirin in Latin America per an earlier contract.[70] Few places in the world would be without Bayer aspirin.

In Australia, G.R. Nicholas' marketing strategy paid off. In 1919, the government fixed the price of "necessary commodities." Aspro became a necessary commodity.[71] In 1927, Aspro Limited was formed in the UK and its factory in Slough, outside London, produced its first tablets. That year, British sales were 10 times higher than those in Australia.[72] In the 1930s, marketers spread Aspro throughout the world: to Fiji, Singapore, Thailand, Borneo, China, Goa, and South Africa, and then north into other African countries.[73]

Chapter 6

Lost Warnings and Loopholes

The initiation of the AAF Rheumatic Fever Control Program brought
to light the fact that the existing knowledge concerning absorption,
distribution and excretion of salicylates was insufficient
for rational therapy.

Paul K. Smith, Helen L. Gleason, D.G. Stoll, and S. Ogorzalek
Journal of Pharmacology and Experimental Therapeutics, 1946

Medicine versus sponging

Before the 1920s, pediatricians were not particularly keen on using any fever reducer for minor childhood illnesses. For example, Columbia University physician L. Emmett Holt, in each edition of his classic book *The Care and Feeding of Children: A Catechism for Mothers and Children's Nurses* between 1907 and as late as 1934, did not mention aspirin (or salicylate). A textbook for physicians, which he wrote with St Louis physician John Howland in 1912, stated "older children, particularly rheumatic, should be treated with sodium salicylate, or aspirin, four or five grains every three hours being given for the first twenty-four hours and then less frequently."[1] In fact, in their books published in 1912 and 1918, Holt and Howland vigorously opposed the use of any of the new fever reducers stating that "too much cannot be said in condemnation of the practice of giving the coal tar products in full doses for the reduction of temperature." Their threshold for treatment of fever was "105 degrees or over."[2, 3] In 1918, New York pediatrician Henry Koplik, considered the most "distinguished pediatrician in America", agreed.[4] He deemed sponging with lukewarm water as the safest and best way to reduce fever and recommended aspirin only for orthopedic pain.[5]

A horrific disaster invites government oversight

As aspirin became a household name via doctors' acceptance, the easily recognized name and symbol, widespread use during the influenza pandemic of 1918, and advertisements, the expiration of Bayer's US patent spawned one of the most widespread and expensive market rivalries of the 20th century. And while the 1906 Pure Food and Drug Act required drug *labels* list ingredients and be truthful, Congress left a huge loophole for advertising. The Act did not apply to brochures, newspaper ads, posters, and later radio ads.[6] Thus, in 1912, for example, the government lost a case against Johnson's Mild Combination Treatment for Cancer because the court ruled therapeutic claims did not fall under the 1906 Act.

Congress stepped up to remedy this problem by passing the Sherley Amendment prohibiting false therapeutic claims intended to defraud.[7] But the onus was on the government to prove that a product was worthless or dangerous *and* an intent to defraud.[8] In 1914 Congress created the Federal Trade Commission (FTC) to address unfair practices. The FTC could battle a claim in court or issue a cease-and-desist order.[9] By 1915, the government had seized 31 falsely and fraudulently labeled medicines.[10] Houchens Medicine Company of Baltimore, Maryland, for example, pleaded guilty as one of its products had been marketed for smallpox claiming "pimples … will be carried off by the medicine." In 1933, the commission launched "the first of a dozen cases against the aspirin makers."[11] More than $750,000 was being spent on ads for Bayer Aspirin, "the Tiffany of analgesics."[12] Others including, for example, Asper-Lax, America's Purest Aspirin, Lord's Aspirin, and Alka-Seltzer were also spending large sums.[13] Claims had been escalating in number and becoming more outrageous. The FTC found "thirteen aspirin makers guilty of false advertising … all were admonished … most for saying that their aspirin was somehow different from that of their rivals." Each promised to stop.[14] Promises, however, often were just that. Skirmishes between the manufacturers tapping into consumer psychology with vague and unsubstantiated terms, such as "better" and "dependable," and the pesky commission trying to take a hard line on "truth in advertising" repeatedly continued. The FTC was no match for industry and barely bridled promotion continued.

Meanwhile, scientific study of drugs was replacing the trial-and-error method. The Food and Drug Administration (FDA) (which had been carved from the Bureau of Chemistry in 1930) created a new Division of Pharmacology in 1935[15] and its own "advertisement" of sorts, a travelling exhibit of problem products that a reporter named the "American Chamber of Horrors."[16] The exhibit included Lash Lure, an irritating dye that caused blindness; Radithor, radioactive radium that was marketed for impotence; and dinitrophenol, a dangerous substance for weight loss that was considered a cosmetic.[17] Pediatricians' concerns about the drugs were also increasing. In 1930 pediatricians split from the AMA and formed the American Academy of Pediatrics (AAP) to become "the voice of child health and protection."[18] At the time the AAP had no role in defining the United States Pharmacopeia (USP), a uniform set of standards for drug quality that the Pure Food and Drug Act had deemed legally enforceable and which was updated periodically by independent physicians and pharmacologists.[19] An AAP committee convened to "reestablish drugs and remedial agents prescribed by physicians ... and put dosage for children on a sound and satisfactory basis."[20] The AMA, however, would not release control of the USP, so the AAP Committee sought to "gather in one place all the pertinent data on pediatric pharmacology." Possibly due to the Depression and the number of drugs useful to pediatricians, it disbanded. "Despite the efforts of the FDA reformers, pediatricians and the AMA Council on Pharmacy and Chemistry, the patent medicine industry flourished in the 1930s."[21]

Then, a horrific disaster forever changed both the government and the pharmaceutical industry. More than 100 people including many children died in agony after ingesting the truly miraculous new antibiotic, Elixir Sulfonamide. The chemist at its manufacturer (S.E. Massengill Company of Bristol, Tennessee) lacked formal training and had unknowingly placed the antibiotic in diethylene glycol, a sweet, easy-to-swallow—but fatally toxic—solvent. Its founder apologized but pointed out that he had not broken any laws. And he was right. He had only misbranded the drug as an elixir. *No law forbade the sale of a useless or toxic medicine, only misbranding it.* The company was fined a mere $26,000.[22] In 1938 seeking to restore consumer confidence, the US Congress passed the landmark Food, Drug, and Cosmetic Act. The Act required the government to approve the safety of all *new* drugs and specifically forbade the sale of any "new drug" that the Food and Drug Administration (FDA) had not declared safe. The Act essentially placed the government in a powerful position—right between the drug companies and the marketplace.

The aspirin manufacturers, however, were off the hook. Aspirin was a "grandfather" drug, not a "new drug," and therefore no safety checks were required. The Act left advertising under the FTC as well which suited the manufacturers. Mann and Plummer noted that *"Business Week* reported, 'business is relieved that the control of advertising reposes finally in the FTC and not the [FDA]; it does not anticipate any big crackdowns from its old friends in the commission offices.'"[23]

Aspirin, likely the most widely marketed drug on the planet, marched on. In 1942 alone, salespeople of Sydney Ross, Sterling's export division in South America, "handed out eighty-one million handbills, twenty-seven million samples, and four million posters. Almanacs, saint's cards, religious posters, paper airplanes … all were plastered with the name of Mejoral [aspirin] and other new Sterling products."[24] And in 1954, as the number of television sets in the United States reached 32 million, aspirin was there.[25] By the mid-1950s, some companies' advertising budgets swelled to over $10 million.[26] Each company "was ready to claim, loudly and, in perpetuity, that its product was faster, safer, more effective. The Aspirin Wars had begun."[27] By 1961, 22 million pounds of aspirin were produced in the United States alone, more than twice the amount a decade earlier.[28] There seemed to be no end in sight. Mann and Plummer surmised that without the marketers, "the drug would never have achieved its monumental success."[29]

Accumulation in adults and then disappearance leaving not a trace (1940s)

Quietly, during the 1940s, Lt. Commander Alvin F. Coburn proved that Langmead's concerns about a danger during the first days of dosing were warranted. Coburn set out to improve upon the salicylate regimen for rheumatic fever. While the new antibiotic sulfanilamide could control the strep infection that initiated the inflammation and thus prevent rheumatic fever completely, it did not affect established illness. Coburn reasoned if salicylate could prevent inflammation, the scarring of the heart might be prevented too. To determine the best dose, Coburn developed a precise measurement of the salicylate level in the blood, an improvement upon previous methods developed during the 1930s.[30] The blood test revealed important information yet, unfortunately, while precise, the level in the blood would prove at times to be devastatingly misleading.

First, in 1943, after Coburn joined the US Navy, he found that for adults it took about three days of regular dosing to reach a steady blood level.[31] In other words, with the same dosing schedule each day, salicylate was accumulating in the blood, and then leveling off. Ten adults receiving 1.6 grams every four hours orally (approximately 160 mg/kg/day for a 60-kg adult) had peak levels on day three or four. A typical patient had levels of 15.3, 23.4, 32.6 and 27.2 mg/dL on days 1–4, respectively. Langmead's 1906 speculation had been prescient.

Coburn also found that once the drug was stopped, the blood level plunged rapidly. As shown in Table 6.1 below, two days after the last dose (in persons receiving 10 grams per day) salicylate is undetectable in the blood in almost everyone. In other words, it left no evidence in the blood that it had been there, possibly explaining why levels were so low in children with Reye's syndrome.

After testing various regimens, Coburn concluded that 10,000 mg (10 grams) (167 mg/kg/day for a 60 kg adult) of sodium salicylate per day, resulting in an average plasma level of 37 mg/dL, controlled rheumatic inflammation. Unfortunately, at that level, toxic symptoms

Table 6.1 The Fall in Salicylate Plasma Levels on Withdrawal of Salicylate Therapy[32]

Case	Salicylate Level in Plasma (mg/dL)		
	During dosing	24 hours after last dose	48 hours after last dose
2	31	10	0
3	27	10	0
4	31	11	0
5	35	10	0
6	38	20	0
7	38	23	0
8	31	9	0
9	40	24	0
10	33	11	0

Note: 10 grams per day is approximately 167 mg/kg/day for a 60-kg adult

such as nausea and vomiting were frequent. Careful monitoring of the patient was necessary.[33]

During the mid-1940s, "massive salicylate therapy," as Coburn's therapy was sometimes called, seemed so promising for rheumatic fever that it was soon tried on children. The studies to follow were essentially "*reverse* dose-response" studies. Instead of starting with a low dose and working up to a higher dose as is done today, the investigators started with a high dose, observed for toxicity, and then lowered the dose.

The method was ill-conceived and the results tragic.

Adult dose schedule dangerous for children with rheumatic fever

The first in the coming series of unfortunate studies of children was conducted by researchers at the Southwestern Medical College in Dallas and published in 1944.[34] Toxicity was observed at doses of 150–170 mg/kg/day. Six rheumatic children also developed a marked prolongation of prothrombin time, a test reflecting liver dysfunction.

(Salicylate's effect on prothrombin, a blood clotting factor produced by the liver, had first been observed in rat studies in 1943.[35]) In 1946, researchers at the University of Utah School of Medicine, using tests of liver function newly developed during the 1930s, found that six adults whose plasma salicylate levels were above 40 mg/dL developed abnormal liver function test results. Now there were two indicators that salicylate affected the liver—prothrombin time and liver function tests.

In 1944, doctors at Cincinnati's Children's Hospital Research Foundation observed signs of toxicity with both aspirin and sodium salicylate at doses between 70 and 280 mg/kg/day, including mild hyperventilation and intense vomiting, which occurred commonly on day 4. In animal studies, they found that bicarbonate generally shortened the duration of poisoning while hypnotic drugs such as barbiturates increased toxicity, leading some to recommend against the use of barbiturates during treatment of salicylate intoxication.[36,37] (Oddly enough, by the 1970s, a barbiturate was sometimes used for treatment of Reye's syndrome.) Others found that the blood salicylate level dropped dramatically after bicarbonate was given for stomach upset and that after it was discontinued, the salicylate level rose higher and higher—demonstrating accumulation of salicylate in the blood.[38]

The most tragic experiment of all, however, was conducted in 1945 in Albany, New York, a few miles from Sterling's giant aspirin factory in Rensselaer. When Dorothy Stevens and Deborah Kaplan at Union University administered the Coburn dose of sodium salicylate to children with rheumatic fever, three developed toxicity and a 10-year-old boy died.[39] After the boy's death, the lab reported his salicylate levels, which had been rising higher and higher (36, 42, 81, and 100.4 mg/dL) over the course of treatment. Stevens and Kaplan concluded that "the dosages and blood levels recommended for young adults under Coburn's program cannot be followed safely in children."[40] In 1948 doctors at the Beth Israel Hospital in New York also found rising blood levels during the first few days of treatment.[41]

In 1946, Yale researchers learned that it took between 15 and 30 hours for the body to remove a dose of salicylate.[42] This fact alone should have led to the logical conclusion that dosing every four to six hours, as was in vogue with other drugs, might lead to accumulation in the body. The researchers however deemed the accumulation on repeated doses "small."[43] To the contrary, Paul Smith and colleagues of the Army Air Force (AAF) School of Aviation Medicine summed up the situation as follows: "[T]he existing knowledge concerning absorption, distribution and excretion of salicylates was insufficient for rational therapy."[44]

And the reports kept coming. Doctors all over the country tried the Coburn schedule with children with rheumatic fever and got poor results. Some vividly described the very early signs of toxic children: a striking apathy, increased breathing rate, seldom smiling, staring ahead blankly, answering questions slowly, and not wanting to be disturbed. The children "hardly ate" and then vomited.[45] Compared with adults for whom the so-called "classic" early sign of salicylate intoxication—ringing in the ears—was common,[46] it only occurred in about a fifth of cases,[47] and children rarely noticed it.[48] At first, the children simply looked ill.

Accumulation in children

In 1947, the *Journal of Pediatrics* published an observation critically important for at-home therapy.[49] Jane Erganian, a recent graduate of the Washington University School of Medicine, and her colleagues Gilbert Forbes and Dorothy Case, all staff of the Department of Pediatrics at the Washington University School of Medicine and the St Louis Children's Hospital, witnessed 13 infants, one after the other, most in a state of collapse, being admitted to the hospital with salicylate poisoning. Two had ingested a rubbing liniment containing methyl salicylate; the others had been treated at home for a cold. Each was younger than 42 months. Their cough and cold symptoms progressed to vomiting, deep rapid breathing, listlessness, semi-stupor, and dehydration. A three-week-old had a bloody nose and stools and bleeding in her brain. Several had seizures and twitching. A blood sample taken from each at hospital admission revealed "high" levels ranging from 39 to 69 mg/dL

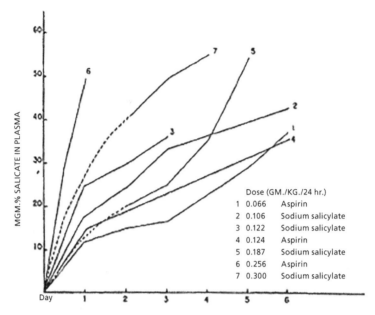

Figure 6.2 Plasma concentration of salicylate with oral aspirin and oral sodium salicylate (divided doses at four-hour intervals).[50]
Reprinted from *Journal of Pediatrics*, *30* (2), Erganian J., Forbes G.B., Case D.L., Salicylate intoxication in the infant and young child. A report of thirteen cases. Copyright (1947) Reprinted with permission from Elsevier.

but four had levels not usually associated with intoxication, only 7 to 21 mg/dL. Salicylate was also present in the spinal fluid of all 10 infants in whom it had been measured. All but one survived after receiving the standard treatment: fluids, glucose, and vitamins C and K.

Erganian asked the critical question. How much salicylate had been given at home? She talked with the parents, consulted with the pharmacists filling the prescriptions, and learned that most had received more than the recommended amount, although two had not. Erganian decided to study the doses herself by conducting an experiment. She administered aspirin or sodium salicylate in various doses for three to six days to seven children ages five to 12 years, measured their salicylate levels, and found they rose higher and higher over a period of several days. *Erganian documented accumulation in the blood, even when the dose was given every four hours at a commonly recommended children's dose of 66 mg/kg/day*, as demonstrated by Child One in Figure 6.2.

One could only conclude that the recommended dose every four hours could be a formula for disaster.

Now three potential factors that could result in accumulation in children had been identified: kidney dysfunction/dehydration, individual differences, and an unknown factor leading to rising levels early in treatment.

Erganian's report was one of the last published in the *Journal of Pediatrics* by the American Academy of Pediatrics, which then launched *Pediatrics* as its official journal.[51] Erganian's data directly refuted the conclusions of the Yale researchers who had studied only one dose a day and concluded that accumulation on repeated doses was "small."[52]

Erganian's report was not included among the 4093 references listed in the 1948 monograph entitled *The Salicylates. A Critical Bibliographic Review*.[53] The monograph's preparation had been "aided by a grant from the Institute for the Study of Analgesic and Sedative Drugs." The institute's roster included Miles, Emerson Drug, BC Remedy, Stanback, Dow Chemical, American Home Products, Sterling, and others.[54] Miles, for example, sold Alka-Seltzer and recommended: "when you need relief with speed ... Alka-Seltzer."[55] The product, a combination of aspirin, sodium bicarbonate, and anhydrous citric acid, was first marketed during the 1930s. During the 1960s everyone knew its brilliant ad: "Plop, plop, fizz, fizz. Oh, what a relief it is."

Early pronouncements stick as dose recommendations for children vary widely

Despite the forgoing reports, one man seemed to reign as the authority on aspirin dosing for children. His name was given only as Archambault and he practiced in the late 1800s during a time when teaching professorships were being established at the prestigious L'Hôpital des Enfants-Malades, the first pediatric hospital in existence when it opened in Paris in 1802.[56] Archambault was likely treating serious rheumatic diseases in children, but his words worked their way into what can only be considered a fog of dosing recommendations for the next 100 years—recommendations that variously used pounds or age as a basis, were applied to common conditions rather than to those studied, omitted frequency and/or duration of treatment, and varied as to any proof of benefit or safety at all.

In the 1800s, doctors generally used rules like the popular Young's Rule to calculate a child's dose based on age in proportion to an adult dose modified by a constant factor.[57] However going into the future for many years Archambault's opinion for salicylate dosing created a mindset that children tolerated high doses of salicylate well. He was not quoted directly. Instead, his protégé Joseph Deseille of the Faculty of Paris penned Archambault's words in 1879: "[V]ery recently, within the Therapeutic Society, our master, M. Archambault insisted on the remarkable tolerance of children for this drug, despite the high doses at which it is administered."[58] Deseille did note: "Any lesion preventing the regular functioning of the urinary tract is a contraindication to a formal administration of sodium salicylate."

For the next 50 years, Deseille's description of Archambault's pronouncement was referenced in important textbooks, including Stanford University's Paul J. Hanzlik's respected 1927 monograph on the salicylates,[59] the 1936 *Manual of Pharmacology* by Torald Sollmann of Western Reserve University in Cleveland, Ohio,[60] (both said the toxic dose is higher than would be calculated for the age), and the first edition (1941) of the classic, widely used textbook, *The Pharmacological Basis of Therapeutics*, by 35-year-old physician Louis A. Goodman and his colleague Alfred Gilman of Yale University. Goodman and Gilman passed Archambault's words to medical students and clinical physicians in the mid-20th century. The text, which sold out in six weeks,[61] echoed Archambault, noting that for acute rheumatic fever, "Children are quite tolerant of salicylates" and added "and require larger doses than calculated by their age or weight."[62] Doctors probably felt comfortable with this opinion after experts at Yale University reviewed Census statistics and found only 66 accidental deaths in children under the age of 14 years during the 10-year period ending in 1943. (Curiously, the 1955 edition of Goodman and Gilman did not address salicylate dosing for children.[63])

While Archambault's words were being memorialized in textbooks, pediatricians debated "drugs versus sponge baths" [64,65]—and provided dosing recommendations. Holt and Howland first mentioned the use of "small doses of aspirin" in 1920 for treating influenza.[66] By 1923, according to William Palmer Lucas, creator of the Department of Pediatrics at the University of California San Francisco, sodium salicylate and aspirin were said to be among the more common drugs used in pediatrics.[67] In his book *Children's Diseases for Nurses*, he wrote the dose was one grain for a six-month old and 3 to 5 grains (180 to 300 mg) for those aged four and five (i.e. a 16-kg four-year-old receiving 180 mg every four hours would receive 68 mg/kg/day).[68] Similar doses were recommended by Charles Gilmore Kerley, a founding member of the American Academy of Pediatrics,[69] and his colleague in their 1924 textbook.[70] In 1928, a physician in Albany, New York, endorsed aspirin for headache or muscle pain in children in his book on infections.[71] In 1930, William McKim Marriot, Professor of Pediatrics at the Washington University School of Medicine in St Louis recommended a frequency of every four hours for infants. The 1933 edition of *Holt's Diseases of Infancy and Children* suggested that aspirin may be given to older children for "colds" [72] while others thought that "Drugs are used chiefly by the ignorant when the family objects to the other measures and demands a drug." [73] The 1950 edition of the Mitchell-Nelson *Textbook of Pediatrics* provided instructions to physicians for mixing a liquid solution of acetylsalicylic acid in limited quantities and recommended the now widely entrenched rule of thumb: one grain [60 mg] per year of age up to age five with no statement regarding frequency or duration (thus a 16-kg four-year-old dosed every four hours would receive 90 mg/kg/day).[74] One undated container of children's aspirin recommended dosing every three hours but no more than five doses in a day.

The dose for a child crept higher in 1959 when an international yard and pound agreement changed the definition of a grain from 60 to

64.79891 milligrams (65 mg), which would increase a dose by 8%.[75] The textbook I used, the 1975 Nelson *Textbook of Pediatrics*, recommended 65 mg/kg/day divided in 4–6 doses with a maximum of 3.6 grams in 24 hours.[76] However, by the late 1970s, according to a survey of 2241 pediatricians, the most common recommendation for a four-year-old child would be one grain per year of age every four hours, or 98 mg/kg/day, an amount more than that given to Langmead's pediatric patient who became toxic and died.[77]

Therefore, a typical dose recommendation for a child generally exceeded the average adult dose of 65 mg/kg/day (i.e. the daily amount if 650 mg given every four hours to a 60-kg adult). Shockingly, it also exceeded some recommendations for rheumatic fever. For example, in 1949 pediatricians reviewing rheumatic fever treatment in the United States reported that their present policy was to use only 0.8 grains [48 mg]/kg/day, and to obtain a blood level with any sign of intoxication.[78] For the specialized treatment of rheumatic inflammation in children, Goodman and Gilman's 1970 text suggested an initial dose of 25 mg/kg/day to be reduced after 1–2 days.[79]

For most of the 20th century, both Archambault's pronouncements that salicylate is well tolerated by children, who require larger doses than their age or weight indicate, and the early dose recommendations seem to have stuck, whereas the concerning reports by Langmead, Lees, Deseille, Blanchier, Hanzlik, and those studying children in the 1940s (e.g. Erganian), as well as the 1959 change in the definition of a dose, were mostly ignored. In addition, frequency varied even though simply changing the frequency of a dose (one grain per year of age) for a four-year-old from every six to every four hours *would increase the total amount from 65 to 98 mg/kg/day*. And duration of treatment was usually not stated.

The medical community generally accepted the dose recommendations in textbooks. And there was little indication they were problematic. Indeed, ushering in the 1950s, Leon Greenburg of Yale University School of Medicine wrote in the *New England Journal of Medicine* that there was a "conspicuous absence of reports of serious poisoning or death, other than allergic poisonings, associated with ordinary therapeutic use of acetylsalicylic acid, even when this use has been continued for a long period." [80]

Amid postwar optimism, by 1948, 10 million pounds (4.5 million kg) of aspirin (four times that in 1929) were being consumed in the United States.[81] By contrast, the population had not even doubled.[82] Americans were spending almost a billion dollars on "packaged medicine ... $135 million went for aspirin and analgesics" in 1951.[83,84] Aspirin, once within the general purview of pediatricians, was about to become the darling of mid-century home therapeutics for children.

It was then that manufacturers had a brainstorm—market a tasty and visually appealing over-the-counter (OTC) aspirin tablet to the parents of all babies born after WWII. Aspirin would soon become the go-to medicine for virtually all postwar Baby Boomers, their Gen X offspring, and some of the Millennials who followed.

Chapter 7

Accidents: Unsupervised Children?

Aspirin: The Major Remaining Menace to Childhood Health
American Academy of Pediatrics, *New York Times*, 1957

Children's aspirin hits the market—toddlers love it

Plough, Inc., a pharmaceutical company in Memphis, Tennessee, was the first to think of all the babies being born after World War II. The 2.6 million babies born in 1940 would swell to 3.6 million a decade later—a million more infants and children needing aspirin annually. Parents, of course, would be the new customers fueling the already soaring aspirin market. Abe Plough who had purchased St Joseph Aspirin in 1920,[1] began marketing a pink, chewable, orange-flavored children's-size aspirin tablet in 1947. St Joseph Aspirin for Children evoked the soothing image of Jesus' caring, earthly father.

Despite the "drug versus sponge bath" debate,[2,3] aspirin had worked its way into the medical armamentarium of doctors and parents alike. Candy aspirin had become available by prescription in 1932.[4] In 1912, University of Illinois physician Bernard Fantus had set forth a list of characteristics for an ideal candy medicine—sweet, attractive, pleasant smelling, free of medicinal taste, rapidly disintegrating, and available in a variety of dosage forms. Fantus had warned physicians to prescribe only an amount that would be safe if taken all at once. Prior to product launch, Plough consulted pediatricians about the dose and the number of tablets in a container.[5] The first bottles, however, contained 50 x 1¼ grain (75 mg) tablets—for a total of 3750 mg, an amount greater than the fatal dose estimated by Hanzlik in 1927. The price was 35 cents.

Advertisements emphasized characteristics parents would appreciate, such as orange flavor and "easy to give." During the fall of 1947, Plough rolled out its coast-to-coast campaign in various newspapers across the country from Austin, Texas, to Raleigh, North Carolina, and Spokane, Washington. According to Plough's ad in the *Lansing State Journal* on 6 October 1947, St Joseph's Aspirin was already "Preferred by Millions, So Pure, So Fast, So Dependable."[6]

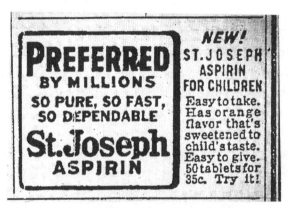

Advertisement, *Lansing State Journal,* 6 October 1947
Courtesy of Consumer Foundation Healthcare

At first pediatricians felt children's-size aspirin was a godsend. Duke University pediatrician and father of seven Jay Arena thought St Joseph children's aspirin "was a tremendous success immediately, because the parents said, 'Oh boy, we don't have to fool around with breaking up this aspirin.'"[7] But, in May 1948, a two-year-old from Durham, North Carolina, downed the entire contents of a bottle and two days later another toddler from Burlington, Vermont, who had taken a similar amount, arrived in a moribund state at Duke University. Both died. The offending sequence of events was predictable. Aspirin was colorful and tasty. Toddlers love anything that looks like candy. The caps were easy to remove. The bottle contained a potentially fatal amount. No warning was posted on the bottle.

According to Arena, he phoned Abe Plough who asked what could be done. Arena suggested a different cap.[8] Plough agreed and his staff came up with 17 different cap closures. Arena, with about 1600 families at Duke and in his practice in downtown Durham, sought to identify a closure that only about 10% of children could remove.[9]

The deaths continued. On 8 February 1950, the *Long Beach Press* reported that two children had been taken to the Seaside Hospital after mistakenly swallowing aspirin.[10] The next month the *Press* reported the death of a 15-month-old Sunland boy who had died "after gobbling a handful of aspirin tablets."[11]

Gentle and safe

Sterling Drug also began manufacturing a children's-size tablet. On 9 July 1950, one of Sterling's early ads for children's aspirin in the *Long Beach Press* highlighted the fact that its tablets were "neither flavored nor colored, so they cannot be mistaken for candy." It also emphasized the "New 2 1/2 grain tablets [half of a regular tablet or ~150 mg] provide proper children's dosages prescribed by your doctor."[12] Sterling's early bottles contained 30 tablets (4500 mg), and, like Plough's, a potentially fatal amount.[13]

Sterling vigorously challenged Plough for primacy of the children's aspirin market. The company had emerged from WWII with "unprecedented profit margins" and was dominating.[14] Its success, like Plough's, was attributed to "its advertising technique which had been perfected during its forty year period of existence," including its thousand-man sales-force who visited small towns distributing tens of millions of copies of hand material and samples.[15] In 1947, Sterling's Bayer Aspirin Division opened the world's largest aspirin manufacturing plant in Trenton, New Jersey. It would produce 60% of US packaged aspirin tablets.[16]

Sterling also advertised directly to drugstores in such magazines as *Chain Store Age*, where an ad in September 1951 stated, "Mothers are talking and buying children's size Bayer … Display Children's Size Bayer in your Baby Needs Department and get those extra 'pick-up' sales."[17] Sterling's omission of flavoring did not last long. By 1952, Sterling had changed its formulation to include flavoring, which it highlighted in ads such as one in the *Reading Eagle* for the new, flavored Children's Size Bayer Aspirin that "tastes so good that children willingly … chew it … drink it … mix it."[18] In 1953, Sterling promoted a striking series of full-page ads for Bayer Aspirin. Popular magazines like the *Saturday Evening Post*,[19] featured toddlers with their mothers, the slogan "Gentle as a Mother's Kiss," and the phrase "so gentle to the system doctors prescribe it even for small children." Aspirin, it said, was "probably the safest of all pain-relieving drugs," which may have been true—if compared with heroin or morphine. These ads did not mention the children's-size product, but the message was clear. Nothing in the ads suggested the dangers within.

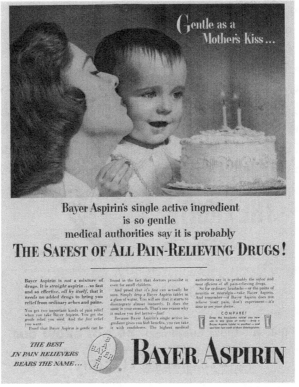

"Advertisement, *Saturday Evening Post*, 1953
Courtesy of Bayer AG, Leverkusen, Germany

Meanwhile, Plough accelerated its advertising efforts. In 1953, Abe Plough told *New York Times* reporter James J. Nagle that his company was doubling its 1953 advertising appropriation mainly to promote St Joseph Aspirin for Children and Mexsana medicated skin cream. [20] During his 45 years in business, Plough had spent $45 million, mostly for newspaper ads. In 1952 alone, he claimed his company had advertised in newspapers with a combined circulation of 42 million, magazines with a circulation of 25 million, radio stations heard in 21 million homes, and TV stations reaching 15 million homes. On top of that, six million St Joseph Weather Chart Calendars and Almanacs were being printed annually. Plough revealed to Nagle that the late C.P.J. Mooney, editor of *Commercial Appeal*, the source of his approach, had told him, "If you never stop telling them you will never stop selling them." Plough's net sales doubled by 1962.[21]

Many new brands now entered the market and industry pelted consumers with advertisements. Two competitors were hot on Sterling's heels. American Home Products had introduced Anacin in 1930. Bristol Meyers, which had introduced Bufferin in 1949, soon added Excedrin.[22] According to Diarmuid Jeffries, "the three producers raised the banners under which (with a few variations) they would fight each other for the next thirty years: Power, Speed and Purity ... [making] a generation of American television viewers wearisomely familiar."[23] Americans could hardly help but see "pounding hammers" as a metaphor for headache and hearing slogans like "Fast, fast, fast relief." From 1951 to 1961, consumption of aspirin increased at four times the rate of population growth.

In Britain, Disprin, a soluble aspirin, was launched in 1948 and, by 1950, Disprin, Aspro, and others were encroaching on Bayer's British market share.[24] Reckett and Colman advertised its "Disprin for children" in the *Journal of Tropical Medicine*.[25]

Image was everything because, well, aspirin is aspirin. The most expensive brand was selling for as much as five times the least expensive brand.[26]

Parents in the dark

Warnings labels were rare for any drug. Not even the highly toxic form of salicylate, methyl salicylate (oil of wintergreen), found in homes as a rubbing liniment, displayed a warning. Methyl salicylate is the most dangerous salicylate by far. Only the miniscule amount used for flavoring can be taken internally. A single teaspoon of a 98% solution contains 7000 mg or 21.5 standard adult aspirin 325-mg tablets.[27] Less than a teaspoon can be fatal for a child.[28] Poisonings occurred after a child drank some of the sweet-smelling oil. While France and Germany required methyl salicylate to be labeled as a poison, the United States did not. The Caustic Poison Act of 1927, which required warnings on certain dangerous household chemicals, did not include methyl salicylate.[29] In 1937, Johns Hopkins pathologist Charles Stevenson pleaded that methyl salicylate be labeled: "Poisonous if used internally."[30]

The 1938 Food, Drug, and Cosmetic Act had been followed by hot debate between the FDA and manufacturers regarding which drugs were safe enough to be directly sold to consumers. In 1951, Congress passed the Durham-Humphrey Amendment which *required* potentially harmful drugs be dispensed with a prescription. One not thus deemed could be sold over-the-counter. In 1954, the FDA finally tackled methyl salicylate by stating it would consider misbranded the label of any container with more than 5% methyl salicylate which "fails to warn that use otherwise than as directed therein may be dangerous and that the article should be kept out of reach of children to prevent accidental poisoning."[31]

In 1951, pediatricians voiced increasing concern with the many new and sometimes dangerous household chemicals, products, and drugs.[32] Pediatrician Robert Warner of Buffalo, New York, sounded an alarm about accidental aspirin ingestions: "[W]e know that the aspirin bottle is one of the chief causes of poisoning ... we give out candy aspirin ... you can't teach a child the difference between one kind of candy and another."[33] The number of children dying of salicylate poisoning was clarified in 1954 when Katherine Bain of the Children's Bureau in the US Department of Health, Education, and Welfare published newly available statistics. The international system for classifying causes of death had introduced E-codes in 1949.[34] E-codes specify the external cause of death (such as poisoning or motor vehicle accident) along with the nature of the injury, its N-code (for example, brain swelling).

The number was surprising. In fact, for the years 1949 and

1950, aspirin and salicylates were *the* leading cause of child death from a drug. Over 100 deaths had been attributed to aspirin and salicylates during 1948 and 1949.[35] Bain astutely commented that the unsupervised child was not the only problem as some poisonings could result from wrong dosage.[36]

The news of the number of accidental aspirin ingestions brought to the public the first general awareness that the popular and effective fever and pain reliever was also a deadly poison. In fact, the aspirin ingestions were a major force behind the creation of poison control centers in the United States. In 1953 the first center opened in Chicago under the sponsorship of the Illinois chapter of the American Academy of Pediatrics.[37] Soon after, centers opened in Cincinnati, Boston, Grand Rapids, and Washington, D.C. By April 1958, there were 128 such centers in 40 states collecting data on toxicity, ingredients, and treatment.

Year after year the poison centers confirmed that salicylates were *the* leading cause of drug death in children.[38] From 1952 through 1956, aspirin and other salicylates were responsible for 389 of the 785 drug deaths in those younger than 15.[39] (By comparison, from 1956–1960, measles caused 450 deaths per year.)[40] On top of that, non-fatal poisonings were many times more common. In New York City alone, for example, an estimated 650 aspirin poisonings occurred during the first 10 months of 1957.[41] The following year the AMA's Committee on Toxicology blamed flavored aspirin, the carelessness of users, and the advertisement "that states or implies a degree of safety not associated with the drug."[42]

The FDA began a campaign to address the accidental aspirin poisonings. While few ads now pictured the aspirin-eating toddlers age group, the idea of a warning on the label generated strong controversy.

Salicylate inhibits ATP production in mitochondria

Meanwhile in laboratories, biochemists were zeroing in on salicylate's effects on metabolism. One of the earliest clues had been uncovered in 1901 when researchers found that salicylate in large amounts increases oxygen use in rabbits. Increased oxygen use is an indicator of increased metabolism, the breaking down of glucose, glycogen, fats, and proteins that fuel the body.[43] Similar results were found in humans.[44]

Always searching for new treatments, doctors recognized an opportunity for a diet drug, and they thought of a chemical cousin to salicylate called DNP (2,4-dinitrophenol). Efforts to make DNP a treatment for obesity illustrate the potential danger of the trial-and-error method of research so common at the time. By the 1930s, when Stanford University researchers Windsor Cutting, H.G. Mehrtines, and Maurice Tainter, who later would become Chairman of the Medical Research Board and Vice President of Sterling Drug, formally described the use of DNP for the treatment of obesity in the *Journal of the American Medical Association*,[45] it had already become a sought-after diet aid. It should have been no surprise that DNP treatment was also potentially fatal. During World War I, French physicians had treated munitions workers exposed to DNP. Toxic amounts caused nausea, restlessness, deep and rapid respiration followed by extreme hyperthermia, cyanosis, hypoxia, and death.[46] Doses higher than about 600 mg were considered far too dangerous for routine use.[47] At first it seemed—at the right dose—DNP was safe and, best of all, recipients lost weight. For those experiencing undesirable "side actions," Tainter recommended maintaining fluid intake, slowly increasing the dose, and "prompt discontinuation at the first hint of an undesirable reaction."[48] Soon after Tainter and colleagues reported that treatment at non-toxic doses resulted in the loss of 2–3 pounds (1–1.4 kgs) per week in 1934.[49] Then, San Francisco physicians spotted six cases of rapidly developing cataracts and blindness in young women using DNP.[50, 51] In 1938 when the Food, Drug, and Cosmetic Act gave the FDA authority, it threatened to prosecute makers of DNP. By mid-1938, the FDA found no interstate traffic.[52]

Understandably, scientists found DNP and salicylate useful for the study of cell metabolism, particularly its dramatic effect on mitochondria, the small organelles inside cells which perform the critical role of burning (oxidizing) food molecules (carbohydrates, fats, and proteins) and capturing the released energy in the chemical bonds of a molecule called ATP (adenosine triphosphate)—a process called oxidative phosphorylation. ATP is essential to life. It contains the life-sustaining energy transmitted from the sun to plants and from plants to humans. *The body uses ATP to power all body functions.* The astonishing quantity of ATP we make to meet our daily needs is difficult to grasp. Professor Bertil Andersson, in his 1997 presentation before the Royal Swedish Academy of Sciences, noted that an adult produces a quantity of ATP about the size of half of his/her own body weight each day and with exertion, many times more![53]

Even more extraordinary is the fact that up to one-third of all ATP formed in the body is used by the so-called "sodium pump" within all cells. This pump prevents cells from swelling by pumping sodium out of cells (perhaps a remnant of our beginnings in the prehistoric sea).[54] The sodium pump is so important that Jens Christian Skou of Denmark, who discovered it in the 1950s, won the 1997 Nobel Prize for Chemistry.[55] One can easily imagine that anything disrupting ATP production could be devastating.*[56]

In 1955, Theodore Brody of the University of Michigan found that salicylate, DNP, and a few other molecules uncouple, that is, disrupt, oxidative phosphorylation, a step in the production of ATP.[57] Uncoupling is like disconnecting an engine from the wheels of an automobile. Stepping on the pedal to provide more fuel will not move the car. The engine just runs faster and hotter until you either run out of fuel or the engine fails. In a laboratory experiment that should have

---

* German chemist Karl Lohmann "discovered" ATP in 1929. In the 1940s, Fritz A. Lipmann proposed that it was "the universal carrier of chemical energy in the cell." Scientists raced to learn exactly how the energy stored in food molecules is transferred into ATP's chemical bonds and found two chemical pathways. The ancient pathway—glycolysis—does not use oxygen and is quite inefficient: only two molecules of ATP are made from each molecule of glucose. The other pathway—oxidative phosphorylation—uses oxygen and is very efficient: for each glucose molecule, 30 molecules of ATP are produced. In 1948, Albert L. Lehninger determined that oxidative phosphorylation and the generation of ATP occur in mitochondria. Five years later in 1953 the Nobel Prize was awarded to Hans A. Krebs for his characterization of the chemical reactions of oxidative phosphorylation, which subsequently became known to every biochemistry student as the Krebs cycle, and to Fritz A. Lipmann for his work identifying a critical co-enzyme.

raised red flags relative to therapeutics, Brody showed that sodium acetylsalicylate depressed the efficiency of oxidative phosphorylation in *brain mitochondria by 25% and in liver mitochondria by 50%*. He also reported that sodium salicylate, aspirin, and methyl salicylate all uncouple oxidative phosphorylation in mitochondria of the liver, kidneys, and brain, like the effect seen with DNP and occurring at levels "comparable to toxic levels" in the intact animal.[58]

Brody stated outright that many of the toxic symptoms of salicylate "over-dosage" could be attributed to the uncoupling of oxidative phosphorylation in mitochondria.

The inhibition of ATP production likely explains florists' 1923 observation that aspirin can revive wilted flowers by causing them to swell, as well as the 1942 finding by Celia Lutwak-Mann, a fellow at Newnham College, Cambridge, that liver glycogen virtually disappeared in rats injected with salicylate.[59]

Despite these remarkable discoveries, industry suggested that the real cause of the poisoning after aspirin ingestions was that parents (who had not been told that aspirin could be a deadly poison) were simply not supervising their children. Sterling Vice President Maurice Tainter even suggested that the children themselves were to blame as they "possibly [had] a psychological drive to attract attention or to frustrate their parents."[60]

FDA embarks on a long road to address accidental ingestions

A child downing a bottle of aspirin was considered an "accident." The problem was the FDA had no authority over accidents. The 1938 legislation only required the FDA to assure that drugs bear warnings against unsafe dosage and against use by children where use would be dangerous. The FDA had to find a way to address the problem. The number of poison control centers was increasing and would reach 500 by 1971.[61] By necessity, the FDA focused on persuasion.

In 1955, it convened a Conference on the Accidental Ingestion and Misuse of Salicylate Preparations by Children to "consider the problem and its solution."[62] The FDA, AMA, American Public Health Association, and AAP weighed in. An advisory group made recommendations.[63] The Federal Register, the US government's record of federal agency rules, executive orders, and proclamations, published recommendations as *Statements of General Policy or Interpretation*, which advised warnings on labels such as "Warning: Keep out of reach of children," dosing standardization, and advice for children under three years, such as: "For children under 3 years of age consult your physician."[64, 65, 66]

Such FDA policy statements are not binding on the FDA or the public.[67] Some manufacturers voluntarily instituted these measures. By 1957 the accidental aspirin ingestion problem—despite the good intentions of an array of committees, government panels, poison control centers, news coverage, "health departments, medical societies, major insurance companies, the American Red Cross, the National Safety Council, and others, including the American Medical Association"[68]—had not been solved. During its spring meeting in 1957, the AAP declared that aspirin was "the major remaining menace to childhood health." Academy leaders called on pediatricians to warn parents to "treat aspirin like a deadly poison."[69] Yet, despite the poisonings, when Asian influenza pandemic struck, aspirin was ready with "fast, safe relief."[70]

The National Clearinghouse for Poison Control Centers, founded that year, began to facilitate the sharing of information. Analysis of almost 4000 detailed reports from 29 poison control centers in various time periods between July 1956 and April 1958 determined that, for all age groups, aspirin was involved in 52% of medication ingestions with accidents the major problem.[72] In 1958, members of the Clearinghouse called for enforcement of precautionary labeling and the use of safety cap closures.[73] Jay Arena later recalled that when the safety closure studies were published,[74] Abe Plough worried about losing sales. Nevertheless, he told Arena, "If it saves the life of one child, I'll do it."[75] And he did. Plough began advertising the safety cap in 1958; Sterling followed within a year.[76] Yet, accidental aspirin ingestions continued to

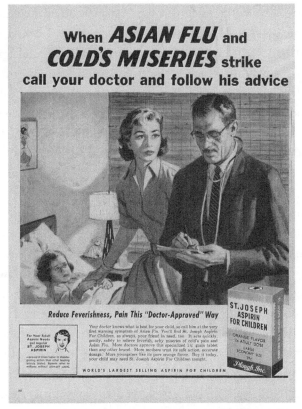

Advertisement, *LIFE*, 2 December 1957[71]
Courtesy of Consumer Foundation Healthcare.

rise. The voluntary approach was simply not working.

From 1960 to 1970, persuasion continued as no law or regulation addressed warning labels or packaging. The 1960 Federal Hazardous Substances Labeling Act authorized the government to require warning labels for hazardous household chemical products but did not include drugs.[77] The consensus was that medicines were better managed under the 1938 legislation (which, please recall, did not cover accidents). President Lyndon Johnson got involved and recommended that the new proposed Child Safety Act of 1966 include a limit on the quantity of salicylate in packages, authorize the FDA to require safety closures, and require a warning label. But the Pharmaceutical Manufacturing Association (PMA) objected, stating these measures would not help because it believed that the primary cause was "parental ignorance, carelessness, or indifference." [78] Industry asked for more time to act voluntarily.[79] The PMA called for studies. The proposed Child Safety Act of 1966 morphed into the Child Protection Act which, when passed, allowed the government to require a warning label on hazardous household items like toys—but again not on aspirin bottles.[80, 81]

Aspirin had fallen or been pushed into the great void between various protection laws.

In 1966, James Goddard, former chief of the CDC, took the reins of the FDA. Journalist Philip J. Hilts wrote: "James Goddard marked the demarcation between the old FDA—that had no MDs, no strong standard of evidence and largely subservient relation with the pharmaceutical industry—and the new FDA that was headed by an energetic doctor, enforced strong standards of evidence and advocated for the public's health." [82] Goddard convened another conference—the Conference on the Prevention of Accidental Ingestion of Salicylate Products by Children—to lay the groundwork for child-resistant packaging. Now, manufacturers agreed to voluntarily restrict the number of 81 mg (1.25 grains) tablets in children's aspirin bottles to 36 tablets (2916 mg).[83] In 1970, Congress passed the landmark Poison Prevention Packaging Act (PPPA). Enforcement was assigned to the FDA until 1973 when it was transferred to the Consumer Protection Safety Commission.[84] Regulations requiring safety packaging for aspirin were issued in August 1972.[85] Between 1969 and 1974, deaths of children less than five years of age involving salicylates and its congeners declined by almost half.[86]

It had been a long road, but thanks to a combination of company volunteerism, FDA policy, and law, by 1978, when I was called about the seven children with Reye's syndrome, most salicylate products carried the warning "keep out of reach of children," were contained in safety packaging, and included a warning to consult a physician for use in children under the age of three. Children's aspirin products were also limited to about 2916 mg per bottle. Childhood aspirin poisoning, which had peaked at a rate of seven deaths per million children younger than five years in the early 1960s, was less than one per million in 1980.[87]

The problem of aspirin poisoning seemed to be mostly solved.

Yet it wasn't. Another epidemic, under the radar of most, was continuing across the United States: "chronic" salicylate poisoning. Chronic was defined as poisoning occurring after 12 hours of therapy. Harris Riley, Jr and Lee Worley, physicians in the Department of Pediatrics at Vanderbilt School of Medicine in Nashville, Tennessee, reported that between 1945 and 1955 more aspirin poisonings had occurred during therapy than had occurred from accidents.[88]

And the seeds of blame had already been sown.

Chapter 8

Poisoning During Home Therapy: Overdose or Wrong Dose? 1940s and 50s

Everything about it is misleading.

John U. Crichton and G.B. Elliott,
Canadian Medical Association Journal, 1960

Infants

At first, doctors prescribed aspirin therapy for minor illnesses at home. Then parents began using tablets purchased over-the-counter. The first reports of salicylate poisoning during treatment at home mainly involved the most vulnerable population—infants (children 12 months and younger).

When a child was diagnosed with salicylate poisoning, clinicians generally assumed that parents had "overdosed" their child. The unspoken corollary assumption, of course, was that the *recommended dose schedule was safe.* An early report seemed to verify this assumption. On 25 January 1936, parents brought an exhausted but restless seven-month-old infant, vomiting and panting "like a dog," to the Vanderbilt University Hospital in Nashville, Tennessee. The doctors diagnosed salicylate poisoning and ordered treatment with bicarbonate, glucose, and a large amount of fluid. The infant survived. The doctors learned that the infant had been given 500 mg/kg/day, an amount well over that generally recommended.[1] In 1937, Katherine Dodd and Ann S. Minot in Nashville, Tennessee, along with Jay M. Arena in Durham, North Carolina, described three cases: a 22-month-old who had ingested methyl salicylate, a seven-month-old whose parents had provided aspirin, and a rheumatic 12-year-old.

The doctors detailed some of the physical effects of the drug.

> The direct effects of salicylate are an increase in the metabolic rate [and its attendant body heat], an increase in the dissipation of heat [panting/ hyperventilating] ... the poisoned subject loses fluid rapidly through vomiting, diuresis [peeing], and sweating because of mental confusion he cooperates poorly in taking fluids even when they are available. With a low fluid intake, the fluid reserves of the body are soon depleted. Dehydration in turn soon places the patient at a tremendous disadvantage.[2]

The doctors emphasized the importance of fluids and noted that the amount of fluid needed is "enormous." They suggested that the poisoning could be avoided with adequate fluid intake.

Many of the earliest reports of poisoning during home therapy involved children in St Louis, Missouri, home state of both Monsanto, one of the largest aspirin producers in the US,[3] and William McKim Marriot, Professor of Pediatrics at the Washington University School of Medicine and Physician in Chief of St Louis Children's Hospital. Marriot's popular 1930 handbook *Infant Nutrition* provided a specific *dose and dose frequency* of aspirin for infants similar to those in early 1920s textbooks.[4, 5] For a six-month-old infant he recommended one-half grain (30 mg) and for a one-year-old child, one grain (60 mg), to be given every four hours. With this recommendation, a one-year-old would receive about 40 mg/kg/day.[6] (Appendix 1) Later editions of Marriott's book in 1935, 1941, and 1947 gave the same recommendation.[7, 8, 9]

In 1942 at Marriott's hospital, physician Henry Barnett and colleagues called attention to the urgent nature of therapeutic salicylate poisoning.[10] They reported four cases in children, ages eight months to five years, during the previous eight years. Curiously, one child had been given less than two times the recommended amount which suggested that the margin between the recommended dose and the toxic one was razor thin. Five years later at the same hospital, Jane Erganian reported 13 children with salicylate poisoning. All but two had been treated for a "cold." Erganian wrote:

> In view of the dangers and the possibility of fatality in infants it is suggested
> that aspirin be given not at all or very cautiously with full awareness of all
> its properties for intoxication. The same possibilities for intoxication in one
> form or another obtain in older individuals, but to a lesser degree.[11]

In 1952, three St Louis infants made national news when the coroner investigated their deaths. They had received aspirin to "bring down a fever." Professor Alexis Hartmann told the *New York Times*, "parents should be wary of giving their young children aspirin or medicines containing it." Another specialist recommended that aspirin not be used for infants under six months of age and only prescribed on an individual basis for older babies. "There should be no textbook dosage," he said.[12]

Doctors however continued to recommend aspirin. And while they may have been precise in their instructions, the commonly recommended dose was simply a guesstimate passed from doctor to doctor, and then from doctor to parent, like a recipe for a good apple pie. The entire contents of the first marketed bottles of children's aspirin were clearly dangerous. But how about half a bottle, a quarter of a bottle, two tablets every six hours, every four hours? No one knew for sure. The 1950 edition of Mitchell-Nelson's *Textbook of Pediatrics* captured the essence of the problem, "dosages of drugs in children are often based on clinical impression rather than on critical investigation."[13] Yet almost all used aspirin. After all, the tablet, one of the few alternatives to time-consuming sponge baths, was easy and modern. Besides, parents had been told that aspirin was genuine and proved safe by millions.[14]

The infant deaths in 1952 marked the beginning of a widening and perfectly legal disconnect between the drumbeat of fantasy advertisements and the nascent but growing knowledge of aspirin pharmacology. No law required manufacturers to read the *American Journal of Disease of Children* or even mention that aspirin could be fatally toxic.

Therapeutic poisoning beyond infancy

In 1953, a cautionary editorial in the *Journal of Pediatrics* drew an important distinction between a one-time ingestion and poisoning from multiple smaller doses over several days.[15] It explained that accidental over-dosage can be "rapidly neutralized" but poisoning during therapy is "quite a different story." The editorial empathized with parents who listen to ads noting they "can hardly be expected to know they are dealing with a drug potentially lethal to infants" and blamed doctors who "should know better." It stated that parents "should be warned never to give aspirin to a baby."

The editorial was one of the first that directly addressed what would commonly be called the *dose schedule* and its components: dose, frequency, and duration. Experts began to tease apart the problem. In 1953, William Hoffman, MD PhD of the University of Illinois College of Medicine, in an editorial in the *American Journal of Diseases of Children* entitled "Pitfalls of acetyl salicylic acid," described the situation. While noting immature kidney function and metabolism in infants he clearly described the potential hazard of four-hour dosing intervals and prolonged dosing:

> With the modern tendency to give drugs every four hours, a second dose of one grain to an infant will cause a pyramiding of the blood level, so that at the end of 24 hours the blood level maybe 20 or 24 milligrams per 100 cc. If the doses are maintained at the same rate obviously extreme toxicity will develop in two or three days. Most pediatricians are not acquainted with this phenomenon and do not realize that this pyramiding takes place.[16]

The following year, Hoffman extended his concern for "injudiciously prolonged salicylate medication to older children."[17] He recognized that "in the more slowly developing intoxication … hyperventilation may not be recognizable." Rather than placing the blame on parental "overdosing," as was common, he explained that dosing every four to six hours could lead to toxic levels and no dose "should be maintained for more than three to five days without either reduction or complete withdrawal."[18] William Wallace of the Western Reserve University soon reminded physicians that dehydration could also lead to accumulation and that impaired kidney function was "a primary contraindication for any continued administration."[19] In 1956, Harris Riley, Jr and Lee Worley echoed Hoffman, and noted that the therapeutic poisonings were marked by "prolonged administration of presumed safe doses."[20] They, like others, alerted physicians of the possibility of accumulation ("pyramiding" as they called it) and stated that the "proper and safe" dose was "controversial."

Nevertheless, by 1957 during the Asian influenza pandemic, although aspirin ads rarely showed infants, one for St Joseph Aspirin for Children touted "safe action, accurate dosage."[21] Others stressed doctor approval. None provided a dosing schedule complete with dose, frequency, and duration.

Is every six hours better?

In 1959, pediatrician Alan Done of Stanford University, considered to be one of the aspirin experts of the day, argued against the use of any drug to lower the temperature in children.[22] In his address at the Annual Meeting of the American Academy of Pediatrics in 1958 and in print in October 1959 he justified this position with the following points: the evidence that fever may be helpful, the lack of evidence that fever up to 104 degrees Fahrenheit is dangerous, the role of fever as a diagnostic clue, the occurrence of allergic drug reactions, the danger of drugs in the home, and the possibility that important symptoms may be masked by treatment. Done offered other means to comfort children with fever such as the avoidance of bundling them up and the use of sponging.[23]

In 1960, he published the famous Done nomogram describing blood levels in one-time ingestions. In 1965, he reiterated previous concerns that a dose every four hours can "result in gradual accumulation to toxic levels." He suggested that doses should be given no more frequently than every six hours.[24] And, in 1971, he published a recognized review on the treatment of salicylate poisoning.[25] He seemed to be aware of all the important facts, but no one could know for sure what had not been studied—the safety of the dose schedule.

In summary, by the 1950s doctors had identified the following factors contributing to toxicity in children—kidney function/dehydration; an individual factor; a danger at the beginning of therapy, and the amount, frequency, and duration of dosing. It is impossible to know how many doctors took notice. What is certain—because children continued to be stricken with therapeutic salicylate poisoning at home during the 1950s—is that this information never reached parents.

A surprising number of poisonings

The numbers of children with therapeutic salicylate poisoning was not insignificant. In the prestigious and widely read *New England Journal of Medicine*, William Segar and Malcolm Holliday of the University of Indianapolis School of Medicine reported a shocking number of children with salicylate poisoning at a single hospital over the six-year period ending in December 1957—49 children and infants under six years of age.[26] Salicylate levels measured in all but two ranged from 18 to 81 mg/dL. Obtaining a history of aspirin use was difficult and, surprisingly, six with salicylate in the blood gave no history of having taken it. Eleven obtained the drug themselves or were fed it by an older sibling and 32 were assumed to have received it by "misguided" therapy, often on the advice of a physician. *At this hospital, therapeutic poisoning was three times more frequent than accidental poisoning.* Thirteen had staggeringly high temperatures, 105–108°F (40.5–42.2°C) measured rectally, causing Segar and Holliday to worry that fever, being a sign of both infection and salicylate poisoning, might invite more treatment with aspirin. This striking temperature elevation is the result in part of increased metabolism* [27, 28]

---

* In 1882, researchers had found a 40% increase in the average heat production in dogs fed 1–5 grams of sodium salicylate. In 1919, Yale University physicians documented an increase in heat production and body temperature in five normal individuals given 1000 or 1250 milligrams (3–4 adult tablets) of aspirin.

Segar and Holliday's widely circulated article was a major call out to the profession. Yet the reports kept coming. In 1959, clinicians in North Carolina and Louisiana described eight children with salicylate poisoning during therapy of upper respiratory infections.[29] In 1960, John Crichton and G.B. Elliot in Calgary, Canada, reported 41 cases of salicylism diagnosed in children less than seven years of age in the four-and-a-half years before June 1960, including 14 who were poisoned during therapy for illnesses such as chickenpox, the common cold, or flu.[30] They believed that salicylate poisoning was so common that "air hunger [hyperventilation] in young infants should be taught as primarily due to salicylate poisoning until proved otherwise." Most of the serious cases were in this group. Frighteningly, *in no case was salicylism considered as the admission diagnosis.*

Crichton and Elliot emphasized that, diagnostically, almost everything about therapeutic salicylate poisoning was misleading. First, another medical condition, usually pneumonia, had been the initial diagnosis. Second, administration was spread over days, obscuring the connection between the drug and the symptoms that followed three to four days later. The time lag in days between aspirin administration and toxic symptoms was not stressed in medical teaching. Finally, many parents believed aspirin was harmless. They wrote, "Extremely persistent questioning was often necessary [to uncover the aspirin use]." Crichton and Elliot believed that a physician prescribing aspirin for a child was unlikely to consider the diagnosis of salicylate poisoning. Salicylate levels had been obtained in only seven and some children had received aspirin in the hospital. They recommended that Canadian health authorities alert "the public that salicylates, especially adult salicylates, are *'potentially fatal poisons for young children.'*" They also called for "more emphatic labeling" and avoidance of aspirin use in children under five years of age.

Nevertheless, these and other ideas for prevention—including spreading doses further apart, limiting the duration of therapy, and withholding the drug from children entirely—remained as suggestions in medical journals.

A television commercial during the 1960s extolled aspirin's "instant flaking action," and noted that aspirin was "recommended repeatedly in public health articles, medical journals, personal consultation."[31] An ad for flavored Bayer Aspirin for Children in the *Catholic Advance* in December 1960 reported doctors' blessings and the "exact amount that doctors prescribe for children."[32] Advertisements that claimed safe doses, doctors' blessings, and the implication that loving mothers provide aspirin to their sick children—without counterbalancing messages about safety—would prove to be a deadly combination for some.

The conundrum of the dose schedule for children

Meanwhile, the FDA explained that if it became "aware that a drug posed a significant hazard, to the public, regardless of its grandfather status (please recall that aspirin was a grandfather drug and no safety checks were required), the Agency will take immediate action to remove it from the market."[33] Unfortunately, the dawning of "awareness" was subjective and slow. One tragic example is that of the groundbreaking drug chloromycetin [chloramphenicol]. In 1950 Australian P.F. Gill reported that infants suffered significant bone marrow depression [where red blood cells are produced] after treatment.[34] Later, even after reports of death from complete bone marrow failure called aplastic anemia were associated with use of the drug, the FDA struggled. As described by Philip J. Hilts,

> The FDA again and again was unable to bring itself to restrict the use of the drug ... [FDA Commissioner George] Larrick testified before Congress that if doctors couldn't sort out what to do on their own then "I'm at a loss." ... In fact, the use fell in the 1970s only after Parke-Davis's [the manufacturer] patent expired, and the company dropped it from its roster of high-promotion items.[35]

Historian Cynthia Connolly found that, from the 1950s through the 1970s, pediatricians sought to address children's dosing issues by identifying needed studies and regulations. Leading academics struggled with potential solutions.[36, 37] Unfortunately, little was accomplished. In 1957, for example, collaboration between the FDA and the USP to improve pediatric dosing ended after USP president Windsor Cutting (the DNP expert) commented, "the difficulty is too great to work out right now."[38] Nevertheless, attempts to improve pediatric pharmacology continued. In 1960, the AAP created the Committee on Drugs (AAP COD). In 1961, the NIH created the National Institute of Child Health and Human Development (NICHHD) which, along with the AAP COD, the FDA, the USP, and several national conferences, continued efforts. Yet by the late 1960s, progress still "seemed stalled."[39] In 1972, the FDA commissioner speaking at the AAP Convention stated the problem needed "immediate attention [as] between 1969 and 1971 more than half of all systemic drugs approved for potential use in children carried a label disclaimer for pediatric use."[40]

Blood levels are misleading

For a physician or the FDA to become aware of a problem like poisoning, it must first be diagnosed. The diagnosis of salicylate poisoning was difficult and often confused with the condition for which it was used. Then a new test made the diagnosis even more problematic. Salicylate poisoning had always been a "clinical diagnosis" based on a history of aspirin use and the observation of the classic signs and symptoms that had been reiterated over and over by various authors including Langmead in 1906, by Dodd, Minot, and Arena in 1937, and in by Riley in 1956. A rather tedious test that involved boiling the urine had often been used to confirm the presence of a salicylate.[41] Then, around the 1950s, a test that measured the amount of salicylate *in the blood* gradually made its way into laboratories.

Here is where a significant problem arose. Many doctors logically assumed that salicylate poisoning was not present if salicylate could not be detected (or was present at a low level) in the blood. Unfortunately, this was not always the case. The fact is that *salicylate poisoning can be present—and even severe—with a very low or zero blood level.* Academic pediatricians serving as the bridge between research findings and clinical practice immediately alerted the medical community. In 1948 Glasgow, Scotland, researchers wrote that the blood salicylate level did not correlate well with toxicity in adults.[42] In 1954, Western Reserve University's William M. Wallace warned, "Severe symptoms at very low blood levels are frequently encountered."[43] Riley and Worley echoed Wallace two years later. [44] In 1960 Done lamented, "Patients have died with salicylate levels of less than 15 mg/dL."[45] In 1965, doctors at the University of Washington in Seattle concluded that a small amount of salicylate could induce hypoglycemia in some infants and that the poisoning could be present with a low blood level.[46]

Researchers identified two explanations for a low blood level in a poisoned child. First, as Coburn had demonstrated, a 48-hour delay between the last dose and the measurement would obviously result in a lower level. Second, blood levels do not necessarily reflect the amount or the effects inside cells.[47] The adult human body contains about 40 liters of water. However, the body is not one big bucket. Water as well as other molecules (including drugs) exist in "compartments." Membranes control the flow of molecules (such as drugs) between the compartments. Blood plasma is one "compartment," but most of the body's water is inside cells where the actions of many drugs take place. (The remainder of the water resides in the area between the cells and the plasma called the interstitium.) In 1914, E. Newton Harvey of Princeton University had found that salicylate (salicylic acid) differs from many other acids in that it enters human cells.[48] This entering (and leaving) proceeds slowly. In 1963 researchers noted salicylate's "slow" distribution in the body's compartments as well as its relatively slowly diffusion into (and presumably out of) the brain that might explain the lag period between dosing and the appearance of toxicity.[49] In 1973 researcher John B. Hill at Becton Dickinson and Company Research Center in Research Triangle Park, North Carolina, discovered that, while blood levels varied greatly in salicylate-poisoned rats, the rats died when the salicylate level reached a narrow critical value in the brain. For this observation, he earned a place in the *New*

England Journal of Medicine.[50] Salicylate death is a brain death. Hill had connected the dots.

If the same were true of humans, factors that enhance the seepage (diffusion) of salicylate *into* the brain cells could play a role. During the 1970s, researchers identified several factors that promote the diffusion of salicylate into cells: higher blood acidity and lower blood protein levels (only salicylate that is not bound to protein enters cells). They also found the total amount of salicylate in the body was greater with larger doses even though blood levels were the same, likely because of protein binding.[51, 52] Alan Done, now working for the FDA, called this finding "an important step in filling the near-void of information … without which we'll continue to rely on grossly inaccurate and arbitrary criteria for pediatric doses, to name just one problem."[53]

However, this information did not reach all and many doctors and parents continued to trust both the product and the dose schedule. Salicylate poisoning, they believed, was a result of "overdosing" and, if instructions were followed, the drug was safe. These beliefs and the misconception that poisoning could not be present with low blood levels led some physicians, when evaluating a hyperventilating, vomiting and neurologically stressed child, to eliminate salicylate poisoning from their list of diagnostic possibilities.

Trust and these beliefs and misconceptions put children at risk of undiagnosed and untreated salicylate poisoning.

PART III

METAMORPHOSIS
1950s–1970s

Chapter 9

An Unfolding Disaster and an Unsuspected Culprit, 1950s

The important thing is not to stop questioning …
It is enough if one tries merely to comprehend a little
of this mystery [of life] every day.
Albert Einstein, *Life*, 1955

Mortimer and Lepow suggest aspirin

In 1954, doctors in Isleworth, England attended to a nine-year-old boy with chickenpox. He had developed a coma and died. At autopsy his doctors found an "extreme degree of fatty degeneration of the liver" and swelling of the meninges (the covering of the brain).[1] Other similar cases involved infants who presented to the doctor with a severe hypoglycemia. The first person to consider salicylate as a possible cause was a young physician in Cleveland, Ohio.

In 1956, 32-year-old Edward A. (Ted) Mortimer, Jr embarked on a seven-year quest to figure out why three infants with chickenpox had died under his care. The infants were between three and six months of age, and their chickenpox had morphed into a sudden, severe, and inexplicable hypoglycemia with intractable seizures. Mortimer, a faculty member at Western Reserve University School of Medicine and an administrator of pediatrics at Cleveland Metropolitan General Hospital, was an insatiably curious clinician with a bulldog personality. His dilemma was that, while every child got chickenpox, death from it was extremely rare. Mortimer and his colleagues reported the illness in an abstract submitted to the 66th Annual Meeting of the American Pediatric Society.[2] While they were not granted a place on the program, their report was published in tiny print in the *American Journal of Diseases of Childhood*. After a fourth child with the same history died, Mortimer and physician Martha Lipson Lepow decided to investigate.

Autopsy reports available for three infants indicated that the "most striking finding" in two was brain swelling and congestion. All had small brain hemorrhages and two had marked fatty metamorphosis (a general term for fat). One was noted to have the type referred to as fatty degeneration.[3]

The fact that riveted Mortimer and Lepow's attention was that only 2% of reported cases of chickenpox encephalitis had a low blood glucose. Perplexed, they talked with the children's parents and learned that three had given 80 mg. of aspirin four to six times a day for several days before the appearance of the hypoglycemia. The fourth too had been given a salicylate.

Mortimer and Lepow hit the library and learned that there was a 20-year record of reports suggesting that salicylate can cause hypoglycemia. First, in 1937, Katherine Dodd, Ann S. Minot, and Jay M. Arena had suggested that dextrose [a sugar] be provided to children with salicylate intoxication because salicylate increases metabolism and fuel such as sugar would be needed.[4] In 1942, doctors in St Louis reported an infant who had developed hypoglycemia after treatment with salicylate.[5] The same year Cecelia Lutwak-Mann of the Biochemical Laboratory in Cambridge observed that rats given large amounts of salicylate became drowsy, began to vomit, twitch, and convulse, and died unless they had been given extra glucose. Glycogen, a molecule stored in the liver that provides energy when glucose runs low, had all but disappeared.[6]

Mortimer and Lepow studied fasted rats. After they found that rats given salicylate had significantly lower blood glucose levels than control rats, they became convinced that salicylates had played a role in the infants' deaths and wrote a full report entitled "Varicella [chickenpox] with Hypoglycemia Possibly Due to Salicylates."[7] Their report was published in the *American Journal of Diseases of Children* in full in 1962 and the accompanying commentary called salicylate "an unsuspected culprit."[8] The article however seemed to receive little play.

Both Mortimer and Lepow went on to hold prestigious academic positions, including service in the American Academy of Pediatrics

(AAP). Mortimer became well known in CDC circles for his participation on a key advisory body, the AAP Committee of Infectious Diseases, known to most as the Redbook Committee, a committee that would become deeply involved with Reye's syndrome during the 1980s.

Similar mystery cases were noted elsewhere. Physicians at the Royal Alexandria Children's Hospital in Brighton called in Professor Sheila Sherlock, a world-renowned liver disease expert. Sherlock travelled 50 miles from London to discuss three curious pediatric hypoglycemia cases with the same "puzzling" clinical presentation and unusual liver findings. Sherlock thinking out loud stated, "The first thing I thought of ... was that the children were poisoned." After more speculation, she came back to poisoning and suggested that, should another case occur, a toxicologist be consulted to look for a "hypoglycemic agent."[9] Then, in the *Medical Journal of Australia*, a pathologist in Melbourne reported 20 more children who had become ill between 1950 and 1961 with acute brain swelling and a "severe and diffuse" fatty liver, some with hypoglycemia.[10] However it would be a report published in *The Lancet* in 1963 that would give the brain swelling/fatty liver/hypoglycemia mystery illness a name.

Australian physicians concerned about therapeutic salicylate poisoning

At the same time, Australian physicians, like those in the United States, were warning that medicines should be kept under lock and key to prevent accidental poisoning.[11] Around 1960, therapeutic salicylate poisoning took center stage when Melbourne city coroner John Pascoe held a disturbing public inquest concerning the death of seven-month-old Alan Geoffrey Botterill (like the inquest held in St Louis in 1952). Doctors testified that, between the Sunday and Wednesday before his death, Alan's mother had given him 12 aspirin tablets for teething difficulty. Royal Children's Hospital assistant medical director John Court told Pascoe "the hospital staff realized, it was extremely difficult for a busy mother to know what to do when a child appeared to be sick or in pain," yet "there was a possibility that a child ill for any reason and particularly one not feeding correctly, might be adversely affected by aspirin." [12] Some sensitive children, he said, "could become very ill or die from the effect of a very small amount." [13] The coroner ruled the death the result of an upper respiratory infection.

Much publicity attended the Botterill case and aspirin's possible role in it. Court later told the press that, between 1952 and late 1959, 31 children had been hospitalized with aspirin poisoning at the Royal Children's and warned that the "indiscriminate use of aspirin tablets, especially for young children, was extremely dangerous." [14] At the time Australians, particularly women, were approaching an "alarming level of pill swallowing and powder taking." [15] Aspirin, phenacetin (an analgesic), and tranquilizers, often in the form of powders, were popular daily remedies. Australians were consuming 400 tons of aspirin a year. [16] Manufacturers for Aspro, Bayer Aspirin, Disprin, and others stoked the buying frenzy with ads in popular newspapers. Nicholas' ads for example even suggested that aspirin be used "in the morning, during the day, and at night," [17] and that it is "particularly valuable for children because of its safety" [18]

Pascoe soon held another inquest. This one concerned the November 1961 death of 18-month-old Steven John Payne. Too distressed to testify, Steven's mother submitted a statement. [19] On 3 November, she had taken the child to the doctor for a stomachache, and then treated the child as instructed. Four days later mother and son again visited the doctor who now diagnosed a nasty head infection. Again, she complied with the orders. Two days later after the child convulsed, she brought him to the Royal Children's Hospital. She had given her son three aspirins (Disprin) a day and then seven or eight tablets in the 24 hours before admission. Hospital physician H.N.B. Wettenhall told Pascoe that, clinically, the cause of Steven's death was salicylate intoxication. Shockingly he added that, between 1957 and 1961, 25 patients had been admitted to his hospital with that diagnosis; 15 were infants. Only eight had recovered, one with "mental retardation." No brand was exempt. Disprin, APCs (aspirin, phenacetin, and caffeine), and Aspro were all involved. Wettenhall summed it up, "You can't

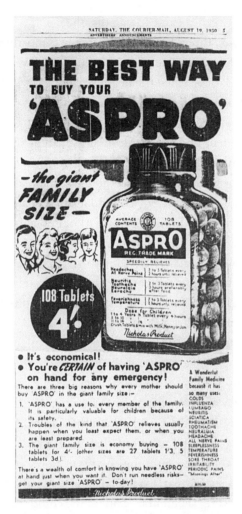

Advertisement, *Courier Mail*, 19 August 1950
Courtesy of Bayer AG, Leverkusen, Germany

predict which children will be affected."[20] Nevertheless, he described two types of children: those sensitive to the drug and those (especially infants under six months) whose kidney function was poor leading to a build-up to "dangerous proportions" after relatively small doses.[21] He believed infants under six months should not be given aspirin at all and, for those between six and 18 months, the maximum should be one tablet every two or three days. [22] The coroner sympathized with Mrs. Payne, "It must have been a terrible hardship for a lovely mother to see her son so ill." [23] Pascoe ruled the death a result of bronchopneumonia *and* a "most unfortunate" accidental overdose. [24]

The day of Baby Payne's inquest, another infant was hospitalized with a chest ailment and an overdose of aspirin at the Royal Hobart Hospital. The infant had been given small doses over several days. The hospital superintendent offered the recommendation that aspirin be given in small doses but not continuously. [25] Doctors were indeed circling the root of the problem, but without specific testing of the dosing regimen, it was impossible to know if a poisoning was the result of individual sensitivity, immaturity, the dosing schedule, a dehydration/kidney problem, or something else. Regardless, the problem was real. That week Dr Elizabeth Wilmot, Director of Maternal, Infant and Pre-school Welfare of the Victorian Health Department, planned a conference to educate 300 infant welfare sisters on the danger of giving aspirin to babies. [26]

Physicians in Sydney, Australia's largest city, were also reporting therapeutic salicylate poisoning. In September 1962, doctors at the Royal Alexandra Hospital for Children in the Camperdown area where R.D.K. Reye was working reported they had cared for 20 children suffering from salicylate poisoning that year alone. Just that week, a child had died. A spokesman for the hospital said half of the salicylate deaths treated were accidental, and half "could be attributed to indiscriminate or injudicious dosing" often upon a doctor's order to give aspirin to a child "every four hours until well" or too frequent dosing being "kept up indefinitely with dangerous results." [27] The doctors clearly understood that *frequency and duration* of dosing were each important.

As the Australian health authorities became involved, the finger-pointing began. One hospital medical director suggested manufacturers revise their label instructions, whereupon the Minister of Health asked the Chairman of the Health Commission to check the labels. [28]

A commissioner claimed the problem lay not with manufacturers, but with "lazy" parents. Mothers, he said, instead of giving simple remedies, such as "a warm bath, or sponging him all over, or a drink of hot milk, to get him to sleep, give him aspirins." He continued, "It is wrong ... parents are just getting rid of their burdens."[29] Another commissioner, who didn't see the need for parents to give their children aspirin at all, thought there was no need to label aspirin as harmful "if they are used properly." One irate mother wrote to the *Herald* and placed blame on doctors who tell anxious mothers to "give aspirin when baby is hot, fretful, and won't sleep."[30] The president of the Victorian Pharmaceutical Society suggested restricting sales to pharmacies.[31] A *Herald* journalist purchased eight different aspirin products and found the majority had no instructions for children other than to keep the pills out of reach and give "as directed."[32] The managing director of the maker of the Aspro brand, Nicholas Pty Ltd, who quite obviously had not been reading the newspapers, told the *Herald* that he believed directions were "adequate" and mothers would not give aspirin to such young children.[33]

In early May 1962, Australian Minister of Health Senator Wade warned that aspirin should not be given to babies.[34] By June a panel of doctors drew up a dosage schedule for children.

- Infants under nine months should not be given aspirin.
- Children two to five years should be given no more than two adult tablets [325 mg] in 24 hours.
- Children over five years should receive no more than three tablets in 24 hours.

In addition, a senior medical director said, if the child was vomiting or had diarrhea, aspirin should not be given without a doctor's advice.[35] The recommendations were posted prominently in the newspaper in a box stating: "Cut this out and Keep it: aspirin dosage."[36] Under these guidelines the daily dose for a four-year-old weighing 16 kg would be 41 mg/kg/day.

In September 1962, despite lingering concerns over the correct dosing schedule, Australia's Health Commission asked 320 makers and importers of aspirin products to adopt the new schedule on their labels.[37] However, two issues had not been resolved. First, some doctors believed that aspirin should not be given at all to children under the age of seven.[38] And, second, physicians still differed widely on the appropriate dosing schedule. Were any of the proposed schedules safe for children? After all, everyone was guessing.

However, physicians in Australia, New Zealand, and the United Kingdom were becoming increasingly vocal about aspirin use for children. In 1964, John Beveridge, Professor of Pediatrics at the University of New South Wales, told reporter Shaun McIlraith that two or three five-grain aspirin tablets can make young children up to about age five slightly sick and four or five tablets can make such youngsters seriously ill.[39] In 1965, F.T. Shannon at Christchurch Hospital lamented, "It is not possible to establish what would constitute a dangerous dosage particularly when continued for longer than 24 hours."[40] In 1966, Brisbane, Australian pediatrician and advocate for children Phyllis Cilento reported in her popular news column "Medical Mother" that she believed the consensus of medical opinion was that aspirin should not be administered for more than two days as it could "accumulate" in the blood and poison tissues—especially the brain. She was concerned that some deaths could go undiagnosed being ascribed to pneumonia or "some obscure infection of the brain."[41]

Scottish physicians deemed the aspirin situation "urgent." Physician J.O. Craig and colleagues noted that at two hospitals for the preschool child aspirin deaths by "faulty therapeutics" were more common than those by accidental ingestion.[42] Craig offered two solutions: withhold the drug entirely from children or discontinue it after two days. Striving to make his point, Craig and colleagues told the *Canberra Times* in March 1966, "Too often, a mother might be to blame. She might be condemning her baby to a slow death by giving aspirin during teething."[43]

The news coverage, both urgent and widespread, in these countries brought therapeutic aspirin poisoning in children to the attention of the public—and mothers—and a chill swept over aspirin use for children. In Australia, "Aspirin fell into disrepute ... and was replaced by equally indiscriminate use of paracetamol [also known as acetaminophen]."[44] In 1965, a New Zealand physician stated that since the press had called attention to the problem in 1962, his impression was "that fewer parents in the Christchurch district give their children aspirin".[45] Australia required a warning about kidney damage on the label of aspirin products that likely also affected sales.[46] By the 1970s, paracetamol sales surpassed those of aspirin in Australia.[47] Paracetamol sales also climbed in Britain, where it had been introduced as the prescription drug Panadol in 1956 and as an OTC drug in the early 1960s. There, sales of paracetamol matched those of aspirin by the early 1970s.[48]

The United States, however, was slow to embrace acetaminophen. Sterling Drug and Bayer Ltd made both aspirin and Panadol. As Johnson & Johnson launched a campaign to boost sales of its Tylenol brand of acetaminophen, Sterling and Bayer decided not to sell Panadol in the United States. According to interviews reported by business historians Mann and Plummer, Sterling executives in charge of Europe and Asia had urged the company's incoming president Mark Hiebert to consider acetaminophen.[49] But Hiebert was frightened by the thought of launching a potential competitor to Bayer aspirin. He thought Bayer aspirin was the American franchise and the base of the company. Thus, Sterling staked its future on aspirin.[50] (Appendix 4)

And aspirin remained the #1 drug for American children until the 1980s.

Chapter 10

Reye's Syndrome and Its Calling Card, 1963

Let us gather facts to get ourselves thinking.

Georges-Louis Leclerc, Comte de Buffon,
Histoire naturelle, générale et particulière,
avec la description du cabinet du Roi, 1749

Headlines were warning about the aspirin therapy poisonings at the Royal Alexandra Hospital for Children in the Camperdown area of Sydney in 1962 as its Director of Pathology, R.D.K. Reye, was preparing to publish a soon-to-become landmark report. The report, written with chief resident medical officer Graeme Morgan and resident pathologist J. Baral, concerned a decade of mysterious child deaths at the hospital. It was entitled "Encephalopathy and Fatty Degeneration of the Viscera[organs]: A Disease Entity in Childhood." [1] Likely because of its rarity, "fatty degeneration" was highlighted in the title. The name Reye's syndrome would soon take hold.

Although the symptoms of Reye's syndrome in infants and children were identical to those of salicylate poisoning, the clinicians at the Royal Alexandra had not diagnosed that. This was not at all surprising as Crichton and Elliot had observed in 1960. In 2008, Jim Baral told me the children were so horribly ill that the last thing on the minds of the young doctors was to ask parents if they had given aspirin. Graeme Morgan sent me a copy of the original handwritten tables that he and Baral had constructed during their chart review. The table showed that doctors had documented that aspirin, and only aspirin, had been given prior to admission in 11 of the 21 children (with the exception that one had been given chlorpromazine).

The Royal Alexandra was ripe with success. Reye's colleague, the world-famous physician Norman Gregg, had recently made the seminal discovery that certain birth defects were linked to German measles (rubella) during pregnancy, and Reye himself had identified tumors under the skin which became known as Reyomas. Reye's days were now spent observing, describing, and coming to conclusions regarding the cause of death. Pathology was the perfect profession for Reye, a reserved man who shunned parties, travel, and even scientific meetings. In his leisure time, he discussed car engines and polished his Jaguar.[2] Ralph Douglas Kenneth Reye was meticulous, organized, and saved his handwritten observations for years. They were later preserved at the Children's Hospital Westmead Archives in Sydney.[3]

In 1951 the body of an infant who had died without a diagnosis had been brought to Reye. The infant had been vomiting and screaming for 30 hours before death and the clinicians asked Reye to examine the tiny body. With great care, Reye gently inserted the sharp scalpel above the navel and drew a long straight pink line on the delicate skin. Using his gloved hand, he examined each organ. Likewise, he studied the infant's brain. He stepped back. What was going on? The liver was slightly enlarged, the cut surfaces pale and moist. And the brain, my God, the brain was swollen to the extent that its convolutions were flattened. He removed small portions of each organ and examined them under the lens of his microscope.

Reye imbedded the tissues in paraffin and froze some. He used a stain to mark fat, a technique infrequently reported before the 1960s. He also employed a stain for glycogen, the molecule that stores glucose as emergency fuel for the body.[4] After tissue preparation, he pulled his chair to the microscope table. One by one he picked up each of the tissues neatly laid on a glass rectangle, turned on the light, slid the rectangle under clamps, and focused the lens. He methodically scanned each slide and described his findings in longhand on paper. The first tissue, then the next, and so on. The appearance of the liver cells was striking. They were filled with fat. The pattern of the fat was unique. In sharp contrast to the large, often single (signet ring) fat drops within the liver cells seen in most liver diseases, these cells showed fatty degeneration. Every cell was packed with tiny fat droplets. He also found the tiny droplets in kidney, pancreas, and heart muscle cells. Even stranger, glycogen was almost completely absent from the liver suggesting some sort of accelerated metabolism.

Fatty degeneration. Reye had seen no case like it since he had become director 10 years earlier. Could an unidentified microorganism have caused the illness? Although possible, this was unlikely. In the end, he, as had the clinicians, concluded the case was unexplained.

Two years later Reye received a second infant. This infant had been diagnosed with rheumatism five days before his hospitalization and given a mixture of sodium salicylate. By the time he was hospitalized, the child had become "restless and irritable" and "did not recognize his parents." With a dangerously low blood sugar level and a temperature of 104°F, (40°C) he too died. Again, fatty degeneration. This time Reye submitted the child's organs for toxicology tests. Nothing turned up. Reye concluded that, given the widespread and uniform abnormalities, it was "unlikely that any viable [living] agent, bacterial or viral, would produce a pattern quite like this." He postulated that an undiscovered toxin had caused a "disordered metabolism in the cells."

After a seventh case, the Institute of Child Health in Sydney and the department of public health in the state of New South Wales became involved. A medical officer visited the homes of the children, interviewed their families, and inquired about illnesses in family members and access to drugs or poisons. Investigators looked for carbon tetrachloride and trichloroethylene compounds, both of which were known to produce coma and liver toxicity. They uncovered no promising leads.

As Reye examined the bodies of more children, his colleagues began calling the illness "Dr Reye's Syndrome." Two-thirds were two years of age or younger. For case after case, Reye carefully documented his observations and filed his notes in his cabinet.

In 1961, 26-year-old pediatric trainee Jacob (Jim) Baral attended his first case, a child with the mysterious condition that doctors at the hospital called "Dr Reye's syndrome." When the child died, Baral felt "haunted" and compelled to learn more.[5] Knowing everything had become an obsessive means of survival. Baral told me that as a child, he had escaped the Krakow ghetto. After the war and time in Israel, his family had settled in Australia. Baral was relieved when he passed his medical examinations and was grateful to be at the Royal Children's. He had tried researching "Reye's syndrome" and found nothing in the medical texts when a colleague directed him to Reye's office. At the end of the hall, Reye's heavy wooden door was closed. Baral walked down the long corridor and, with apprehension, knocked. To his relief the pathologist warmly welcomed him. As he entered, Baral felt a sense of sanctum sanctorum. Sun streamed in the window. Ensconced in the large, paneled office, Reye was at home. He swiveled his chair from his desk to his microscope and showed Baral the cases. His collection was impressive.

Soon the idea of writing a report emerged. The two men began sifting through the information in search of an explanation. When Reye invited Baral to train under him, Baral gratefully accepted, although he thought they made something of an odd couple. Reye, the son of a German immigrant, tall and athletic, according to Baral, was known as the "bronzed Apollo of the Great Barrier Reef." Baral was short and studious. Although Baral spoke several languages and had taught himself to read English, the prospect of writing a report with Reye filled him with anxiety. Fortunately, Graeme Morgan, the young Chief Resident of the hospital, would also participate. For almost a year, Morgan and Baral met regularly at Morgan's kitchen table overlooking Sydney Harbour. The two young men read every chart and recorded every finding by hand in tiny print while Reye drafted the pathology section of the report. In 2009, Morgan, reflecting on their work, credited the completion of the paper to Baral's continuous encouragement.

Reye and colleagues' report described 21 children who had become ill between 1951 and 1962.[6] The illness was marked by an initial period when the children did not seem very ill, often with symptoms of a cold. Then an abrupt deterioration occurred. Hyperpnea (rapid or deep breathing) was "the commonest" breathing abnormality and vomiting, "severe" in most, was "a constant symptom." Finally neurologic symptoms such as seizures, stupor, or coma set in. Half had a "wild delirium" with screaming, irritability, and violent movements. Convulsions if present were difficult to control.

The children were in severe stages upon arrival at the hospital. All but two were already in a coma. Consistent observations were vomiting often progressing to a stage in which black vomitus ran "effortlessly from the mouth," abnormal breathing, and a low sugar in the spinal fluid. Ketones were noted on the breath or in the urine of 12 children. Low sugar in the blood was found in some and abnormal liver function tests in all of those tested. One child with a normal blood sugar had none in his spinal fluid. Seventeen died. The average survival after hospital admission was only 27 hours. The four who survived recovered rapidly. In short, the illness was rapid and terrifying.

Brain swelling and fatty degeneration seemed to define the illness. Reye wrote:

> The brain was always swollen ... In the liver it is the uniformity and the completeness of the fatty change that is such a striking feature; every cell in every lobule is packed fatty droplets ... Few conditions resemble the fatty degeneration syndrome at all.[7]

Yes, fatty degeneration was unusual and because Reye had done tests beyond those done by many pathologists, he had seen it. At the time, only a few very rare conditions were known to cause fatty degeneration—fatty liver of pregnancy, tetracycline and carbon tetrachloride poisoning, and Jamaican vomiting sickness, a disease peculiar to the island of Jamaica that resulted from ingestion of a certain fruit. The children had none of these. A few rare genetic disorders of metabolism called "inborn errors of metabolism" were also known to cause fatty degeneration. These are manifested mostly in infancy and are often recurrent.

Reye and colleagues likely did not possess the 1954 edition of the textbook *Legal Medicine Pathology and Toxicology* by Thomas Gonzales, Chief Medical Examiner of New York City, and his colleagues. The Chief Medical Examiner had compiled a list of deaths from salicylates for the period 1918 through 1951: 46 accidental and undetermined fatalities as well as 22 suicides. On page 824, Gonzales noted that "fatty degeneration of the liver" (and the kidney) was a finding in salicylate toxicity.[8] Had Reye known this, he may have added it to his list of possibilities.

Reye, Morgan, and Baral's report was published in the highly regarded and widely distributed medical journal *The Lancet* on 12 October 1963. The accompanying editorial offered a clear opinion that the illness was caused by a potent toxic agent.

> The rapidity of the clinical deterioration, the severity of the vomiting, the altered blood in the gastric contents [there was often blood in the stomach], and the profound cerebral involvement all suggest a potent toxic agent. The degree and extent of the fatty infiltration of the liver and the speed of its development can scarcely be explained in any other way.[9]

The editorial also deemed the illness a "new syndrome."

Immediately, physicians around the world recognized they had been treating children with the same condition. Lord W. Russell Brain and Dr Donald Hunter fired off a letter to *The Lancet*'s editor indicating the condition had been around for quite some time.[10] They seemed amazed (and somewhat annoyed) that "Dr Reye and colleagues report as though it were a new clinicopathological entity and in an annotation you call it a challenging and dramatic 'new syndrome.'" Citing their own paper written with Hubert Turnbull in *The Lancet* in 1929, they believed that "credit of recognizing this should go to Turnbull." Reye and Morgan replied that they were "not convinced" and politely stated that if it could be proved that the syndrome occurred before 1951, the etiologic agent might be better identified.

Reye's report did not include photos of the liver cells, but soon medical journals published photos of fatty degeneration, the multitude of tiny fat droplets inside every liver cell. Now the collection of symptoms and pathology findings had a name. Doctors began diagnosing "Reye's syndrome" for children with the typical symptoms *and* the finding of fatty degeneration of the liver on biopsy or at autopsy. During the 1960s, the diagnosis of Reye's syndrome became a snap after a new blood test for liver dysfunction became widely available for pediatric cases and doctors no longer had to examine the liver itself.

Reye's report was a double-edged sword. For clinicians, once the diagnosis of Reye's syndrome had been made, did they really need to think of anything else? On the other hand, Reye's detailed description of the pathology findings changed the brain-swelling illness from a vague collection of signs and symptoms to a condition with a very specific calling card—fatty degeneration.

The meticulous work of Reye, Morgan, and Baral put the brain swelling illness on the map. Reye and his colleagues hoped that others would investigate cause, prevention, and treatment. At the time they had no way of knowing that the illness was responsible for untold numbers of deaths, illnesses, and disabilities in children around the world.

Chapter 11

Mother, The Perfect Scapegoat, 1960s

The search for a scapegoat is the easiest of all hunting expeditions.

Widely attributed to Dwight D. Eisenhower,
President of the United States

The 1962 Kefauver Amendment

A medical tragedy in the early 1960s spawned a new wave of government regulation. In 1961, as related by Philip Knightly and colleagues in *Suffer the Children: The Story of Thalidomide*, 33-year-old obstetrician William McBride of the Crown Street Women's Hospital in Sydney agonized over three infants born with flipper-like appendages and bowels that did not open to the outside.[1] Why, he asked, were Baby Wilson, Baby Wood, and Baby Tait, all delivered in a two-month period between May and June 1961, born with similar severe birth defects? McBride's mental "control group" consisted of all the babies he had delivered. The probability of the random births of three such babies at the same time was almost nil. These defects were rarely seen once in a lifetime. McBride reviewed the patients' records and discovered that the only drug each of the mothers-to-be had taken early in pregnancy was Distaval. Distaval, a drug that he himself was prescribing upon the recommendation of a sales representative, was also known as thalidomide.

Grünenthal, a German pharmaceutical company, had developed thalidomide as an over-the-counter sedative in the late 1950s and had distributed it around the world. By the time the company removed thalidomide from the market, it was too late for more than 12,000 babies around the world. Thanks to FDA reviewer Frances Kelsey the drug was not marketed in the United States and no more than 40 "thalidomide babies" likely occurred there. "If the drug had made it to the American market by its target date, it has been estimated that an additional 10,000 babies might have been born grossly deformed from the drug."[2] The reign of "medical opinion by experts" was about to be replaced with actual testing and government approval.

On 10 August 1962, photos of the children were printed in full pages in *Life* magazine to underscore the nonchalant way the industry was "testing" drugs on humans.[3] On 2 October 1962, the US Congress took aim at the appalling deficiencies in the industry's system of evaluating drugs and unanimously passed the landmark Kefauver-Harris Amendment to the 1938 Food, Drug, and Cosmetic Act. The amendment created another giant hurdle for the free-wheeling industry. For "new drugs," companies would now be required to use qualified experts and controlled trials to prove that their drugs were *both* safe and effective. Prior to this legislation, drugs could be marketed 60 days after a marketing application—if the FDA did not object. And now, the FDA would be required to affirmatively approve applications for "new drugs," *both* prescription and—*for the first time*—over-the-counter (OTC) drugs that had come onto the market after 1938.

At first, it looked like aspirin, an "old or grandfather drug" marketed before the 1938 Food, Drug, and Cosmetic Act, would be unaffected by the 1962 amendment. It had already mostly avoided the 1906 Pure Food and Drug Act, the 1927 Caustic Poison Act, the 1938 Food, Drug, and Cosmetic Act, the 1951 Durham-Humphrey Amendment, the FDA's 1954 methyl salicylate policy, and the 1960 Hazardous Substances Act. However, although it would avoid the upcoming 1966 Child Protection Act, aspirin would soon get caught up in the new evaluations.

In 1966, when the FDA began to review the 4000 "new drugs" approved with safety data alone between 1938 and 1962, it stepped onto a sticky wicket. Some had ingredients that had been marketed before 1938 and some of these ingredients were being sold in an estimated 500,000 OTC drugs. To bring order to the review, FDA decided to study ingredients. There were fewer than 500 of these.[4] Aspirin was about to receive a comprehensive review, one that would drag on *Bleak House* style for many years.

How salicylate accumulates

To comply with the new requirements of the Kefauver-Harris Amendment, scientists needed tools to evaluate safety and efficacy. One was pharmacokinetics, a branch of pharmacology, which seeks to understand the movement (kinetics) of a drug through the body. Specifically, it involves four processes: how a drug is *absorbed* from the stomach or from an injection site, *distributed* into different areas of the body, *metabolized* (broken down), and *excreted* (eliminated). A burst of pharmacokinetic data on many drugs followed. Now some observations and speculations about aspirin could be explained.

Through the 1960s, Coburn's and Erganian's demonstration of accumulation was confirmed and reasons for accumulation were reported both at meetings of experts and in publications. For example, in 1962, the Empire Rheumatism Council, with the support of the Nicholas Research Institute Ltd, sponsored the first large international symposium on "Salicylates" in London.[5] Seventy-six scientists and physicians, including American aspirin expert Gerhardt Levy of the State University of New York at Buffalo, and many aspirin industry representatives including those from the United States, England, and Switzerland attended.[6] Alan Done reported that the half-life (the time needed to eliminate half of the drug from the body) of salicylate varied "inversely with age among patients with salicylate intoxication" and that salicylate lasts longer in the blood of young animals compared with older ones.[7, 8] (In 1968, a study of salicylate in puppies and other young animals found diminished metabolism.[9]) Meanwhile, Levy gave a single dose of 1000 mg of aspirin to healthy adults and found that it took between 2.55 and 8.5 hours to reduce the body content by 50%, similar to an earlier finding in 1959.[10]

Also, at a symposium sponsored by the Association of Medical Advisors in Pharmaceutical Industry in London, Nicholas researchers again reported accumulation of salicylate in adults.[11] Specifically, the

Nicholas researchers found that doses of 1000 mg every six hours resulted in progressively higher blood levels until the seventh dose.[12] This regimen, 67 mg/kg/day for a 60-kg man, approximated the regimen being recommended for children.

Why does accumulation occur? In groundbreaking and separate studies, researchers at the Nicholas Research Institute and Gerhard Levy in Buffalo found the metabolism of salicylate differs from that of most other drugs.[13] Most drugs are metabolized by a process called *first-order kinetics:* as the dose increases, metabolism of the drug increases. Thus, no matter how large the dose, the drug will be gone from the body in four-to-five half-lives.

However, salicylate—and alcohol, for example—do not work this way. Larger doses increase the half-life. This *zero-order kinetics* begins at a dose of only about 300 mg in adults. Zero-order kinetics occurs because the rate of metabolism of salicylate is constant. Specifically, aspirin, after being rapidly converted to salicylate, is metabolized into four main metabolites. Between 1965 and 1972, researchers in England and the United States determined that the two main metabolites— salicyluric acid (SU) and salicyl phenolic glucuronide (SPG)—are formed at a constant rate.[14, 15, 16, 17]

Simply put, if the amount of drug ingested exceeds the rate of its metabolism, the drug accumulates as would water in a sink if the drain is too small. Therefore, accumulation depends on each component of the dose schedule—dose, frequency, and duration. An increase in any of the three components can lead to accumulation. Like alcohol, too much, too fast, or too long, and you are intoxicated. A small change could be critical. Levy found that small increases in dose could lead to large increases in the amount of drug in the body.[18]

Some studies suggested that certain individuals have particularly slow metabolism that may be genetically based.[19, 20] Levy and Jaffe noted the prevalence of slow metabolizer status was unknown. "There is a reasonable likelihood that some salicylate intoxications resulting from therapeutic use of this drug may be due to 'unusually slow elimination of salicylate.'"[21] In 1977, Furst and colleagues at the

University of California, Los Angeles would find significant differences in metabolism between identical and fraternal twins suggesting a genetically determined variation in metabolism which would explain why peak levels vary among individuals.[22] Their data also suggested that SU and SPG increased over the first three days of treatment explaining why levels peak at around three days.

No longer a guess, a supposition, or a one-time observation, accumulation at recommended doses was now recognized as an indisputable fact. Factors contributing to accumulation now included kidney function/dehydration, individual rates of metabolism, age as well as dose, dose frequency, dose duration. Possibly channeling concerns about the effects of dehydration, some ads such as one in the *Ladies Home Journal* added the importance of fluids in 1962.[23]

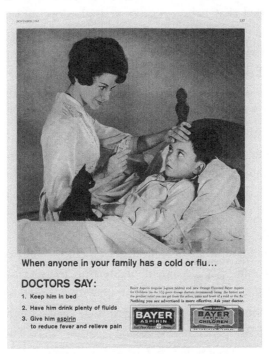

Advertisement, *Ladies Home Journal*
Courtesy of Bayer AG, Leverkusen, Germany

Aspirin experts now fell into two schools. In 1964 Levy and a colleague suggested the then radical idea of individualizing salicylate therapy rather than using a one standard-dose-fits-all approach.[24, 25] Researchers who had found a wide range variation of blood levels at five days—4.4 to 33 mg/dL—among inpatients with rheumatoid arthritis given doses of 50 mg/kg/day also recommended individualizing therapy.[26] Of course, individualizing therapy would open a can of worms as this approach would not lend itself to easy dosing with over-the-counter preparations at home. With absent pharmacokinetic studies, the other approach was to take a guess at what regimen would avoid the significant accumulation. The latter approach continued.

During the 1960s, pediatric textbooks such as *Pediatric Therapy* edited by Harry C. Shirkey[27] and *Current Pediatric Therapy* edited by Sydney S. Gellis and Benjamin M. Kagan [28] continued to suggest daily amounts of 65 mg/kg/day and 90 mg/kg/day respectively. Shirkey, however, added that babies receive a single dose and "Therapeutic toxicity is best prevented by limiting continued dosing to older children and by limiting dosage in younger children to a single prescribed dose."[29] Shirkey lamented that children differ in "drug absorption, distribution, storage, degradation, conjugation [metabolism], and excretion ..."[30] (Appendix 1)

The pharmacology data was likely a thorn in the sides of the manufacturers. Complicated adjustments to account for these issues would surely put a damper on sales. Industry appeared to prefer the dialogue on accidental poisoning—mother must be to blame.

User error?

In a 1969 monograph, *Aspirin in modern therapy*, Maurice L. Tainter, DNP expert and Vice President of Sterling Drug, maker of Bayer Aspirin and Bayer Children's Aspirin, and Alice J. Ferris of Sterling's Winthrop Laboratories claimed "overdosage, generally administered by a well-intentioned but overzealous parent, may lead to serious consequences."[31] They noted that, of 463 poisoned children discussed in 17 published reports, 42% were "victims of therapeutic excess." Doses they mentioned for children were the doses commonly recommended. They were aware of the issue of duration of therapy as they wrote "*continued administration* [emphasis added] should be considered only for the older child or where, in the judgment of the physician, its use is indicated by the nature or severity of the illness."

Tainter and Ferris devoted an entire chapter to "Adverse Reactions to Overdoses." Use of the term overdosage is where the problem of therapeutic poisoning became dangerously obscured by linguistic imprecision. In common usage, overdosage means an amount more than that recommended. An unfortunate (and fallacious) belief then followed—that a poisoned child must have been given more than the recommended dose. They may have believed this as they disagreed with the "common concept the children are abnormally sensitive to aspirin" writing that "a careful search of the published literature has not uncovered data to prove this assumption"—a statement indicating a stunning ignorance of published reports.

Tainter drove the "overdose" scenario hard and repeatedly suggested mother had "overdosed" her child. He was no lightweight.[32] A former professor of pharmacology at Stanford University, Tainter had academic clout. He had worked his way up the academic ranks at both Stanford and the College of Physicians and Surgeons Medical School in San Francisco and in 1951 he had received an honorary doctoral degree from Rensselaer Polytechnic Institute. He served as a professor at Albany Medical College, Director of Research at Winthrop Chemical Company, and Founding Director of the Sterling-Winthrop Research Institute. He also served in 1955 as President of the New York Academy of Sciences and was on the editorial board of several pharmacology journals. In other words, his résumé was impressive.

In June 1966, Tainter attended the Conference on the Effects of Chronic Salicylate Administration sponsored by United States National Institute of Arthritis and Metabolic Diseases (NIAMD) of the NIH in New York City. NIAMD had become aware of evidence concerning the effects of "chronic" salicylate use, especially in children, and possible bone and teratogenic effects (affecting the embryo) in animals. *Chronic was defined as treatment for more than 12 hours.*[33] Forty-three experts in rheumatology, research, and pharmacology registered for the meeting including attendees from universities throughout the United States, Canada, and the United Kingdom.[34] Government scientists from the FDA, the Federal Trade Commission (FTC), and the NIH were also present. Private business participants included representatives from La Wall and Harrison Research Laboratories, Inc., the US Vitamin and Pharmaceutical Corporation, the Warner-Lambert Research Institute, and Sterling Drug. A doctor summarized the session on potential fetal effects by concluding in an almost futile tone: "Salicylates given under certain circumstances, to certain animals, can be teratogenic [causing a birth defect]."

The attendees also discussed the serious problem of poisoning during therapy, including vast differences in individual salicylate levels, the impaired metabolism of the young, an observation that bed rest slows elimination, and the longer half-life in children. Yet they repeatedly used the baffling term, "therapeutic overdosage." Tainter proclaimed that the poisonings were "frequently caused by parents making mistakes in dosing."[35] Alan Done seemed to back him up saying that "serious" poisoning is most frequent in children "inadvertently overdosed by parents."[36] After these pronouncements, the discussion reached a dead end.

The conferees, top-notch experts in salicylate, let the topic of "therapeutic overdosing" lapse. They then moved on to a discussion of children and adults with rheumatic diseases. The topic of the vastly more common "chronic" aspirin therapy—treatment of colds, flu, and fever with over-the-counter aspirin in children—simply drifted away.

Tainter seized another opportunity to blame mother. In his testimony before Congress during consideration of the proposed 1966 Child Safety Act, Tainter chose to paint a vivid scenario of mothers overdosing children:

> Another very serious problem that is not written about much, for fairly obvious reasons, is that from 14 to 74 per cent of the aspirin poisoning cases are due to the administration of overdoses by the mother, either on her own, or on the recommendation of a physician ... she misunderstands the doctor and piles the dosage in, or what was an initial large beginning dose

is continued. The therapeutic overdosage is a very large factor of the entire poisoning syndrome.[37]

The manufacturers largely opposed the proposed Act, as did the AMA, which apparently either confused the accidental poisonings with the therapeutic poisonings or bought the blame-the-mother argument.

It was easy to blame the mother. After all, mother was giving the medicine. An advertisement for Bayer Aspirin for Children during the 1960s pictured the charming child actress Linda Risk with a teddy bear saying, "My mother gives me Orange Flavored Bayer Aspirin for Children. That's because she loves me!"[38] And no one could know for sure how much aspirin mother was giving at home.

Joan Beck, a pioneering science columnist for the *Chicago Tribune*, wrote about the situation in her nationally syndicated column "You and Your Child" in 1967. Her assessment was almost perfect.[39] She reported,

[W]hen a youngster gets overdoses [the imperfect part] of aspirin as a treatment, the problem may go unsuspected until too late to save his life … the aspirin may begin to pile up in his body … can reach a danger point … An infant should not be given aspirin for more than two days. And he should get liberal amounts of liquid all during this period.[40]

Nevertheless, use of the vague and undefined term "overdose" continued to support the dangerous mindset that overdoses could be avoided simply by following instructions. The term overdose obscured the fact that the dose and frequency combination being used could result in accumulation and was the very one recommended for children at home. Nevertheless, for many doctors and parents alike, aspirin seemed safe, effective, easy to give, endorsed by experts, and a necessity for loving parents. In 1972, Plough distributed the 50th Golden Jubilee Edition of the St Joseph Family Calendar featuring ads for St Joseph Aspirin for Children. Now, parents could see the ads every day right on the walls of their kitchen.

As I learned about aspirin poisoning, the pillars propping up the idea that Reye's syndrome and salicylate toxicity differed crumbled. Reye's syndrome had not arisen in the 1960s at all but could be traced to the 1920s when pediatricians began embracing salicylates. Doctors often missed the diagnosis of salicylate poisoning because, as Crichton explained, "everything about it was misleading." Low blood levels could occur during severe salicylate poisoning. And finally, concerns about the dosing schedule were valid.

Chapter 12

Algorithm Think: If It's One, It Can't Be the Other, 1960s

The obscure we see eventually,
the completely apparent takes longer.

Aphorism quoted by Peter D. Mitchell, Nobel address, 1978

Early reactions to Reye's 1963 report

After Reye's report, descriptions of the syndrome appeared in reports from such diverse places as Johannesburg in South Africa, Auckland in New Zealand, Edinburgh in Scotland, and Czechoslovakia. Doctors had, over the same period, seen cases like Reye's and had been just as perplexed.[1,2,3,4,5] H.L. Utian and colleagues at the Transvaal Memorial Hospital for Children in Johannesburg, South Africa, for example, had encountered 14 such children. Most were infants with an initial upper respiratory infection followed by the "explosive" disorder. The clinicians had considered salicylate intoxication but had dismissed it because they had "never obtained a history of poisoning" and the blood salicylate level "was never raised to more than mild-moderate levels."[6] Utian's report set the stage for the many that followed—aspirin was not to be seriously regarded as a possible culprit.

There were two notable exceptions. In May 1965, H.M. Giles of Selly Oak Hospital in Birmingham, England, wrote to the editor of *The Lancet* stating, "I would like to suggest that salicylate might be involved … Most if not all of the features can be produced by salicylate." He noted his own difficulty obtaining a history of salicylate use. "The true incidence of administration may well be high since in three of my own cases only close and direct questioning elicited the fact that it had been given."[7] Several months later, Trevor P. Mann at the Royal Alexandra Hospital for Sick Children in Brighton, England, concluded that salicylates must surely be viewed with suspicion in what he called the wet-brain/fatty liver syndrome, as well as the chickenpox encephalitis with hypoglycemia syndrome.[8]

The purported first case of Reye's syndrome in the United States was in a six-month-old infant, who had died at the University of Minnesota in 1963; both viruses and toxins had been considered as causes.[9] In 1965, doctors described five Connecticut and Rhode Island children who had become ill with the clinical pattern of Reye's syndrome during 1963. Tests for toxins only revealed a small amount of isopropyl alcohol (a compound used for disinfection).[10] These initial cases were followed by similar ones in Oklahoma City, Oklahoma,[11] and Cleveland, Ohio.[12] In 1966, doctors from Scotland, Czechoslovakia, and New Zealand reiterated some of Reye's especially disturbing findings: onset after an initial common, trivial infection,[13] low blood and spinal fluid glucose levels,[14] low blood-sugar levels resistant to glucose infusions,[15] seizures even when blood-sugar levels were normal,[16] extremely swollen brains,[17] and in some survivors, severe mental retardation or epilepsy.[18] One group reported an adenovirus in the liver.[19] They speculated the illness was viral in origin.[20] Many noted aspirin had been given to some of the children and one specifically noted that medicines given had been "in amounts generally regarded as harmless."[21]

Again, and again, aspirin was considered and dismissed. In 1967, for example, physicians in Washington, D.C. seemingly unaware of accumulation and toxicity at low levels, dismissed salicylate poisoning in a three-year-old because the patient had received only "small amounts" and the salicylate level was low, only 8 mg/dL.[22] The following year, after Duke University researchers learned that only four types of viruses had been found in brain tissue among 82 cases of Reye's syndrome, they focused on toxins. Yet they too concluded (except for isopropyl alcohol) that no historical or chemical evidence of "salicylates, barbiturates, hydrocarbons, lead, arsenic, or other toxic substances" had been found.[23]

The first large case series of "Reye's syndrome" from a single hospital (besides Reye's) was authored by Chief Resident in

Pathology M.G. Norman and his colleagues at the Hospital for Sick Children in Toronto in 1968. Norman searched the hospital's the previous 15 years of autopsy records and found 21 children with fatty liver between 1954 and 1966. The children, all younger than nine years, were ill for about four days before the onset of vomiting and a rapid decline. Curiously, among Norman's cases, 9% had juvenile rheumatoid arthritis, a disease routinely treated with aspirin. [24] Several had previous medical conditions including rheumatic fever, nephritic syndrome, scarlet fever, and bronchitis. Because the children usually hyperventilated and six of them had vomited coffee grounds-like material (often a result of bleeding in the stomach)—both signs of salicylate poisoning—doctors had checked the blood for salicylate. For the 10 tested, the level was below 25 mg/dL. Norman noted: "no common single drug was administered to every child." He speculated, "If salicylates were the cause, it is difficult to understand why this syndrome was not recognized in greater numbers earlier than in the 1960s." [25] Norman did not realize that most of cases in Reye's original report had occurred during the 1950s, the first decade children's aspirin was widely advertised or that a low blood level was meaningless in the setting of therapeutic poisoning.

And so it went. Clinicians reported cases and offered speculations about the involvement of aspirin.[26,27,28,29] In 1969, among 33 cases of Reye's syndrome in Canadian centers within the previous several months, none had "a clinical history of ingestions or exposure to toxic agents."[30] In 1970 and 1971, cases were reported from such diverse areas as Arkansas,[31] Oklahoma,[32] Washington, D.C.,[33] Buenos Aires,[34] Perth in Australia (reporting on cases before 1967),[35] and a United States airbase in Japan.[36] A Johns Hopkins Hospital physician echoing the thoughts of numerous others wrote that many of the children had been treated with salicylates, penicillin, or tetracycline, and "finding one of these compounds in blood or tissue is of questionable significance."[37]

Doctors looked for salicylate poisoning and, after their evaluations, concluded the children did not have it.

Clinical giants spar

Sometime during the 1960s, Ted Mortimer came to believe that aspirin played a role in Reye's syndrome. The infants he had reported in 1962 had brain swelling, tiny fat droplets in the liver (fatty degeneration), and hypoglycemia; they essentially *had* Reye's syndrome. Mortimer thought aspirin was a key factor and never let it go. Yet as powerful a voice as Mortimer had, he faced deeply entrenched acceptance of aspirin manifested, for example, in the person of well-known and admired Boston pediatrician Sydney S. Gellis. Gellis gave voice to the status-quo viewpoint that aspirin did not cause Reye's syndrome and reflected the opinions of the many doctors who had comfortably recommended aspirin for children and could not imagine it responsible for so devastating an illness.

Gellis, the "quintessential pediatric generalist," was the "go-to guy" at the Boston Children's Hospital during the 1950s. His gift was the ability to apply a "multitude of research articles" to the practice of pediatrics. When he died in 2002, his obituary noted, "A better clinical teacher did not exist."[38] Most closely associated with the Floating Hospital of Children at Tufts, Gellis was known to have "strong opinions about almost everything and was not afraid to be wrong." Experience and opinion alone carried much weight during the 1950s. Gellis opined that aspirin might worsen Reye's syndrome but did not cause it.

In 1967, Gellis, then Pediatrician-in-Chief at Tufts New England Medical Center, discussed a case at the Massachusetts General Hospital.[39] It was an honor to be a discussant there as these conferences were published the prestigious *New England Journal of Medicine*. The case was that of a six-year-old boy who had died after the onset of chickenpox. The boy had developed continuous vomiting, deep, irregular breathing, low blood and spinal fluid glucose levels, blood in his stomach, acetone on his breath, an enlarged liver, and an abnormally high liver enzyme levels. His blood salicylate level was only 6.5 mg/dL. He died after three days in the hospital.

As master clinician, Gellis' task was to propose a diagnosis. He offered three possibilities: a complication of chickenpox, an unrelated condition such as hepatitis, and Reye's syndrome. Gellis' final diagnosis was Reye's syndrome, which he characterized as "a complex syndrome with several viral etiologies." He mentioned Mortimer and Lepow's 1962 report linking aspirin to a similar illness and then—without offering a shred of evidence—offered his opinion: "I doubt that salicylates constitute a primary etiology in this syndrome; rather, I suggest that they accentuate the underlying basic process." A pathologist confirmed that the boy had Reye's syndrome.

A physician attending the conference pointed out the child was one of five similar cases seen during the past year. One had been exposed to measles, one to mumps, and three had upper respiratory infections. In four, severe vomiting beginning within 72 hours of the infections was followed by changes in mental state. Four of the children survived, although one had severe, permanent brain damage. The physician was surprised that such a large amount of fat could accumulate in the liver so quickly.

Gellis became intrigued by Reye's syndrome. As editor of the 1967–1968 *Yearbook of Pediatrics*, he selected D.M.O. Becroft's report for review.[40] Becroft's cases of Reye's syndrome, Gellis said, were not dissimilar to those of Mortimer and Lepow. In the mode of either-or thinking, Gellis asked Mortimer if his diagnosis of chickenpox could be mistaken and if the patients could have had Reye's syndrome instead. Mortimer responded in characteristic fashion. "Anyone who says these infants didn't have varicella is out of his chicken-poken mind ... *The most important question, then, is whether there is a relationship between salicylates and Reye's syndrome.* [Emphasis added] It is our belief that in many instances salicylates do play an etiologic [causal] role in the syndrome." [41]

Mortimer was crystal clear. Unfortunately, he had no direct proof, no smoking gun, and no statistical backing. The strength of his conviction did not sway his colleagues who were relying on the strength of their own convictions. It was an unwinnable battle between clinical giants. Gellis did not further acknowledge Mortimer's ideas and wrote, "[T]he clinical picture strongly suggests viral infection rather than toxic agents as the likely etiology." [42]

Clinicians continued to discuss the role of salicylates. In 1969, St Louis doctors discussed the death of a 20-month-old toddler with Reye's syndrome. The medical students had dismissed salicylate poisoning because the blood salicylate level was zero. The students, like Gellis, assumed that if it was one, it couldn't also be the other. Yet John Kissane, Professor of both Pathology and Pediatrics, was frustrated.

> After the exhilaration of making that diagnosis, I wish to point out that this is really no comfort to anybody; we have no idea what Reye's syndrome is, into what category of disease it belongs ... our department has expressed the view that this is an intoxication of unknown etiology. [43]

Ted Mortimer entered another debate in 1970, this time with Diane Pross and colleagues at Duke University Medical Center who had reported the case of a nine-month-old baby with Reye's syndrome in *Pediatrics*. [44] The infant was well until three days before hospital admission when he developed a fever and runny nose and was treated with two "baby" aspirin every four hours. Despite vomiting, the aspirin was continued. The day before admission, he awoke with a high fever, agitation, and vomiting coffee-ground material. His liver tests were abnormal. At Duke his salicylate level was 25 mg/dL. His physicians treated him with dialysis, and three days later he was eating and back to normal. Pross and her colleagues searched the literature and found that *of 46 children under two years old with Reye's syndrome only two had survived*. Pross noted, without citing a reference, that abnormal tests of liver function were "not usually found" in salicylate intoxication. Nevertheless, she mused, "In the present patient it is not possible to distinguish clearly between salicylate intoxication and Reye's syndrome. Similarly, it must be considered that the dramatic response to dialysis might have been due to removal of salicylates." Ed Shaw of the Department of Pediatrics, University of California, San Francisco, shot a letter to the editor of *Pediatrics* stating with clarity that the infant had received "an inappropriate, huge, and unnecessary dose of 150 mg of aspirin every 4 hours for 3–4 days." He argued "that aspirin might have been a cause or even *the* cause of Reye's syndrome." [45]

A letter by Mortimer was even more urgent.[46] The Pross report, he said, prompted him "to beat a drum that I have beaten noisily on previous occasions." He pleaded with those who saw patients with hypoglycemia and other manifestations of Reye's syndrome to ask the family specifically about "salicylates and dosage, and to draw a salicylate level on admission." In response, Pross stated aspirin had not been given to all children, levels were never more than "mild to moderately elevated," and profound liver failure is quite unusual in salicylism. This astonishing exchange of opinions in *Pediatrics* highlighted both why Mortimer believed aspirin had a significant role in Reye's and why others did not. The debate continued.

Gellis never wavered. In 1971 in the *Yearbook of Pediatrics* he wrote, "Reye's syndrome seems to be at a dead end for the present from the point of view of etiology."[47] In 1972, he wrote, "We can only conclude there are multiple causes."[48] In 1977 he wrote, "Well, there you have it, or at least parts of it. In summary, we can't do much with the apparent causes of Reye's syndrome."[49] In 1978 he wrote, "we are still no closer to the answers to this disorder than we were 5 years ago."[50] In 1979, Frank A. Oski and James A. Stockman of the State University of New York Upstate Medical Center took over the editorship of the *Yearbook*, but even then Gellis was not done letting his opinion be known. He was about to jump into the thick of it.

Some had suggested that Reye's syndrome was not a single illness. However, Peter R. Huttenlocher of Yale University put that idea to rest in 1969. In one of the first analytic studies on Reye's syndrome, he compared the liver function test results of children with Reye's syndrome to those with many other conditions characterized by encephalopathy such as anoxic (lack of oxygen) encephalopathy, encephalitis, bacterial meningitis, brain abscess, and brain tumor. He *concluded that abnormal liver function in a child with encephalopathy usually indicated Reye's syndrome.* Unfortunately, he had not studied salicylate poisoning. Huttenlocher concluded that almost all acute toxic brain encephalopathies with abnormal liver tests in children were, in fact, "Reye's syndrome."[51]

Another influenza pandemic, Reye's syndrome, and mitochondria

The Hong Kong influenza pandemic of 1968–1969 attracted many academics to the study of Reye's syndrome. Reports emerged from Boston, Chicago, Cincinnati, Cleveland, Columbus, Denver, Memphis, New Haven, Rochester (Minnesota), Pittsburgh, Nova Scotia, St Louis, and Toronto, as well as the CDC in Atlanta and as far as the Southeast Asia Treaty Organization (SEATO) in Thailand where a brain swelling illness was receiving special recognition in Udorn, Thailand. Thai locals called it "Udorn encephalopathy." Parents reported their child had been well until he developed a fever, convulsions, and coma. Self-treatment with herbs and modern nonprescription medications was common.[52] Autopsy findings were typical of Reye's syndrome. Spot surveys revealed the illness was also occurring in Bangkok, Khon Kaen, and Chiang Mai and probably accounted for many deaths in children in these regions. The cause of "Udorn encephalopathy" was a mystery. In 19 of 21 villages surveyed between two and eight cases were estimated to have occurred each year for the past two years. Many more cases likely occurred because only one in 10 children reached the hospital.[53]

The United States had been using the Thai Air Force base since 1964. Curtis H. Bourgeois and colleagues at the Southeast Asia Treaty Organization (SEATO) Medical Project and the Udorn Provincial Hospital studied the records of 139 children, most between the ages of one and seven, who had been admitted to the hospital between 1967 and 1969 including 113 deaths. The researchers concluded that "all causes except toxins and viral infections" had been eliminated and conjectured that "the worldwide distribution [of Reye's] would rule out all but the most common manufactured products." They proposed that aflatoxin, a fungal toxin, be considered because of similar pathology findings[54] and speculated that compounds like cyanide, which inhibit the production of ATP, cause changes in the nervous system like those seen in Reye's syndrome.[55]

And they did something new. They used an electron microscope to visualize the fine structures inside the liver cells of the children and were struck by obvious abnormalities in the mitochondria, the small organelles where life-sustaining ATP is made.[56] The list of molecules known to inhibit ATP production in mitochondria was short. It included DNP, phenol, and salicylate—structurally similar compounds. Sterling's Maurice Tainter took notice. In 1969, in the monograph entitled *Aspirin in modern therapy*, Tainter and his colleague Alice J. Ferris noted Brody's 1955 discovery that salicylates are powerful inhibitors of mitochondria's ability to produce ATP.[57]

Shortly after, Arnold Silverman and colleagues in Colorado suggested that decreased ATP production might be responsible for the symptoms of Reye's syndrome and that aspirin could cause it. "Aspirin capable of uncoupling oxidative phosphorylation, results in decreased ATP production. Many of the findings of Reye's syndrome could fit into this mechanism."[58] He further mused, "One has the feeling when treating these patients that a 'total body uncoupling' at the cellular level has occurred and, though unproved, may result from defective ATP."[59] Researchers in Cincinnati agreed that Reye's syndrome looked like an "uncoupling illness."[60]

Between 1962 and 1979, Mortimer, Giles, Mann, Shaw, McAdams, Hilty, and now Silverman had expressed their suspicion that aspirin may be the culprit in the brain swelling/fatty liver illness called Reye's syndrome. But their thoughts remained in print in medical journals.

Chapter 13

A Gordian Knot, 1970s

It was six men of Indostan, to learning much inclined,
who went to see the elephant (Though all of them were blind),
that each by observation, might satisfy his mind.

Telling of an Indian parable, widely attributed to
John Godfrey Saxe

Reye's syndrome entered the 1970s as a mysterious illness with few treatment options and took its place among the top causes of death in children.[1] At the same time, published reports of childhood therapeutic aspirin poisoning decreased. A review of salicylate poisoning in *Pediatrics* in 1974 mainly referenced reports from the 1950s.[2]

Three expert groups dismiss aspirin

Despite speculation about the role of aspirin in Reye's syndrome by Mortimer, Giles, Mann, Shaw, McAdams, Hilty, and Silverman, experts at several highly respected institutions made assertions that seemed to close the door on the idea that aspirin was involved. These assertions, based only on observation and not formal comparative research, became dogma for the next decade.

First, the Viral Diseases Branch of the Center for Disease Control (CDC) pronounced that it could find no evidence that aspirin was involved in Reye's syndrome. Studying medicines had been a side issue of the study that spawned this statement. In 2009, Thomas Glick, the study's first author, told me that he had been interested in Reye's syndrome since he had attended to a six-year-old girl in the emergency room as a medical student at Harvard. The girl had an "extraordinary delirium" just four days past her first rash of chickenpox. When he later joined CDC as an EIS officer, his supervisor who had collected a few cases out of interest told him to go, "Do your stuff, it's not gonna cost a whole lot of money, I'll support you in it." Glick recalled, "So, as these little micro epidemics came up, we started the surveillance system." Glick and CDC colleagues reported their findings in *Pediatrics* in 1970. They had developed "case definition" criteria to determine which children would be included.[3] CDC's definition required the presence of an acute onset encephalopathy and liver involvement *with no other reasonable explanation*. In other words, according to CDC's definition, if the child was diagnosed with salicylate poisoning, he or she did not have Reye's syndrome and could not be included in their study—even if the child had brain swelling and fatty liver. Implicit in the exclusion of children with salicylate poisoning was that salicylate was not a factor in Reye's syndrome. (The same issue arose in 2020 when Chinese authorities first used a case definition that included both a respiratory illness and contact with the Wuhan market, a definition that CDC Director Robert Redfield correctly pointed out would potentially miss a larger number of non-market cases.[4])

Although Reye's syndrome was not a reportable disease like measles, CDC had collected reports of 62 children with the illness since 1967. Glick's report was one of the first large reports summarizing epidemiologic characteristics of the illness. The prodrome was an upper respiratory illness in 48, chickenpox in seven, and either gastroenteritis, multisystem complaints, or a rash in the others. One child had had both smallpox and typhoid vaccinations five days before. Younger patients were more likely to have low glucose levels in the blood or cerebral spinal fluid. Only 15 (24%) had survived.

A medical epidemiologist had investigated 48 "to some degree" and, for 21, the home had been inspected. Only 69% of the 48 cases were known to have taken a salicylate. The report concluded: "Considerable negative epidemiologic evidence in the present series of cases indicates that most, if not all, cases of Reye's syndrome in the United States are etiologically unrelated to exogenous toxins or common medications." The authors however noted that a viral illness, particularly influenza B, was associated with Reye's syndrome. While the study design was not intended to be definitive regarding the role of either an infection or medication use, this study was quoted repeatedly as evidence both *against* the role of salicylate and *for* an association with influenza B and chickenpox—even as these infections were also absent in many cases.

The second report emanated from the pathology department at the Cincinnati Children's Hospital Medical Center (CHMC).[5] At the time, pathologists relied on the light microscope and special stains to identify fatty degeneration. But in the early 1970s researchers at the CHMC had become interested in the new field of electron microscopy (EM). In addition to fat, they could now see changes in mitochondria which suggested to them "a chemically mediated and potentially reversible mitochondrial injury." They speculated none of the toxins considered by Becroft in 1966 and Bradford in 1971—both of whom had considered aspirin—were known to cause a similar lesion in mitochondria. They were partly correct. Aspirin was not *known* to cause these mitochondrial changes—however, no one had looked, which was an oversight given Brody's 1955 discovery of its profound physiologic effect on mitochondria. In 1973, the Cincinnati researchers went further. In an abstract in the journal *Gastroenterology*, the CHMC researchers opined that certain brain disorders, including salicylism, influenza encephalitis, varicella encephalitis, and others were "clearly distinguishable" from Reye's syndrome by liver biopsy. They presented no data.[6]

In 1972, a third report described an investigation by David W. Reynolds, a CDC EIS officer stationed in Oklahoma, respected pediatrician Harris Riley, Jr, and others. During our conversation in 2007, Riley remembered Abe Plough, as a promoter who had even visited the home of his parents, the owners of the Harris and Riley Drug Company in Tupelo, Mississippi. At age 32 Riley had been the youngest chairman of the Department of Pediatrics at the University of Oklahoma.[7] He was an expert on salicylate having written a widely quoted review in 1956.[8] The 1972 report involved 11 Oklahoma children who had died of Reye's syndrome. After casting a wide net looking for the cause, they noticed the children had all received aspirin yet, they too concluded they had found no evidence for intoxication or drug overdosage. Then, like the 1970 CDC paper, because eight cases had occurred around the time of an influenza B epidemic, they reported a relationship between Reye's syndrome and influenza, particularly influenza B.[9]

The same year in an editorial review in the *Journal of Infectious Diseases* (*JID*), Riley curiously failed to mention that hyperventilation (rapid or deep breathing) was a key finding in Reye's syndrome.[10] The omission was puzzling because hyperventilation is also a key feature of salicylate intoxication.[11] (Please recall in the late 1800s Bayer's Heinrich Dreser had dismissed aspirin as a potential product because it caused panting in dogs.) Few other childhood illnesses (beside pneumonia) present with hyperventilation. Nevertheless, Riley emphasized the role of infection in his review.[12]

These pronouncements from the three groups of experts not only confirmed what many physicians were already thinking but also defined the status of salicylate as a causal factor for the next 10 years. Salicylate poisoning and Reye's syndrome were distinctly different illnesses.

The search for a cause

Having dismissed aspirin, researchers considered other possible causes. Understandably, they focused on virus infections. Influenza type B virus, which occurs annually and usually affects children, was the chief suspect. In 1971, CDC reported that 36 children in New England and New York had been hospitalized with Reye's syndrome in January and February and in an editorial note in the *MMWR* noted: "From the minimal laboratory data available, it seems likely that in many cases in the present outbreak, the antecedent illness may be influenza B infection."[13] In addition, 14 cases were identified in Chicago during an influenza B outbreak in 1971.[14]

In 1973, influenza B moved center stage. Scientists were predicting outbreaks of a new influenza B variant, and the CDC and the AAP proactively encouraged doctors to report Reye's syndrome. The response was shocking. *In one week, 70 cases of Reye's syndrome were reported from 14 states.* The *New York Times* featured Reye's syndrome for the first time on 24 February 1974.[15] It stated 379 cases, including the deaths of 157 children with Reye's syndrome, had been reported to the CDC between mid–December 1973 and 30 June 1974.

The numbers were alarming. CDC researchers scrambled to uncover more clues and noticed two patterns. About two-thirds of the cases reported since 1967 occurred in clusters. The cluster children were older, with a median age of 11 years, and usually had an initial upper respiratory infection. The other pattern was that of sporadic cases in children with a median age of six years. This pattern was associated with many viruses, most commonly chickenpox.[16] The fact that different viruses seemed to precede the explosive symptoms of Reye's syndrome remained a vexing mystery. Reye's syndrome was occurring after influenza A infection too, as documented in 1969, the year of the Hong Kong influenza pandemic.[17] Neurologic disorders like those seen in Reye's syndrome had been reported earlier during the 1957 Asian flu pandemic.[18, 19, 20] Could these have been Reye's syndrome? During the winter of 1977/1978 while influenza A (both H3N2 and H1N1) was circulating, CDC again received an increase in Reye's syndrome reports.

CDC estimated that during influenza A years, Reye's was occurring at about half the rate as during influenza B years.[21] The accuracy of the rate difference is questionable however as the "outbreak" of Reye's syndrome during the 1973/1974 influenza B season may have been amplified by the intense effort to encourage reporting. Despite the strong association with influenza, children with Reye's syndrome had many other types of viruses before the onset of vomiting, including adenovirus type 3; coxsackie A, A9; coxsackie B, B4, B5; Epstein-Barr; ECHO (enteric cytopathic human orphan) virus 2, 3, 8, 11; herpes simplex virus; influenza A; influenza B; parainfluenza; polio type 1; reovirus 1, 2; rubella; rubeola; vaccinia; and varicella-zoster virus.[22]

If a virus was responsible for Reye's syndrome, where was it when Reye's syndrome struck? CDC's David Morens and Gary Noble noted the evidence that "active influenza is a regular occurrence during Reye's syndrome is inconclusive."[23] Darryl C. Devivo and James P. Keating of St Louis Children's' Hospital aptly agreed calling the "relationship between a viral infection and Reye's syndrome 'obscure.'" [24]

Researchers were intrigued by other observations. For example, sibling cases had to be a clue but what did they reveal?[25] In one study, no genetic markers were found.[26] In the mid-1970s, a potentially meaningful but inexplicable phenomenon was noted. The age of patients was changing. Many were now older—10 years of age and older whereas early reports were generally of children younger than eight, with most under three years of age.[27] Neurologists at the Mayo Clinic in Rochester, Minnesota, confirmed the phenomenon.[28] Between 1956 and 1967, the children they studied were under four years of age but between 1968 and 1971, all were between 10 and 15 years of age. By 1977, many were teenagers. For example, in February 1977, a 16-year-old Ossining boy was the fourth youth in the previous two weeks in northern Westchester County to be stricken with Reye's syndrome.[29] How could this age shift be explained?

Researchers also looked for clues by studying subcategories of cases: infants, adults, race, varying socioeconomic groups, endogenous fatty acids, abnormal response to infection, increased blood ammonia, and endotoxins.[30, 31,32, 33, 34]

Toxins were considered because fatty liver is "a frequent accompaniment" of a toxic substance.[35] Reye himself had noted the similarity to Jamaican vomiting sickness and tremetol poisoning, poisoning from milk produced by a cow fed on snakeroot or rayless golden rod. Pesticides created headlines in the mid-1970s after children living in heavily sprayed areas in Canada came down with Reye's syndrome.[36,37] Phenothiazines, a frequent treatment for vomiting, were always considered too, as were salicylates. Yet no single agent seemed consistent with all the observations, and every agent seemed to be plagued by one or more problems: not every child had been exposed; the amount of the toxin was "low," the blood levels were "low;" or the pathology differed.

The confusing mix of possibilities was further complicated by the fact that Reye's syndrome sometimes occurred in conjunction with conditions other than infections: mental retardation, leukemia, juvenile rheumatoid arthritis, rheumatic fever, sickle cell anemia, nephritic syndrome, and juvenile diabetes.[38] A comprehensive summary of Reye's syndrome by DeVivo and Keating reflected the disheartening situation.[39] All proposals for the cause were speculative. It seemed that anything was possible.

Cincinnati physicians on the trail

In 1970, at a case conference, University of Cincinnati Chief Pathologist A. James McAdams noted outright the similarities between salicylate poisoning and Reye's syndrome. "You can debate, as you will," he opined, "whether aspirin is actually an agent of toxic hepatitis but clinically and pathologically the only obvious difference between Reye's syndrome and salicylism is the positive incrimination of salicylate in the one." Pediatrician William K. Schubert, director of the clinical research center, added that chemical toxins and drugs including salicylate would be looked at during studies. The conference discussion appeared in the *Journal of Pediatrics.* [40]

Two years later, young internal medicine physician Calvin C. Linnemann arrived at the University of Cincinnati as a new faculty member excited by the opportunity to study Reye's syndrome. When I interviewed Linnemann in 2007, he told me that he had learned about Reye's syndrome as a CDC EIS officer stationed at the Louisiana health department during the 1960s and knew that CDC generally viewed Reye's syndrome as an infectious disease. In fact, he had told Schubert that it was "clear" that Reye's was some sort of infection. Ever the patient pediatrician, Schubert kindly told him he was "wrong." After all, Schubert said, exchange transfusions [and not antibiotics or antivirals] were being used as therapy because it was caused by some sort of toxin. Nevertheless, Schubert encouraged him to study it all he wanted.

By early 1974, Linnemann and colleagues from the Department of Medicine along with Associate Professor of Pediatrics John Partin and Schubert reported the findings of a study of 24 children with Reye's syndrome.[41] After trying every method they knew to find a virus in the liver and brain and finding none, they had decided to ask the parents about exposures. The information they collected revealed two things. *Every child had taken aspirin, and some were on chronic aspirin therapy.*

Linnemann's study was the first of a substantial size to show that 100% of children with Reye's syndrome had indeed taken aspirin. The children had taken aspirin for an average of 3.7 days—almost the exact same number of days as those in the Arizona study. Available levels averaged only 12.3 mg/dL. Only three had levels greater than 20 mg/dL. Two had histories of unusual aspirin ingestion—one often took aspirin for chronic headaches, and one had received excessive amounts. That year in Columbus, at the first meeting ever held on Reye's syndrome, Milo Hilty speculated on a possible role for aspirin.[42]

By 1975, Linnemann and his colleagues had extended the study to include 58 children. Still, almost all had taken aspirin.[43] In addition, seven had unusual aspirin exposures (including three children with juvenile rheumatoid arthritis). While the salicylate levels were not unusually high and some were zero, many of the children had discontinued aspirin because of vomiting. The researchers pointed out that aspirin was toxic to the liver, associated with hypoglycemia and depressed cellular immunity.[44, 45, 46]

Linnemann soon found himself on the same trail as Mortimer, Giles, Mann, Shaw, McAdams, Hilty, and Silverman. Soon Jon Dean Waldman and colleagues at Northwestern University pointed out what many clinicians seemed to have forgotten—*that a low salicylate level was not a reason to rule out salicylate intoxication because salicylate levels decline rapidly once the drug is stopped.*[47] Waldman declared: "The controversy of the relationship of salicylate intoxication as a possible etiologic factor in Reye's syndrome is reiterated. A blood salicylate concentration of 11 mg/dL thirty hours after cessation of aspirin therapy strongly suggests that the patient had had salicylate intoxication."

Why had clinicians ignored this fact for so long? Several psychological realities may explain. Physicians treating a devastating and rapidly evolving condition are juggling many responsibilities—the needs of the ill child, the expectations of concerned parents, and the desire to declare a diagnosis. In a time-sensitive situation like this, biases may quickly come into play including a narrowing of vision and attention to only selected information (aspirin is safe), premature termination of the search for evidence, cognitive inertia (satisfaction with the simplest and first diagnosis), wishful thinking, repetition bias (repeated reports that aspirin was not involved), group think (everyone agrees aspirin is not involved), and an underestimation of uncertainty.[48] And of course there was the idea that aspirin poisoning was generally due to an "overdose by mother."

Nevertheless, reports of Reye's syndrome in children on recommended doses of aspirin were increasing.[49] These cases only stoked the dilemma of the role of aspirin in Reye's syndrome and, as the cases piled up, there seemed to be no way of resolving it. Clinicians now became confused when a child meeting the criteria for Reye's syndrome also had taken *large* amounts of aspirin or had a high (> 25 mg/dL) blood level of salicylate. Physicians at the Bergen Pines County Hospital in Paramus, New Jersey, faced just this situation.[50] An 18-year-old girl with acute viral hepatitis, signs and symptoms of Reye's syndrome, and a recent cough with malaise began vomiting and complaining of a headache, ringing in her ears, and diminished hearing. Her parents had been concerned about her aspirin use. When she began hallucinating, screaming, tearing her hair, and biting herself, she was admitted to the hospital where her serum salicylate level was high, 40 mg/dL. She gradually improved. A liver biopsy showed both viral hepatitis and fatty degeneration. The physicians asked: what was the diagnosis—hepatitis, salicylism, Reye's syndrome, or all of them?

Physicians at Stanford University related a similar story.[51] Two siblings, ages seven and nine years, after being treated with aspirin for upper respiratory infections were admitted to the hospital with acute encephalopathy and salicylate levels in the toxic range (50 and 40 mg/dL). The doctors estimated that the children "may have received as much as 80–150 mg/kg/day." One died and the autopsy showed marked cerebral edema and tiny fat droplets throughout the liver cells. The doctors wrote, "The role of aspirin as a cause of both acute encephalopathy and hepatic dysfunction has now been well established, but its importance as an etiologic or contributory factor in the pathogenesis of Reye's syndrome remains to be determined." The doctors seemed to believe it had to be one or the other.

Then, in 1975, Finnish investigator Matti Sillanpää and colleagues reported a most informative event—a case of Reye's syndrome unfolding in the hospital before their eyes. The teenager was being treated with aspirin for fever and swollen joints at a dose of 82 mg/kg/day divided into three doses (Appendix 1).[52]

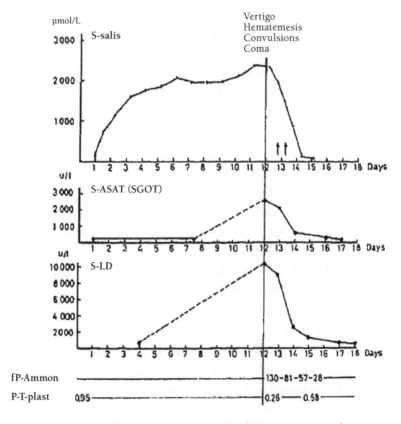

Figure 13.1 Serum salicylate concentration (S-salis), S-LD, S-ASAT, fP-Ammon and P-T-plast during the critical days of salicylate treatment.[53]

Sillanpää M., Mäkelä A., Koivikko A., *Acta Paediatrica Scandinavica*, 1975

Copyright © 1975. Reproduced with permission from John Wiley and Sons.

After developing a runny nose and a fever on day 8, she became suddenly confused. The aspirin was stopped on day 10, yet she became restless and delirious with deep respirations. She vomited blood, lost consciousness, and convulsed. Her liver function test results were abnormally high. The doctors exchanged five liters of her blood twice. After 60 hours of coma, she suddenly awoke. *Her liver function abnormality and the salicylate level peaked at the onset of coma* as shown in Figure 13.1. The illness was clearly salicylate intoxication, but was it Reye's syndrome too? Was it both? Or … were they the same?

Some parents in the United States had begun buying the new pain and fever reducer, acetaminophen, mainly Tylenol. OTC Tylenol elixir for children had been launched after Johnson & Johnson had purchased its maker McNeil Laboratories in 1959. The company released a chewable form for children in 1972. (Appendix 4) Aspirin use was very slowly declining but not soon enough to affect a case-control study that Linnemann performed in the mid-1970s and did not report until 1981.[54]

Linnemann studied five patients with biopsy-proven Reye's syndrome and seven control subjects with only a viral illness. All twelve had used aspirin. The only logical conclusion was that aspirin use was ubiquitous. However, Linnemann did not give up. He decided to test the hypothesis that salicylate and a virus interact to produce Reye's syndrome.[55] He gave one group of ferrets both influenza virus and salicylate and another group only salicylate, and guess what happened? All the ferrets—even those without the virus—developed moderate to severe fatty changes in the liver. Linnemann's team however concluded that the liver pathology differed from Reye's syndrome despite some similarities (such as glycogen depletion, fatty changes, and enlarged pleomorphic mitochondria as well as depression of several enzymes known to be depressed in Reye's syndrome).

As Linnemann labored over his "aspirin–virus" hypothesis, two new publications seemed to exonerate aspirin. First, researchers, in a study too small to be definitive, suggested amino acids differed between children with Reye's syndrome and those with salicylate intoxication differed.[56] Another report claimed mitochondrial enzymes differed.[57]

In 1977, CDC suggested that while aspirin "may not be an important contributor," only a case-control study could definitively answer that question.[58] Curiously, cases now averaged 11 years of age. The average time from the beginning of the antecedent illness to vomiting was 4.1 days and time to hospitalization was 5.7 days, numbers almost identical to those for the Arizona children, which were 4.4 days and 5.9 days respectively.

FDA focuses on drugs including aspirin

Ted Mortimer was likely behind the first trace of an idea that eliminating aspirin use in children might eliminate Reye's syndrome. In April 1974, a year after the Freudenbergers' daughter Tifinni died, representatives of the FDA and the prestigious AAP Redbook Committee, including Mortimer, reviewed information on Reye's syndrome gathered that winter during the influenza B outbreak and issued this statement: "Particular attention should be paid to exposure to toxic substances or drugs such as ASA [aspirin]." The statement was published in the AAP's newsletter, *News and Comment,*[59] and in a statement by the AAP Redbook Committee in *Pediatrics* in January 1975.[60]

In January 1976, the FDA again called upon experts. The Bureau of Drugs convened a Neurologic Drugs Advisory Committee Panel on Reye's syndrome to focus on phenothiazines.

Sydney Gellis presided. Two documents summarized the meeting. The minutes reported that 28 committee members, consultants, and FDA staff attended the meeting including aspirin experts Alan Done and Sumner Yaffe and pediatrician John Partin.[61] A lawyer stated that a study had shown a "highly statistical relationship" between Reye's syndrome and phenothiazines. A doctor reported a study of 38 children with Reye's syndrome between 1958 and 1968 that he had conducted under contract with the FDA. After having "problems finding an appropriate control group," he reported medication use in cases: only 68% used phenothiazines, 34% aspirin, and 42% penicillin. CDC's Lawrence Corey noted that 51% of children with Reye's syndrome had used phenothiazines and 78% had used aspirin. Someone mentioned the Cincinnati data indicating that almost 100% of the children had used aspirin. The discussion drifted to aspirin. A pediatric pharmacologist pointed out that aspirin could form toxic metabolites and individuals varied in the ability to metabolize the drug. (Bingo!) One aspirin expert at the meeting expressed surprise that "aspirin was present in such high [blood] concentrations." (Bingo #2) A Reye's syndrome expert offered the opinion that, since there was evidence to indicate that Reye's syndrome was a disease of the mitochondria, one "should not give affected children aspirin." (Bingo #3) The discussion then continued like waves upon the shore progressing and receding as the committee's focus shifted back and forth to the role of phenothiazines and tried to make sense of observations which could not be anchored to any probability without a comparative study. The second document signed by Sydney Gellis recommended changes to package inserts for phenothiazines (another meeting on this topic was held later[62]) and suggested for the Committee's consideration "the importance of notification of physicians that salicylates and acetaminophen are potential hepatotoxins and should be avoided in children whose symptoms and signs may suggest early Reye syndrome or other hepatic disorders. Tepid water sponging is a safe, effective alternative."[63]

Twelve months later in December 1976 an article was published in the FDA *Drug Bulletin*, "Reye's Syndrome: Etiology Uncertain But Avoid Antiemetics in Children." The article explained that the committee had concluded that evidence was "insufficient to show that anti-emetics (drugs to treat vomiting), aspirin, and acetaminophen are clearly causally related to RS, although this possibility cannot be eliminated." It recommended against the use of antiemetics, aspirin, and acetaminophen in children whose symptoms suggest Reye's syndrome because they might adversely affect the course of the disease.[64] It contained no statement about the hepatotoxicity of salicylates or acetaminophen.

By the summer of 1979, I had completed the case-control study and was wrestling with safety concerns uncovered in my reading.

PART IV

BUILDING A CASE
1979–1980

Chapter 14

The Telltale Tiny Fat Drops, September 1979

When we meet a fact, which contradicts a prevailing theory,
we must accept the fact and abandon the theory, even when the theory
is supported by great names and generally accepted.

Claude Bernard, *An Introduction to the Study of Experimental Medicine*, 1865

Public health and personal concerns seemed to multiply during the summer of 1979. My mother-in-law Beth Pinkston was dying of cancer in Prescott, and we visited often. The retired radiologist had practiced prior to stringent radiation standards. Concurrently, over 1800 people were reporting illnesses after camping in western Arizona. I travelled there with a team and determined the source was water connected to an irrigation system. Hepatitis was occurring at daycare centers. A girl acquired plague above the Mogollon rim. Colorado River rafters became ill. Staph broke out in a nursing home. And, most important, as always, was my infant, my husband, and dinner.

With George Ray's encouragement, I drafted a manuscript describing the case-control study and the information I had found on aspirin. I included as co-authors staff of the Arizona Department of Health Services who had assisted in the investigation: Lee Dominguez, who had conducted the interviews with me; Dora Woodall, who had handled the virus work; and serology specialist Warren Stromberg. I asked George Ray to be a co-author.[1] I decided I would submit the report to *The Lancet* where Reye had published his 1963 report. In mid-September I mailed the draft to CDC for formal review.[2] CDC's scientists and editors and then the journal's editor and its independent reviewers would critique the manuscript. I was confident they would find any major and potentially embarrassing flaws. That week researchers in the Viral Disease Division eliminated one of the

153

proposed causes of Reye's syndrome, the mold aflatoxin. A case-control study showed no connection between the two.[3]

I had by now uncovered evidence that dispelled the first four assumptions used to dismiss aspirin as a cause of Reye's syndrome (as summarized in Chapter 11). Two were left. Did salicylate produce fatty degeneration of the liver? Was the FDA overseeing aspirin?

Do salicylates affect the liver?

I first tackled the question of fatty degeneration. During the 1940s and 50s researchers had found indicators of liver damage such as changes in prothrombin [4] and liver enzymes during salicylate use.[5,6] In 1960, in the prestigious journal *Nature*, scientists at King's College Hospital reported that rabbits fed salicylates developed marked increases in liver enzymes at salicylate blood levels above 30 mg/dL and two of six rabbits had cloudy swelling and fatty infiltration of the liver. At the time it was known that cloudy swelling of organs and cells, the result of "imbibition [taking in] of water," commonly precedes fatty degeneration.[7]

Pediatricians began routinely using liver tests during the 1960s[8] and had reported case after case of liver damage during aspirin treatment of rheumatic diseases.[9,10,11] In 1974, Hyman Zimmerman of the Veterans Administration Hospital in Washington, D.C. suggested that problematic doses generally ranged from 3 to 5 grams per day [50–83 mg/kg/day for a 60-kg adult].[12] Astonishingly, this amount was being recommended for children.

The author of a 1974 editorial in *The Lancet*, who seemed to be unaware of accumulation with small doses, wrote that "no evidence exists that much smaller doses of salicylates [blood levels smaller than 25 mg/dL] such as are commonly taken for minor symptoms in the form of aspirin have a serious effect on the liver."[13] The absence of evidence, however, is not evidence of absence. Researchers soon filled the void.[14,15,16,17,18,19,20,21,22] Aspirin indeed could affect the liver after only a few days of therapy at levels less than 25 mg/dL and a general dose-response relationship existed. The good news was that once aspirin therapy was discontinued the liver damage subsided and, interestingly, the elevated levels of liver enzymes could return to normal even if aspirin use was continued.[23] This was explained by the 1977 observation that metabolism of salicylate increases with continuous aspirin use.[24, 25] Curiously, in 1977 an expert panel commissioned by the FDA for unstated reasons decided that a warning about the liver changes was "not warranted."[26] If doctors were not aware of aspirin's effect on the liver, would they even consider it as a cause of Reye's syndrome?

Do salicylates cause fatty degeneration?

The heart of the matter seemed to be determining if salicylate can induce fatty degeneration. If it did, weren't Reye's syndrome and salicylate poisoning identical? I quickly learned that pathologists use several terms to describe fat in cells. Fatty infiltration and fatty metamorphosis mean fat drops of any size. Fatty degeneration describes small fat drops. Special stains are needed to see fatty degeneration, and many pathologists seemed satisfied simply using the more general terms. Precision is critical here because fatty infiltration/metamorphosis is relatively common; fatty degeneration is rare.

Cincinnati experts Bove, McAdams, Partin, Partin, Hug, and Schubert had described an extremely important, and not generally appreciated, phenomenon. *Early on the characteristic lesion of Reye's syndrome—fatty degeneration—was almost impossible to see in a liver biopsy unless liver tissue is prepared in a very specific way.* They called it "masking of lipid." Without a fat stain the cells would at first appear almost normal and then become foamy with vacuoles (microvesicles which appeared like holes) "... *despite existence of abundant lipid [with fat stain].*"[27]

Notwithstanding a wide variety of staining practices, physicians had already reported fatty degeneration in association with both methyl salicylate and salicylate poisoning. In 1937, for example, Melbourne physicians Stanley W. Williams and Rona M. Panting of the Children's Hospital described reports of "fatty degeneration" from France and

Scotland.[28] One 10-year-old child had received five days of treatment and at autopsy had "fatty degeneration of the liver."[29] In 1948, Yale's Gross and Greenburg listed nine references in the French, German, and American literature citing reports of fatty degeneration with salicylate use.[30]

Most reports involved the deadly methyl salicylate used in the popular rubbing liniment oil of wintergreen. As far back as 1926, physicians performing autopsies of children who had died of poisoning by methyl salicylate had found fatty degeneration.[31,32,33,34] In fact, a physician at Johns Hopkins *found 30% of 13 cases had fatty degeneration of liver cells.*[35] In 1943, 76 cases of methyl salicylate poisoning were reported in the *New England Journal of Medicine* where the pathology findings included swelling and fatty degeneration of the liver.[36]

Reports of fatty degeneration, specifically with aspirin, had begun to appear before Reye's report. In 1945, physicians Mary Maher Troll and Maud L. Menten of the University of Pittsburgh and the Children's Hospital of Pittsburgh reported autopsies of a two-and-a-half-year-old and an 11-year-old (one suffering a cold, the other rheumatic disease) who had received aspirin. Hepatitis was described in one and fatty degeneration of the liver and kidneys in the other.[37] In the late 1940s, doctors at the Jewish Hospital in Philadelphia reported autopsies of a five-month-old and a 54-year-old.[38,39] The liver of each showed hydropic (swelling) degeneration and that of the adult also showed fatty degeneration. In 1959, swelling of the lungs and fatty metamorphosis of the liver of the small droplet type was noted in a nine-month-old who had been given aspirin.[40] Finally, Mortimer and Lepow's 1962 report described brain swelling and "marked" fatty degeneration of the liver, which they associated with aspirin use.

Two years after Reye's report in *Poisoning, Diagnosis and Treatment*, physician and professor at the University of Zurich, Sven Moeschlin, wrote that in salicylate poisoning the "parenchymatous organs [liver, kidney, heart] revealed cloudy swelling and fatty degeneration."[41] The 1969 edition of *Diseases of the Liver* edited by Cincinnati physician Leon Schiff noted that "among the chief causes of such fatty metamorphosis in early life … certain poisonings, notably aspirin and carbon tetrachloride."[42] In 1969 and 1970 respectively, while neither mentioned fatty degeneration specifically, Sterling Drug' Tainter [43] and Yale's Goodman and Gilman's pharmacology text[44] reported "fatty infiltration" could occur in severe salicylate intoxication. Others noted findings such as mild inflammation or a problem with the liver cells, which was variously described with artistic words such as lobular disarray, smudged cells, or ballooning.[45] A few other reports did note fat, but the descriptions were vague.[46,47]

The presence of fatty degeneration during aspirin poisoning seemed like an open-and-shut case, but there was one problem. These reports conflicted with the conclusion of the Cincinnati experts who had stated that Reye's syndrome and salicylate poisoning could be differentiated with a liver biopsy. What was going on?

Experts waffle

During the 1970s, pediatricians at the Children's Hospital Medical Center (CHMC) in Cincinnati had risen to the pinnacle of expertise of Reye's syndrome pathology. CHMC has a stellar reputation. Its forerunner the Children's Hospital Research Foundation (CHRF) had been incorporated in 1883 by citizens who wanted a place for sick children. Albert Sabin developed the oral polio vaccine there. In 1962 the NIH had encouraged the institution to establish a new Clinical Research Center. The tradition of CHMC was that no child would be allowed to die without an explanation.[48]

The CHMC doctors were recognized as *the* experts on the liver pathology of Reye's syndrome after they published the first electron micrographs of liver cells of children with Reye's syndrome in 1971. In 2011, John and Jacqueline Partin told me that in the mid-1960s, William Schubert, director of the research center, and pathologist-in-chief A. James McAdams, had become excited about the new field of electron microscopy and sent young pediatrician John Partin to Johns Hopkins as a post-doctoral fellow in cell biology. When he returned, he began seeing children with unexplained encephalopathy, "some with elevated aspirin levels," he recalled. It was "natural for us to establish a more accurate diagnosis." Research assistant Jacqueline Partin, Partin's wife, developed expertise in the tissue preparation.

As soon as the Partins examined liver tissue from children with Reye's syndrome, they saw that something was very wrong with the mitochondria. The implication of this finding was enormous because mitochondria perform vital metabolic functions, including conversion of the energy in food to ATP. The Cincinnati investigators concluded that pathways involved in the generation of ATP might explain observations in Reye's syndrome.[49] Others found decreased activity of mitochondrial enzymes in children with Reye's syndrome.[50] The Partins later described Reye's syndrome as "a terrible disease affecting picture perfect children in a ravaging and uncontrollable storm of disordered cell function" and that the lack of information had left them "deeply frustrated." (In 2001 experts in toxicology and cell biology Lawrence Trost and John Lemasters of the University of North Carolina at Chapel Hill wrote, "it is now widely accepted that most, if not all, metabolic alterations in Reye's syndrome reflect a primary mitochondrial injury."[51])

Beginning in 1971, Cincinnati researchers wrote a series of reports with excellent descriptions of liver tissue visualized with both the standard light microscope and the new electron microscope. Their first paper followed the brief report by researchers who had observed changes in mitochondria in Thailand[52] and was published in the *New England Journal of Medicine*.[53] Partin, Partin, and Schubert examined liver tissue from 10 consecutive children with Reye's syndrome, at three different time points during the illness. They concluded that liver cells were universally affected by a process that results in mitochondrial swelling and "small droplet" fat accumulation. Four stunning photographs called electron micrographs (EMs) of liver cells greatly magnified revealed multitudes of massively swollen and misshapen mitochondria inside every cell.

The swollen mitochondria took on bizarre shapes like amoebas, as shown in Figure 14.1. The matrix, the material inside the mitochondria,

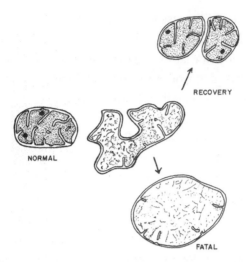

Figure 14.1 Schematic Representation of Liver Cell Mitochondria in Reye's
syndrome
From *New England Journal of Medicine*, Partin J.C., Schubert W.K., Partin J.S.
Mitochondrial ultrastructure in Reye's syndrome (Encephalopathy and
fatty degeneration of the liver), Vol. 285, p. 1339.
Copyright © 1971 Massachusetts Medical Society.
Reprinted with permission from Massachusetts Medical Society.

was greatly expanded. The researchers also saw changes in other
organelles,* and varying degrees of depletion of glycogen (the storage
form of glucose). As the electron microscope became more available
through the 1970s, others documented similar findings.[54,55,56,57] Of great
interest was that the abnormal mitochondria improved quickly, within
days, and returned to normal in those who survived as though they
had been attacked and recovered. Partin and colleagues concluded that
the injury in Reye's syndrome was *chemically mediated and potentially
reversible.*[58]

The electron microscope was a research tool and not widely available
so it could not generally be used for diagnostic purposes. I could not

---

* Changes were seen in other organelles involved in metabolism, including a
proliferating endoplasmic reticulum (structures in the cytoplasm involved
in the synthesis of proteins or the metabolism of fats) as well as increased
microbodies (an organelle that performs many metabolic functions).

find a single EM of liver tissue from a child or adult with salicylate poisoning. I did find a just-published report by researchers from Utah and Seattle who found that increasing amounts of salicylate placed on rat liver cells resulted in worsening liver cell function, and that the cells exposed to a level of 40 mg/dL examined under an electron micrograph had "mitochondrial swelling, disruption of the inner mitochondrial membrane, loss of mitochondrial cristae, vacuolization, and lipid [fat] accumulation."[59] The findings resembled those described by Partin and colleagues. (Later I found a 1976 report from Tel Aviv University describing mitochondrial injury in a child treated with aspirin therapy for rheumatoid arthritis with a "safe" salicylate level.[60])

In 1972, Schubert, Partin, and Partin reported that EMs of liver cells of children with Reye's syndrome differed from those of other illnesses including lack of oxygen, iron deficiency, partial starvation, protein deficiency, intoxication with aflatoxin and several others. This supported Huttenlocher's conclusion that Reye's syndrome was a unique and specific condition.[61] Salicylate poisoning was not mentioned.

They also examined brain cells with the electron microscope and observed the cells were even more swollen than generally seen with lack of oxygen.[62] There, too, mitochondria inside the neurons were "universally injured."[63] No fat accumulation was seen, which was not surprising because the brain gets most of its energy from glucose, not fat. Partin and colleagues suggested the damage observed with Reye's syndrome also differed from that in cases of liver encephalopathy or experimental ammonia intoxication.[64]

Sometime during the 1970s, the Cincinnati researchers noticed that most of 30 consecutive children with Reye's syndrome seen at their hospital between late 1963 and early 1972 (about half of whom had died or suffered severe brain damage) had salicylate in the blood but only nine had levels greater than 20 mg/dL.[65] They began to speculate on the role of aspirin, and here is where things became cloudy.

First, in a 1973 abstract in *Gastroenterology*, Partin, Partin, and Schubert *declared* that salicylism (and several other conditions) were "clearly distinguishable" from Reye's syndrome by complete analysis of a liver biopsy.[66] Soon after, they began to waffle. For example, in 1975 Schubert wrote in an editorial in the *Journal of Pediatrics* that "some" cases of salicylate intoxication were "distinctly different" from Reye's syndrome by both light and electron microscopy and that these were of the "large-droplet type." The reference for this statement was the 1973 abstract. [67]

In 1974, at the first national conference on Reye's syndrome in Columbus, Cincinnati's Kevin Bove talked about Reye's syndrome. Bove was a card-carrying pathologist having received certification by the American Board of Pathology in Anatomic and Clinical Pathology.[68] Bove reported that "some" children with salicylate intoxication did indeed have fat in the liver (two of five studied as well as "five of seven in whom salicylate contributed to a fatal outcome"). He stated that the "pattern" differed from that in Reye's syndrome. [69] Bove hypothesized that "high levels of salicylate may aggravate … RS without being instrumental in its causation." At the same time, like Reye, he noted that only three other conditions were known to cause "severe diffuse fatty metamorphosis of the microvesicular type."[70] In 1975, in an editorial in the *Journal of Pediatrics*, Schubert recommended a liver biopsy be done in order to make an accurate diagnosis specifically noting that salicylate intoxication could be differentiated by its "large droplet" fat.[71] Once again, his reference for this statement was the 1973 Partin abstract, which had given no specific data.

The mixed messages surrounding the presence or absence and character (large or small drops) of fat in the liver in salicylate poisoning likely stemmed from several facts. First, liver biopsies were generally not done for any reason in children before the 1960s.[72] Also, as Schubert told me later, biopsies were rarely done when they knew the diagnosis. By 1975, the Cincinnati researchers seemed to have reported only one child with a high salicylate level and that child, they said, did not have the mitochondrial lesion of Reye's syndrome.[73]

Notwithstanding this lack of clarity around the pathology of salicylate poisoning, by the mid-1970s, academic physicians in

Cincinnati and St Louis advised in medical journals that the pathology of Reye's syndrome could be differentiated by examination of a liver biopsy.[74,75] Later, Boston academic Frederick Lovejoy told me that at the time he had believed this.

Reconciling the old reports stating that salicylate poisoning could be accompanied by fatty degeneration and the opposite opinion of the experts seemed impossible. Lipid stains were needed. The experts had written "precise diagnosis requires lipid stains that usually cannot be obtained from stored tissues."[76] In other words, tissue had to be fresh or frozen. Where could I find liver tissue from a child with salicylate poisoning? I was stuck.

Enter the frozen collection of the Armed Forces Institute of Pathology

I contacted Lyle Conrad, Director of the Field Services Division, my boss in Atlanta. I pictured him with his thick glasses, hair askew, leaning back in his worn leather chair behind his huge desk piled high with papers. "Lyle, the missing piece. I only have case reports from the literature. Without more evidence, the Arizona study won't carry much weight on its own."

Lyle thought awhile and replied, "You might want to call the Armed Forces Institute of Pathology (AFIP) in Washington, D.C. They keep specimens from all sorts of diseases."

"AFIP?" I had never heard of it. "Really?" I asked both skeptically and hopefully. I had exhausted all options. Why not give it a try?

The AFIP, I imagined, would be a non-descript federal building housing jars of organs and freezers filled with tissues. There would be banks of file cabinets stuffed with documentation of the circumstances leading to the tissue owner's current location. This was a last-ditch effort. The AFIP, in fact, a triple service agency in the Department of Defense, had been collecting specimens since its inception in 1862. Its tissue repository, which contained over three million specimens, was considered a "national treasure."[77]

Using a directory of federal offices, I located the AFIP Department of Drug-induced and Environmental Pathology and on 19 September 1979 dialed the phone number of the department chairperson. To my surprise, the chairman himself, Dr Nelson Irey, answered. I told him what I was looking for. "We might have some specimens from children with aspirin/salicylate poisoning," he told me. "I'll let you know."

Just five days later Irey sent me a letter. When I saw the return address—Armed Forces Institute of Pathology—on the envelope, I ripped it open and unfolded the paper inside. Words, phrases jumped off the page: "in all 11 cases ... the livers showed microscopically fatty changes in the form of small cytoplasmic fat vesicles."

In other words, the children with salicylate poisoning at the AFIP had fatty degeneration. Over the years many researchers believed that Reye's syndrome was some sort of intoxication. I was now convinced that toxin was aspirin.

The AFIP had 13 reports of children with salicylate intoxication in its files: four were the result of accidental ingestions; eight occurred during therapy; and one was both. The majority had been treated with aspirin. This seemed to be the largest group of children with salicylate poisoning ever autopsied and collected. Being a "case series," it added evidence to the case reports. Upon detailed review, all had salicylate levels that ranged from 30–120 mg/dL. Ten had microvesicles in the liver cells. All six liver biopsies stained for fat *were positive*. Other findings included cerebral edema, pulmonary edema and congestion, and bronchopneumonia.

The AFIP data gave me a reason to push for early release of the Arizona case-control study results. To that end, on 28 September 1979, I submitted a summary abstract for consideration for presentation at the Late Breaker session of the Epidemiology Exchange of the American Public Health (APHA) meeting in New York City in November 1979.[78] Health professionals from around the country would be attending. The abstract concluded:

> It is postulated that salicylate, operating in a dose-dependent manner, possibly potentiated by fever, represents a primary etiologic agent in Reye's syndrome.

I was suggesting that aspirin was the direct cause of Reye's syndrome. The words of June Aprille, a young researcher at the Shriners' Burns Institute at Massachusetts General Hospital and the Harvard Medical School encouraged me. She had done sophisticated work with mitochondria and the blood of children with Reye's syndrome and had suggested a role for salicylates, "any factor may be synergistically important … salicylates may have such a role." [79]

The Presiding Officer of the late breaker session, physician Michael Gregg, now Deputy Director of CDC's Bureau of Epidemiology and editor of CDC's *Morbidity and Mortality Weekly Report* (MMWR), received my abstract. He had been Director of the Viral Diseases Division from 1967 to 1976, during which time he had overseen Reye's syndrome activities, including the reports that aspirin was not involved.[80,81] In 1977, Gregg, along with other CDC investigators, had explored the aspirin question in 379 cases of Reye's syndrome reported to the CDC in the mid-1970s. They had found that aspirin had been given to 78% of the 175 cases for whom this information was recorded. They speculated that more might have taken aspirin but, in the end, they concluded that aspirin "may not be an important contributor" and only a comparison study will further "elucidate the role of salicylates." [82] The Arizona study was a comparison study. I was certain Gregg would be interested.

On 8 October, Gregg replied. My presentation would not be accommodated.[83]

I was stunned, but not enough to pull back the draft manuscript which was in CDC's hands. In it the highly probable link was accompanied by an explanation of how differentiating between salicylate poisoning and Reye's syndrome is difficult and a recommendation that the pharmacokinetics of aspirin in children be investigated. The manuscript had a red flag statement, one that likely generated both great concern and incredulity: "[T]he amount of salicylate taken by these children is not in the dose range generally considered to be toxic."

The implication was that commonly used doses were causing Reye's syndrome. In other words, the most frequently used medication for children, the one doctors and parents embraced for over half a century as a comfortable household remedy, could also be—at the usual doses—a deadly poison.

In September Senator John Melcher of Montana had entered the Reye's Syndrome Act of 1979 (S.1794) into the Congressional record and asked the CDC and NIH to prepare a full report on Reye's syndrome.[84] One investigator estimated the annual cost of acute care for children with Reye's syndrome to be between $25 and $37 million. The Act would mainly establish up to three research centers and provide funding for a three-year program of grants and studies for the illness. Representative Geraldine Ferraro of New York introduced a similar Bill in the House. Dr Wallace Berman, Chairman of a Multi-Center Study Research Group supported by the NRSF (Michigan), immediately wrote to Vander Jagt concerned the Act would direct funding away from the collaborative study he was spearheading.[85] Berman's group had plans for a meeting in Columbus in October and representatives from 14 children's hospitals or major medical hospitals had agreed to participate.[86] At the same time, the Ohio foundation, now with 48 chapters in 21 states and Canada, continued to keenly focus on spreading the word about the syndrome and announced new chapters in 10 areas.[87] In November, *Family Circle*, a popular family magazine, featured an article that proposed three theories regarding the origin of Reye's syndrome: an allergic response to a virus, a genetic metabolism disorder, and an environmental trigger. Aspirin was not mentioned.[88]

Meanwhile, advertisements continued to encourage mothers to use aspirin. Sterling's ad for Bayer Children's Aspirin in *Good Housekeeping* recommended its product "when mother has to be the 'doctor'." [89] The ad was ironically reminiscent of the Congressional testimony in the 1960s that had blamed mothers for toddler aspirin ingestions.

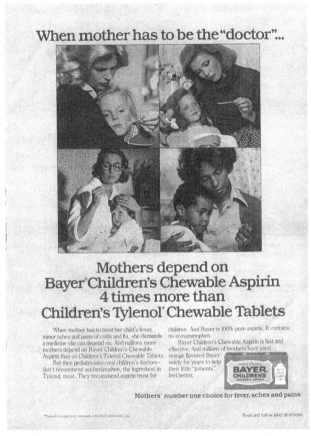

Advertisement, *Good Housekeeping*, March 1980[90]
Courtesy of Bayer AG, Leverkusen, Germany

Approximately one child was dying of Reye's syndrome every day. The pressure of the unknown had been disconcerting. The pressure of knowing was worse. The only relief would be publication.

Chapter 15

Now What?

The mind likes a strange idea as little as the body likes a strange protein
and resists it with similar energy …
If we watch ourselves honestly, we shall often find that we have begun to
argue against a new idea even before it has been completely stated.
Wilfred Trotter, *The Collected Papers of Wilfred Trotter, FRS*, 1941

I needed CDC's approval to publish the Arizona case-control study. The general feeling at CDC was that while the idea was intriguing, the data were limited, and conclusions difficult to draw.[1] Schonberger felt if the results were to be accepted, they would have to be supported or refuted. That meant that others would have to replicate the findings by collecting data, analyzing it, and subjecting the new data to scientific scrutiny. At the time, aspirin was on the verge of a rebirth. Researchers were conducting large studies to determine its benefit in preventing the primary killer of adults in the United States—heart attacks. Sterling Drug was planning an application to the FDA to allow it to market aspirin for the prevention of second heart attacks. The dose needed would be a small fraction of the amount being used for aches, pains, and fever in children. One dose later suggested for prevention of heart disease was 2.7 mg/kg/day.[2] (Appendix 1)

Research groups studying Reye's syndrome were naturally focusing on their areas of expertise. The chairman of the scientific board of the NRSF of Ohio, a basic scientist, was interested mainly in biologic mechanisms, and the chairman of the multi-center treatment trial, a clinician, was focused on treatment. Two recent well-attended medical conferences on Reye's syndrome—one at Ohio State in 1974 and the other in Halifax, Nova Scotia, in 1978—barely mentioned aspirin. Surely all of this was on the minds of the CDC reviewers as the draft Arizona manuscript circulated for review.

While the iconic status of aspirin likely helped fuel skepticism about the Arizona study, other factors may have been playing out as well. CDC had just experienced a major public humiliation that may have left some wary. In 1976, fearing a swine flu pandemic comparable to that of the deadly 1918 Spanish influenza, CDC had recommended mass vaccination for the entire country. But when the swine flu did not materialize, and the vaccine was linked to Guillain-Barré syndrome, a terrifying ascending paralysis that works its way up to the respiratory muscles, CDC was chastened. CDC's director, David Sencer, a man greatly admired and respected, had lost his job. Schonberger had completed the critical assessment that linked Guillain-Barré with the influenza vaccine.[3] He had watched some of the best people at CDC struggle with questions of how to act and when.

Public health decisions always rest on a knife-edge of time—too slow and people might die, too fast and people might die. The trick is to use the right amount of data to make the right decision at the "right" time. And that is never easy.

Finally, unspoken differences in the status of EIS officers may have influenced CDC staff. Simply put, there were two classes of officers—house officers and field officers—and the investigations by house officers were thought by some to be better. After all, house officers had easy access to resources and worked under the eyes of experienced supervisors. The Arizona study had been conducted by a field officer. During the 1960s, George Johnson who had conducted the first investigation had mused, "I drove through the mountains to Charlotte, North Carolina, wondering all the while if my investigation could measure up to those of the confident Ivy League men in the choice surveillance section jobs in Atlanta."[4]

The tension between headquarters and the field was collegial yet real. When I spoke with J. Lyle Conrad in 2011, he explained that Alexander Langmuir, the creator of the EIS, had been a field guy. During the 1960s when the CDC received a large grant to study measles, Langmuir wanted to create a Field Services Division, just like the other five divisions: Bacterial Disease, Viral Disease, Parasite

Disease, a field office in Kansas City, and Chronic Diseases. Langmuir got 20 extra EIS positions and asked Conrad to start recruiting staff. When only 10 had signed up, Conrad went to Washington to cull prospective field officers from a list of interested applicants saying, "Call them ... offer them Arkansas ... offer them Colorado." The push succeeded. The EIS Class of 1966 had 20 "field officers."

When Langmuir retired in 1970, anthrax expert Phil Brachman took over as Director of the Bureau of Epidemiology, a position he held until 1981. The Bureau of Epidemiology oversaw all the divisions. According to Conrad, for the first three or four years of Brachman's tenure, his philosophy was clear. Field officers only investigated "outbreaks;" house officers investigated real "epidemics" and field investigations did not even make it into the Bureau's summary reports. As far as Conrad could see though, house officers spent a lot of time writing. Conrad's point was the men and women in the "house" were investigating a hundred "epidemics' and those in the field were doing 1000 "outbreaks" a year (he tallied the outbreaks from monthly reports). Luckily, according to Conrad, Joe Giordano, Brachman's deputy, came to his assistance saying, "[T]hose officers in the field ... It's all part of the same problem. They're not different. They're in fact better."

Despite this collegial banter, the reality was that the work environment and the opportunities *were* different. The house concentrated expertise in one or several areas and the field offered broad experience. House officers had immediate access to experts, statisticians, laboratories, and libraries and could easily dive deeply into the heart of a problem. Field officers, on the other hand, had the advantage of being unconstrained by preconceived ideas but had to fend for themselves. Both are needed when facing a deadly illness.

In October 1979, I attended the National Institute of Occupational Safety and Health course in Atlanta and gave Schonberger and Gene Hurwitz, the EIS officer working on the Ohio case-control study, the questionnaire from the Arizona study.[5] I returned to Arizona to find an ever-growing list of bread-and-butter public health projects— meningitis, *Giardia* (a type of parasite) infections in a day care center, and a mobile home park built on the former site of an asbestos-processing factory. I discussed hepatitis control in Yavapai County, helped plan a day care center workshop, and made plans for a study of pelvic inflammatory disease.

I asked to present the Arizona study at the 1980 EIS Conference, a public meeting held in Atlanta at CDC each year in April. Somehow Ted Mortimer learned about the Arizona study and wrote to me that he was bothered by the possible interaction with a virus yet felt the idea was "intriguing and worthy of further pursuit."[6] I began a collaboration with the AFIP to formally study the tissues of the children with salicylate poisoning with the goal of publishing the findings.

In November, CDC Director William H. Foege, responding to a communication from Michigan Congressman Guy Vander Jagt, wrote that CDC was working to improve its surveillance system. From 1977 through May 1979, the agency had received 792 reports related to Reye's syndrome, including 70 from Michigan since 1 January. Foege told Vander Jagt that CDC was available to work with his state.[7] By December, the study team in Ohio had almost completed a year of enrollment. It modified its questionnaire to better clarify the role of medicines given during the prodromal stage—a sign that Schonberger's team was becoming serious about the possibility that Reye's was linked to a pharmacologic toxin. Around the same time, I received word that CDC had approved the manuscript and immediately mailed it to *The Lancet* for consideration.

On 1 January 1980, I noticed an obituary in the *Arizona Republic*. It read "Brenda Dee Moore Newman, 13, who came here in 1970 from Wisconsin and was an eighth-grade student at Arroyo Elementary School, died of an illness on December 29, 1979 in Good Samaritan Hospital."[8] Within days, I received the official report of Newman's death: Reye's syndrome. My heart sank. Newman's death shook me.

I quickly drafted a new protocol for an evaluation of future Reye's syndrome cases in Arizona, narrowly focusing on the relationship between the salicylate dose, the serum level, and the severity of Reye's syndrome. On 4 January 1980, I sent the protocol to pediatricians at the three large Arizona hospitals likely to see cases.[9] Each agreed to measure salicylate levels for new patients with Reye's syndrome. In addition, staff at Maricopa County Hospital and Tucson Medical Center agreed to report cases. Salicylate was soon found in the blood of every child with Reye's in Arizona. The last dose of aspirin for the first three new cases had been two-to-four days before.

On 17 January 1980, I called the FDA to get more information about aspirin and was referred to Charma Konner in the Over-the-Counter (OTC) Division. She explained to me that the FDA had commissioned a draft report of proposed rules for aspirin. It was dated 1977 and covered internal analgesics, antipyretics, and antirheumatic products. It was the first time I heard about this monograph. She promised to send it.

CDC was meeting roadblocks. In late February 1980, EIS Officer Cornelia Davis, who was in Schonberger's branch, complained that while CDC had asked 400 hospitals for information on Reye's syndrome, only a third had replied. Three states had reported most of the cases: Ohio 100, Michigan 22, and Minnesota eight. Ohio and Michigan were the states where the parent advocacy groups were the most organized.[10] Davis told *Science* reporter Gina Kolata that the CDC's best incidence estimates were one to two cases per 100,000 children under 18 years, but that only 16 states then had laws making Reye's syndrome reportable. CDC, she said, had no promising leads.[11]

Schonberger had now begun to uncover data casting doubt on the connection with aspirin. It was natural to look for disconfirming evidence and there seemed to be plenty of that around. In mid-February he sent me drafts of two reports. A CDC officer found no aspirin ingestion for three cases of Reye's syndrome in Tennessee. According to Schonberger, the officer who had investigated the cases was "absolutely convinced" no aspirin had been available to these children. Another investigation of 36 cases in 1971 had found salicylate use in 29 cases.[12]

In late February I again received crushing news. The editor of *The Lancet* had decided not to publish the Arizona study report.[13] My sense of urgency increased. I sent the manuscript to Jerold Lucey, editor of

Pediatrics, the journal of the American Academy of Pediatrics (AAP). The same month the NIH finalized a report on Reye's syndrome activities for the Senate Appropriations Committee. The committee, at the urging of the Michigan foundation, had asked for a list of all activities funded by each Institute, recommendations for research, and suggestions for increasing public awareness. [14] The NIH reported that, during 1979, NIH funds for Reye's syndrome spread across many departments totaled almost $10 million. The NIH experts had concluded that Reye's syndrome was a "severe toxic disorder ... with ... no clear understanding of the pathogenesis or etiology." CDC reported spending $65,000 on Reye's syndrome during the four years prior to September 1979 in addition to $176,570 for the Ohio study and a study on aflatoxin. [15]

Funds however were not the only problem. Rather, as John Dieckman had realized, no single group was dedicated to Reye's syndrome. It was an orphan condition, a side project. Dieckman was right to press for more. And the worrisome headlines kept coming.

Schools for 12,000 Shut in Michigan Due to Flu
("and a related disease called Reye's syndrome")
Associated Press, 25 February 1980 [16]

Reye's Syndrome Stalking Children Again but
Death Rate is Lower,
Arizona Republic, 28 February 1980 [17]

15 in State Struck by Reye's Syndrome Since January 1,
New York Times, 2 March 1980 [18]

In March the perplexing findings of EIS officer John Sullivan-Bolyai and colleagues were published. [19] Of 54 children less than one-year-old with Reye's syndrome, more than 48% were black compared with older children of whom 8% were black. Also, the majority were males. Reye's syndrome was now being reported in older children and adults as well. [20] [21] University of New Mexico School of Medicine researchers reported two fatalities in adults with proven influenza. [22] The researchers reviewed 30 fatal encephalopathy cases with proven influenza and found that most of the cases had brain edema and more than half had evidence of liver dysfunction or fatty degeneration. They suggested that cases diagnosed as influenza encephalopathy might indeed be Reye's syndrome, thus raising the idea that many cases of Reye's syndrome might never have been diagnosed at all.

The March/April issue of *Forensic Science International* carried the first report of Reye's syndrome in Denmark.[23] The four-year-old girl had been on long-term salicylate therapy for rheumatoid arthritis when she died after a trivial infection. The authors noted that several cases of Reye's syndrome had been reported in children on salicylate therapy with rheumatoid arthritis and that "the literature gave [this connection] little credit." The high rate of Reye's syndrome in children on long-term aspirin therapy was begging for attention.

Around the same time, Cincinnati's William Schubert was concerned. Since the second week in December 40 children with Reye's syndrome had been admitted to his hospital.[24] Most had vomiting and liver damage *without* neurologic signs, again suggesting the occurrence of many more cases than had previously been suspected. CDC did not count these cases because its case definition required brain dysfunction. Schubert concluded that the number of cases depended on how hard you looked for them.

On 11 March 1980, Ray Hime gave another heartfelt presentation to parents in Silver Bell. The age of children with Reye's had risen dramatically. The median age was now 11 years with most children in the 12 to 15-year-old age group. How could the age of the cases have changed? Hime's map of cases reported to the CDC, for the four months prior to 31 March 1980, showed 429 cases. All around the country, parent members of the foundation were giving talks just like his.

Chapter 16

The FDA's 1977 Draft Monograph—*Shh*

[T]he Panel believes that government requirements for inclusion of
warnings and cautionary language are inadequate, particularly as to
possible effects of this advertising upon children.

Over-the-Counter Drugs. Establishment of Monograph for OTC Analgesic,
Antipyretic and Antirheumatic Products, Proposed Rule
Federal Register, 8 July 1977

Charma Konner of FDA's Over-the-Counter Division promptly mailed
the *proposed* monograph to me. The monograph was a "proposal to
establish conditions which over-the-counter (OTC) internal analgesics,
antipyretic and antirheumatic drugs are generally recognized
as safe and effective and not misbranded" based on the panel's
recommendations.[1] Within the hundreds of pages of miniscule print, I
located text showing that the expert panel had issued recommendations
regarding aspirin labels, some of which involved children's dosing.

The FDA had developed the monograph system to address its
new responsibilities for OTC drugs defined in the 1962 Kefauver
amendment. When FDA learned the daunting fact that as many as
500,000 OTC drugs were in existence, it hired the National Academy
of Sciences and the National Research Council to perform preliminary
assessments. These bodies concluded that more than half of all OTC
drugs *did not work at all.*

In 1972 the FDA Commissioner finalized a regulation concerning
its plan to assess the remaining OTC drugs and their labeling.
Independent advisory panels would prepare monographs on 26 classes
of active ingredients. The monographs would serve as guidance for the
FDA and the manufacturers for the categories of safety, effectiveness,

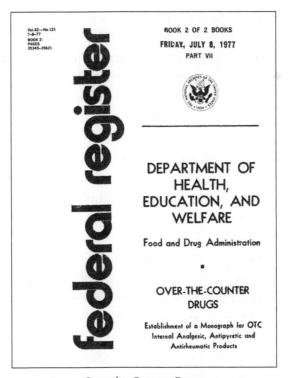

Over-the-Counter Drugs
Establishment of a Monograph for OTC Internal Analgesic,
Antipyretic, and Antirheumatic Products, 1977

and branding.* All 26 monographs were to be completed by 1974—12 years after the Kefauver amendment was passed.

Aspirin fell to the OTC Internal Analgesic and Antirheumatic Ingredients Panel.[2] The Commissioner of the FDA appointed the panel's seven members (the chairman died in 1976 and one member resigned in 1977) leaving five to complete the enormous task. Its task was to evaluate analgesics (pain relievers), antipyretics (fever lowering drugs), and antirheumatic agents. As aspirin was a "grandfather" drug—one

---

* Category I drugs were ingredients and uses generally recognized as safe and effective and were not misbranded; Category II drugs were those that were not generally recognized as safe and effective or were misbranded; and Category III drugs were for conditions for which the available data were insufficient to permit current classification.

marketed before 1938—its manufacturers had had "no obligation to prove it safe or effective. Rather, the burden of proof in a court of law had rested with the FDA."[3] The FDA now adopted the position that it would consider grandfathered drugs misbranded if their manufacturers did not follow the provisions in the *final* monograph.[4] The rulemaking process had three steps: a proposed monograph, a tentative final monograph, and then a final monograph.

The panel first convened in October 1972 and divided the active ingredients into two categories, salicylates and non-salicylates. Forty-one companies submitted data on 50 ingredients in marketed products.* All who requested an appearance before the panel were afforded the opportunity. More than 50 persons appeared. The panel thoroughly reviewed the literature, listened to testimonies, and considered data submitted through 22 November 1976, including submissions from industry such as Bristol-Myers Co., Dow Chemical Company Research Center, McNeil Laboratories, Miles Laboratories, Monsanto Industrial Chemical Company, Plough Inc., and Sterling Drug.

Five years later, in July 1977, the panel completed a detailed report.[5] It contained a litany of concerns about aspirin, its unusual pharmacokinetics, imaginary illnesses such as "file cabinet headache," advertising, and dosing instructions for adults and children.

The draft monograph first focused on claims for use and safety. Some were deemed too ambiguous, such as "jumpy nerves" and "fretfulness."[6] The panel concluded that a general indication statement for analgesics and antipyretics should be: "For the temporary relief of occasional minor aches, pains, and headache, and for the reduction of fever."[7] The panel also recommended that all references to arthritis and rheumatism be relegated to the FDA Category II (not generally recognized as safe or effective or misbranded) and that safety warnings be increased.

---

* Salicylates included aluminum aspirin, aspirin, calcium carbaspirin, choline salicylate, magnesium salicylate, salsalate, and sodium salicylate. Non-salicylates included acetaminophen, acetanilide, antipyrine, codeine, iodopyrine, phenacetin, quinine, and salicylamide.

The panel considered various adverse effects including those involving the liver and wrote: "In view of the recent findings which have confirmed that aspirin causes a reversible hepatitis, especially in children and adults with systemic lupus erythematosis or rheumatoid arthritis and for other reasons ... the Panel concludes that arthritic patients should not be self-medicating without medical supervision." While the panel recommended that health professionals be alerted to the need for periodic liver tests, it wrote: "An OTC liver warning for this group is therefore not necessary."[8]

Despite published reports suggesting that aspirin might be involved in Reye's syndrome, the panel did not mention it.

The panel expressed considerable concern with advertising, especially "certain aspects of commercial advertisements of OTC medicines that urge the consumption of these drugs without directing attention to adequate warning" of the hazards of potential immediate and long-term use.[9] The panel believed "government requirements for inclusion of warnings and cautionary language were inadequate particularly as to possible effects of advertising upon children."[10] It asked the Federal Trade Commission to more effectively regulate advertising.

Importantly, the panel struggled mightily with dose. It found that the public believed the dose of aspirin was "two tablets." Yet, on review, they learned that while most tablets contained 325 mg, some contained as much as 650 mg. To make matters worse, two systems of weight—the old apothecary system based on grains (gr) and the new metric based on milligrams (mg)—were being used and the United States Pharmacopeia XIX permitted that a quantity of available aspirin in a tablet range from 5% above or below that stated.

The bottom line was that a five-grain aspirin tablet could contain anywhere from 285 mg to 340 mg. The panel noted this difference could be a particular problem for children because a small (20%) increase in dosage could cause a large (40–60%) increase in the blood salicylate level over time. Because of these observations, the panel recommended that all products containing aspirin, acetaminophen, or sodium salicylate be standardized to contain either 325 mg (five grains) per dose for adults or 80 mg (1.23 grains) per dose for children less than 12 years of age, and that labels clearly state the amount.

The panel report also tackled the trickiest problem of all—*the dosing schedule*—and nailed the essential issue. *For aspirin, frequency and duration are as important as dose amount.* It recognized the unusual and complex pharmacokinetics of aspirin and that even small increases in dose "may exceed the capacity of the metabolizing systems and cause inordinate increases" in the blood level.[11] It also recognized that a significant proportion of serious salicylate intoxications, including deaths, were caused by "inappropriate" multiple dosing. (It did not use the term overdose yet used the term inappropriate in a setting where appropriate had not been determined.) These intoxications, it said, are claimed to be more severe and to occur at lower plasma salicylate levels compared to toxicities resulting from a large single dose.[12]

The panel struggled with determining an "appropriate dosing schedule," especially for children, and had to revert to the old method—ask the experts. A representative sample of recommendations based "on many currently marketed products for OTC use," suggested a dose of 162 mg every three hours [or 81 mg/kg/day for a 16-kg four-year-old child].[13] A survey of 2241 pediatricians revealed the schedule preferred by the majority was 65 mg (one grain) per year of age every four hours as needed, or 98 mg/kg/day for a four-year-old child.[14] Industry proposed a slightly different schedule.[15] Its dose for the same child would be 76 mg/kg/day. The panel finally decided that dosing based on body surface area (using a formula that considered body weight and height) was preferred and would provide a reasonable margin of safety.[16] The panel's revised schedule would provide 75 mg/kg/day for a four-year-old child.[17] All of these were in the ballpark of the amount that had been used for decades.

Industry and the panel agreed on a frequency interval of four, rather than the three hours that some recommended. (Appendix 1) However, in the end, the dosing schedule was so entrenched that the difference between the dosing schedules recommended on labels, the one proposed by industry, and one recommended by the panel was small.

The panel, however, made one additional recommendation—a limit on the duration of the course of treatment. It proposed that for fever, the product *should not be used for more than three days,* and, for pain, not more than five days, recommendations similar to that of Australian and Scottish doctors a decade earlier.

The panel's monograph was of unprecedented scope and detail, but nothing could remedy the fact that the recommendations were not based on actual testing of aspirin use in children in real-life OTC treatment situations. The panel's work was a doomed game of catch-up to understand the path of a drug through the body and its effects.

As the draft monograph (also called 'proposed rule') entered a comment period, the manufacturers inundated the FDA with reports defending their own products and attacking rivals. Plough, Inc. and Sterling Drug each submitted comments. Some saw an opportunity for preemptive marketing. Johnson & Johnson, makers of children's acetaminophen, suggested that the following warning be required for aspirin products: "Do not exceed recommended dosage because serious potentially life threatening, body chemistry changes, respiratory failure, coma, convulsions, and cardiovascular collapse may occur."[18]

According to J. Richard Crout, Director of FDA's Bureau of Drugs from 1973 to 1982, no one

> envisioned the difficulty of rulemaking over every one of these ingredients and their labeling, and the squabbling that would occur, the number of comments that would come in, and the work it would take to resolve all those comments ... the OTC Steering Committee was in the Commissioner's office. What the mistake was, was to put too many details of decision making at the level of that steering committee, and then have the head of the OTC review ... come back to the bureau and expect to implement it. Because [the heads of the Steering Committee] were both new to the bureau and were not scientists, they basically couldn't penetrate the bureau. So, there was a disconnect, a cultural and an allegiance disconnect, between the OTC Review and the rest of the reviewing divisions.[19]

In 1974, the FDA Bureau of Drugs had reorganized. It now included a Drug Monographs office, yet the delays continued.[20]

In 1979, Alan Done, now Director of Clinical Pharmacology and Toxicology at Wayne State University and the Children's Hospital of Michigan, Sumner Yaffe of the University of Pennsylvania and the Children's Hospital of Pennsylvania, and John Clayton of Plough, Inc. in Memphis, Tennessee, published the industry's pediatric dosage recommendations in the *Journal of Pediatrics*.[21] They recognized the medical literature contained "scant information about salicylates, particularly at therapeutic levels in children" and also the unique characteristics that contribute to so-called pyramiding. They noted that aspirin poisoning in children occurs "when inappropriate doses are administered." The undefined term "inappropriate dose," seemed to be replacing the word "overdose." Both terms however represented a dangerous obfuscation of concerns about the children's dosing schedule that had been expressed by concerned physicians for many years.

The monograph, which had been entered into the Federal Register on July 7, 1977, was not final.

Chapter 17

Replication—The Ohio and Michigan Studies

[W]e got a Reye's syndrome case that came in four hours ago.
And we were there, boom.

Frank Holtzhauer, Epidemiologist, Ohio Health Department,
describing the Ohio Study, 2008

Two new case-control studies that would be known as the Ohio study and the Michigan study were about to produce results. The Ohio study had been organized after the disastrous swine influenza program had been halted and Schonberger decided to use the funds earmarked for influenza to study Reye's syndrome. His division partnered with the Ohio Department of Health to perform a case-control study. When I first spoke with Schonberger in April 1979, the study had been in progress for four months. Now in early 1980, Ohio had collected over a year's worth of data. Yet neither the Arizona nor the Ohio or Michigan studies were the first case-control studies to address Reye's syndrome.

Several had been conducted between 1973 and 1977. For example, in 1976, Frederick Ruben and colleagues in Pittsburgh together with researchers at the University of Michigan and CDC found 67% of 24 children with Reye's and 56% of 16 controls had received medication including aspirin during the past.[1] In 1977 Lawrence Corey and his CDC colleagues including Michael Gregg reported no differences in medication use between cases and controls.[2]

A more recent case-control study (unpublished) came about by chance. When I spoke with him years later, Frank Holtzhauer, a disease investigator in north-east Ohio, recalled performing his routine weekly review of death certificates in early 1977 and realizing he had been turning over card after card that read: "Cause of death,

Reye's syndrome." Thirty-two cases were reported in Ohio between 2 October 1976 and 4 April 1977. Concerned, he called his supervisor, Ohio State Epidemiologist Thomas Halpin, and a chain of calls began. Halpin relayed the observation to CDC and to EIS officer James Marks, who was stationed in Ohio. Marks had never forgotten his first-hand experience with the devastating syndrome during his pediatric training in San Francisco. An official CDC investigation was ordered, and, on 17 March, EIS officer John Sullivan-Bolyai travelled from Atlanta to Columbus.[3] Sullivan-Bolyai and staff from the Ohio Department of Health canvassed all large Ohio hospitals likely to admit pediatric patients (those with more than 500 beds or more than 40 pediatric beds) and found 190 cases between 1973 and 1977. Their findings, later published in the *American Journal of Epidemiology*, included a temporal relationship of Reye's syndrome and influenza B and varicella, an increased risk for black infants compared with white infants, sibling cases, and repeat episodes.[4]

During our conversation in 2008, Holtzhauer told me that he and Sullivan-Bolyai had also conducted a "field test," a case-control study. The two men worked weekends at Holtzhauer's home in Cayuga Falls. Just as Reye's protégés Morgan and Baral had done two decades before, they worked at a kitchen table. They developed a questionnaire, calling it their "fishing expedition" and asking about exposures: carpet cleaners, pesticides, and medications. They selected controls from the children's classrooms. Holtzhauer also remembered: "It was wintertime … pristine snow that morning we finally had the data … we had no computers … had all these line listings … with names down the side and checkmarks … it was a Sunday … we couldn't get into the office … all over my living room floor, a sea of line listings. And when we worked the numbers, it came up with aspirin … I have nothing written down. Then John started to make the calls … from then my memory gets fuzzy."

The official report of the investigation written by Sullivan-Bolyai, Schonberger, and Gregg stated there were 11 case-control pairs, and concluded, "the lack of sufficient numbers in this pilot study precluded any further analysis." Years later, neither Sullivan-Bolyai nor Schonberger recalled the aspirin finding. The report, however, recommended a larger case-control study.[5] Shortly afterwards, CDC began that study—the Ohio study. It would become one of CDC's most scrutinized studies.

John Sullivan-Bolyai was the physician who had called me in December 1978.

Ohio goes full steam

The Ohio Department of Health in Columbus was a few blocks from the vast 22-acre site of the deteriorating Ohio Penitentiary in downtown Columbus. In the late 1970s, the area was undergoing revitalization, with construction of a Hyatt Regency hotel, a convention facility, and the Nationwide Plaza.[6] The offices of Disease Prevention, however, were in a typical nondescript government building at 35 Chestnut Street. Its façade, however, belied the dedication, drive, and youth of the staff within. Thomas Halpin, chief of the Division of Preventive Medicine and Ohio's State Epidemiologist, was a quiet, devoted pediatrician with, it was said, a bear-trap memory. Sullivan-Bolyai thought of him as a standout public health physician. Halpin called on Holtzhauer to get the study started. The job seemed "massive" to the young man— communications with CDC, setting up an internal group, designing a rigorous protocol, and hiring and training staff necessary to conduct the study and gather the data. In 2009, Holtzhauer recalled with pride, "Ohio really wanted to do a good job on it."

NRSF (Ohio) parent-advocates John and Terri Freudenberger were invited to the study meetings. Their awareness campaign had created a powerful network that enhanced the study's system for finding cases. According to Terri Freudenberger, the Ohio foundation donated 10,000 brochures to the Ohio State Health Department in November and December 1979 and the Cincinnati and Dayton chapters respectively distributed 135,000 and 40,000 Awareness Bulletins through the schools. "It would be hard to imagine a Reye's syndrome case, at that time, slipping through," Holtzhauer told me. Ohio State

University biostatistician Dick Lenese aided with the study design, and his doctoral student Janet Rice did much of the quantitative work. "I'm sure there were very learned folks at CDC who were saying, 'We're gonna do this right.' … There was engagement," Holtzhauer recalled.

The first person Holtzhauer hired was a young woman of deep faith. Lois Hall told me she had wondered if divine intervention had brought her to the project. In September 1978, as the 23-year-old university biology graduate dreamed of attending medical school, a med-school interviewer asked her why. She had answered, "To help people, of course." Although she was not admitted, she was now given the opportunity of doing just that—a job at the Ohio Department of Health. In June 1979 Bob Campbell joined the team. An energetic physician with a master's degree in preventive medicine, Campbell had performed research in Vermont analyzing the relationship between ski injuries and equipment. Halpin, Holtzhauer, Hall, and Campbell had several things in common. They were young, smart, and articulate. Each could have done better financially yet each had chosen public health. They loved the job. They took it seriously. They wanted to do good things. They wanted to help people.

Schonberger assigned Eugene (Gene) Hurwitz, an in-house EIS officer in the Viral Disease Division, to the Ohio study. Adolfo Correa-Villaseñor, a field officer assigned to Ohio, assisted. Hurwitz had earned his medical degree from St Louis University and had just completed a residency in pediatrics when he joined the CDC in the summer of 1978. In 2008, Holtzhauer recalled, "I know there were others, but Gene I remember … Gene probably never really got as much acclaim as he deserved because he was really into this. This was his life." According to Holtzhauer, "We went from the bare bones … [epidemiology] to a Cadillac design. We had the money … we had everything … The protocols were all written out. Our people were trained. It was very, in my mind, quite rigorous … how proud we were that we could get these calls. We got a Reye's syndrome case that came in four hours ago. And we were there, boom."

By April 1980 the Ohio group had collected medication data on 91 children with Reye's syndrome and their controls.

Michigan legislature demands action

At the same time, Michigan had either become a hotbed of Reye's syndrome or Dieckman's efforts vis-a-vis the Michigan foundation were simply uncovering cases. The foundation had spawned a grassroots movement. Art and Dana Allen had joined after their six-year-old daughter had died in 1979. She had chickenpox and had become "violently ill, vomiting and gradually losing interest in her surroundings." They took their daughter to the Detroit Children's Hospital where a few days later she died.[7]

The case-count in Michigan did not escape the eyes of the public. Fear and outrage were roiling when new EIS field officer physician Ronald Waldman arrived in Lansing in the summer of 1979. Fresh out of Johns Hopkins with a master's degree in public health, he had a new hand-held Hewlett Packard calculator in case he needed to calculate the "probability" that something he saw was a fluke. Waldman had already accomplished a lot. After finishing a residency, he had joined the WHO Intensified Smallpox Eradication Programme, which had been launched in 1967 as part of a vast effort to relieve the world of the ancient scourge. He then joined the CDC and during the next two years continued his international work traveling back and forth to Somalia during refugee tragedies. Conrad, his boss as well as mine, told me Waldman was seldom where he was supposed to be. Before Waldman left for Lansing, I had tracked him down and asked him to keep his eyes and ears open for clues to a possible link.

At the same time, in Ann Arbor, University of Michigan Mott Children's Hospital pediatrician Joe Baublis, one of the few dual-degree clinical researchers around, obsessed over Reye's syndrome. In 2006, his wife Joan told me that Baublis had taken a staff position at Mott and earned a PhD in virology after the family returned from a stint with the Air Force in Japan. He saw his first Reye's case in the mid-1970s and then the numbers grew. While caring for Reye's syndrome children from all over Michigan, Baublis was also managing the virology laboratory and working on a grant to learn more about the disease. He traveled around the state giving presentations to parents so they would be able to get their children into treatment as fast as possible, and this generated more diagnoses. It was exhausting, but he kept going.

Baublis was always looking for a common thread. One of his theories was a possible link to bat guano. Some of the children lived west of Ann Arbor in a rural area where there were many old houses with bats. Perhaps fleas or mosquitoes were vectors. He had wanted to go there with Joan, a nurse, and test the guano. According to Joan, in 1977 he was fatigued with an ever-increasing caseload and his phone was ringing off the hook. Yet Baublis thought constantly about Reye's. "I know it is right there," he told her over and over, grasping his hand in front of him as if catching the answer.

Michigan was reeling from another highly political public health disaster putting the population on edge. Michigan health officials had recently announced the results of a multimillion-dollar study of possible health effects of polybrominated biphenyl (PBB), a chemical often used as a flame retardant that, six years earlier, had accidently been mixed with livestock feed. The study indicated the unnerving fact that all Michigan residents exposed to the chemical might still have it in their body.[8]

Waldman spent his first few months dealing with typical, mostly food-related illnesses. In February 1980, however, his attention turned to Sherwood, a village of 400 residents in south-west Michigan. The previous November, seven-year-old Holly Burgett and her six-year-old brother had both died of Reye's syndrome in the tiny village. Now, eight-year-old Michael Duttlinger was stricken. On Thursday 21 February, the day after Michael's burial, 900 people gathered in a small gymnasium in Union City. Parents from Battle Creek about 25 miles north, where two more children had died just the previous week, attended. Michigan officials had counted 18 cases of Reye's syndrome since 1 December 1979. State and federal officials were there to talk about what they knew. According to the *Ironwood Daily Globe*, "What they know is not much."[9] Fearful and frustrated, Michael's mother insisted, "We have got to shut them down," she said. "We can get that school fumigated."[10] Most parents kept their children home. The next day the district closed four schools for the remainder of the week. On 1 March 1980, an ad in the *Ironwood Daily Globe* noted that the Pamida Discount Center offered a coupon for St Joseph Children's Aspirin— two 36-count containers for only 69 cents.[11]

It was the worst kind of tragedy—children dying unexpectedly and suddenly. Later, in 2011, Waldman recalled, "[I]t got bad in Michigan that year. The culminating event was that Ken Wilcox [Dr Kenneth R. Wilcox, Jr, Chief, Bureau of Disease Control and Laboratory Services] got called in. I went with him downtown to the legislature. And they just read the riot act … the charge to the state health department was to find the cause of this disease and stop it." Waldman felt the state officials had been wary of him, a "fed," but he soon won them over. The CDC and Johns Hopkins had trained him well. And although Conrad had observed that Waldman was never where he said he was going to be, this time Waldman was in the right place.

Waldman set up a surveillance system and by March he had a case-control study up and running. He chose 25 school-aged children with Reye's syndrome from the Lower Peninsula and 46 classmate controls who had been absent with similar prodromal illnesses during the same time. The children ranged from five to 16 years. The questionnaire consisted of a "shotgun" list of 73 potential exposures. Personnel from the Michigan Department of Public Health and the University of Michigan schools of Nursing and Public Health conducted the face-to-face interviews, an average of 6.5 weeks after the onset of the illness. The questions on medications were open-ended. "Did you give any medication for fever? For headache?" The families were asked to show bottles or containers if available and give the brand name. For the cases, only the medicines given between the onset of the prodrome and the protracted vomiting of Reye's syndrome were studied.

By early April, states with active surveillance (where officials look for cases) had reported many cases. Ohio 134, Michigan reported 69, and

Minnesota 23.[12] Waldman's team completed the case-control study in April 1980 as reports of deaths from Reye's syndrome kept coming in.

The April 1980 EIS Conference, Atlanta

An article in *Better Homes and Gardens* in February 1980 emphasized early diagnosis for Reye's syndrome. The same month, Ari L. Goldman of the *New York Times* reported that the current flu outbreak was at an epidemic level and that emergency rooms were "jammed from morning to night, and doctors were recommending fluids, rest and aspirin." [13]

I was anxious to get the data out during my presentation of the Arizona study at the April EIS Conference in Atlanta. This would be the first public disclosure of the aspirin link. I was not yet aware of the results of the studies in Ohio or Michigan. Shortly after the conference program listing my talk, "Reye's Syndrome Associated with Salicylate Consumption," was distributed. I received a letter from William Schawo, president of a new Reye's syndrome foundation based in Denver, Colorado, asking for information.

Before traveling to Atlanta, I visited the AFIP on the campus of the Walter Reed Medical Center in Washington, D.C. Conrad had convinced Brachman to release funds for my trip. There I met with Floribel Mullick, a young pathologist whom Irey had chosen to work with me and who later became director of the institute. She seemed meticulous and pleased to collaborate. We made preliminary plans for formally studying the tissue samples of the children who died of salicylate toxicity.[14] I noticed I had lost interest in coffee, my go-to beverage. This had happened once before when I was pregnant. I was thrilled as I flew to Atlanta.

The conference commenced with welcomes by Brachman and Director William Foege. My presentation was scheduled on the last day. The conference presentations covered myriad topics including, among others, the lack of association between multiple sclerosis and pet dogs, Legionnaires Disease in attendees of an American Legion conference in Philadelphia, and *Salmonella* infections from homemade ice cream, as well as investigations conducted overseas.

Immediately before my presentation, Ohio EIS officer Adolfo Correa-Villaseñor presented preliminary data from the Ohio study. The data offered several surprises. First, the fatality rate of 70 cases was only 6%. Ohio, it seemed, was uncovering large numbers of mild cases, suggesting that case numbers in the United States could well be in the thousands. Next, Correa-Villaseñor presented data on 43 cases and 48 controls. The cases had used salicylate significantly more often than had the controls.[15] Ohio had replicated the Arizona finding.

My report was next. As I climbed the steps onto the stage, I noticed the audience had thinned out. I presented the data in the prescribed 10-minute format, every word chosen for clarity and impact. Significantly more of the Reye's children had taken a salicylate than did controls; they had taken larger doses, and the amount correlated with disease severity. My final words were: "We present the hypothesis that salicylate causes or contributes to the cause of Reye's syndrome."[16] I waited. Then, quiet applause. A few people told me it was a nice paper.

Meanwhile, Waldman and the Michigan staff had completed a case-control study of 25 children with Reye's syndrome.[17] Most had an upper respiratory illness prodrome, one had chickenpox, and one had GI symptoms. They had drilled down to the ingredients in all the medications. A packet of Goody's powder contained aspirin. Pepto-Bismol contained salicylate. Waldman had spent many tedious hours in his basement apartment entering all the data into his calculator by hand. After the data were finally all in, he chose a matched case-control statistics analysis program, inserted the card into his calculator, and pressed go. The results, he recalled when we talked in 2011, "blew his mind." "[W]e had a very long questionnaire … And we asked them everything. And I swear, Karen, that although I knew of your interest and everything, when we did the analysis, it just blew my mind how strongly—I mean it was *only*—it was aspirin."

Only two medicines were used statistically significantly more often by the cases than the controls—vitamins and aspirin. For aspirin, the values were 96% versus 65% of the controls. For acetaminophen, the use was reversed. Waldman later recalled, "I was stunned. I was absolutely stunned." According to Waldman, Michigan began "pressuring him to get something in the *MMWR* [*Morbidity and Mortality Weekly Report*] ... They wanted the announcement to come from the feds." But Waldman was unsure. After all, this was *aspirin*, and he was a new epidemiologist. He worried. But Michigan wanted federal officials to take some ownership of the data and its implications.

Waldman later reflected on the day he considered the highlight of his EIS experience. In April 1982, he brought the Michigan data to Atlanta. He witnessed first-hand what appeared to be skepticism that formed the dominant opinion "about the whole topic." He also felt "there was a lot of skepticism that I could have done a study that would be meaningful in any way." Nevertheless, he persisted. "I remember meeting with Walter Dowdle [Director of the Center for Infectious Diseases] who said, 'Okay, I want you to make a presentation to me.' I agreed. We went down to Auditorium C ... and I got up at the podium. Dowdle sat in the back row ... And I gave the presentation, which was between 10 and 15 minutes. And he asked a few questions. He came up to the front of the room and he shook my hand and said, 'I'll support you all the way.'" Yet even with this third study with the same result, uncertainty remained.

After all, it was aspirin.

Chapter 18

Enough, Summer 1980

Knowing is not enough, we must apply.
Willing is not enough; we must do.
Widely attributed to Johann Wolfgang von Goethe

A letter to the Director of the Field Services Division

When I returned to Phoenix after the EIS conference, I found a letter from Jerold Lucey on my desk. Lucey had accepted the manuscript describing the Arizona study and had slated it for publication in *Pediatrics* in the December 1980 issue. My first thought was that December was eight months away. Meanwhile, I read in the *Arizona Republic* that CDC had told the press that cause of Reye's syndrome is still a "mystery."[1] In May, however, Schonberger briefed CDC's Advisory Committee on Immunization Practices that a study in Arizona had shown a statistical connection between Reye's syndrome and the ingestion of aspirin and noted a lack of widespread agreement in the medical community.[2] Little additional press followed. The year 1980 would turn out to be a banner year for Reye's syndrome. Over 500 children were reported to CDC, more than any year on record.

Between studies of *Giardia* in water, a respiratory illness in White River, an outbreak of gastrointestinal illness at a hotel, and Borrelia infections as well as work on recommendations for safe Colorado River trips, I followed the medical literature and grew increasingly distressed with the silence concerning the three studies. In an article in the *New England Journal of Medicine*, Pennsylvania State University College of Medicine physician Elliot Vessel asked: "Why are toxic reactions to drugs so often undetected initially?"[3] He observed that during pharmacology courses in medical schools, students get the message that "in almost all patients each drug has a single, well-established group of therapeutic and adverse effects. In practice, however, many patients do not experience either the anticipated therapeutic or toxic effects." He noted the importance of factors that can either increase or decrease the rate of a drug's effects and toxicities including genetics, metabolism, elimination, kidney function, the disease state being treated, and others. Vessell's article only increased my concern about the delay. Elimination of aspirin, it seemed, would eliminate the illness. Aspirin for everyday illnesses in children was simply not essential. The path seemed simple. For whatever reason, CDC was struggling with concerns about the veracity of the aspirin connection. In June, a CDC report entitled, "The Epidemiology of Reye's syndrome: A review—with emphasis on recent observations" did not mention aspirin.[4]

On 23 June, I wrote a letter reminding Conrad, my ever-supportive boss in Atlanta, that the Arizona study would be published in *Pediatrics* in December and pleaded with him to do something.

> I am convinced that the hypothesis that salicylate is the direct cause of Reye's syndrome is both biologically plausible and consistent with what is known about the drug and the disease. I think that CDC should make a prompt and intensive effort to either prove or disprove this hypothesis. Perhaps the most reasonable way to do so is by having all parties with data on the subject meet, share data, draw conclusions if possible, and /or design a definitive study. I do not think CDC can allow another Reye's syndrome season [more cases occurred in the winter] to go by without resolving this issue.[5]

The letter outlined possible mechanisms including the problem of accumulation, which by then I had become aware:

> [O]ne does not have to delve very far into the salicylate literature to learn that the relationship between toxicity and blood level is poor, that therapeutic dosing is responsible for most salicylate-related deaths in children today, that the unusual pharmacokinetics of salicylate predispose to the accumulation of toxic amounts of salicylate in the body at close to

therapeutic doses, that individual differences in capacity for salicylate metabolism have been observed, and that concomitants of viral illness such as fever, dehydration, and acidosis lower the toxic threshold of salicylate.

I included a copy of the Arizona study and a line listing of 21 consecutive Arizona cases with salicylate consumption histories and blood levels.

Conrad never let grass grow under his feet.

Four days later, in a memo to his boss Brachman, Conrad wrote: "As you can see from the attached letter from Dr Starko, and a copy of her paper which is about to be published, we need to consider further action, soon."[6] He suggested Gregg host a working group of interested people, including Halpin from Ohio and Correa-Villaseñor who was now at Johns Hopkins, to make a decision as to what we should plan for the next [flu] season. Conrad had really come through. On 24 June I wrote to Gerhardt Levy, one of the foremost aspirin experts in the United States[7] and encouraged CDC to ask him to consult.

In late June, the NRSF (Ohio) now with 77 chapters in 28 states held its Sixth Annual Meeting at Georgetown University.[8] President John Freudenberger announced that awareness of the syndrome was increasing, and articles had recently appeared in *Newsweek*, *Time*, *Good Housekeeping*, and *American Baby*. Montana Senator John Melcher spoke to the 350 participants gathered at the prestigious National Press Club and expressed hope for more federal involvement. Paul Coates of the Children's Hospital of Philadelphia received the annual research grant for his work on lipid metabolism. Congressional award recipients included Melcher, who was working on a statute (S. 1794) for government funds for Reye's syndrome research and Geraldine Ferraro of New York for supporting Reye's funding legislation. Chairman of the Foundation's scientific board Dennis Pollack presented an award for the establishment of a NRSF (Ohio) Research Laboratory to Ohio State researcher Brian Andresen, who was working on markers for early diagnosis. A scientific session included speakers from the United States, Canada, and Malaysia. Former EIS officer George Johnson now of Fargo, North Dakota, discussed his study of the 1960s. The meeting glittered with flags, banquets, and celebrities. CDC's Villaseñor-Correa's attended but his abstract did not mention the Ohio aspirin data.[9]

CDC finally released the Arizona data. In July 1980 Gregg, editor of the *MMWR*, published abbreviated results.[10] Schonberger had written the report plainly entitled "Follow-up on Reye syndrome—United States." The report began by reporting that 304 cases from 37 states and the District of Columbia had been reported to CDC in the five months ending 30 April 1980. Only 22% of those with known ages were less than four years old. The cases peaked at the same time as reports of isolation of influenza B virus in the WHO collaborating laboratories. The case-fatality rate was 23%. The article noted associations with both influenza B and influenza A. The next paragraph cautiously reported the results of the Arizona study, and concluded, "Further investigations are needed to more clearly define the possible role of salicylate use and toxins in the pathogenesis of Reye syndrome." The article did not mention the Ohio study or the Michigan study, or the multiple strands of evidence pointing to aspirin laid out in my paper and letter.

Toxic shock syndrome

At the same time, CDC was right on top of another problem. In late 1978, University of Colorado infectious disease pediatrician James Todd had reported a seemingly new and unusual illness in children less than 19 years old characterized by a sudden onset of high fever, a sunburn-like rash, peeling skin, and multiple-organ failure.[11] He called it toxic shock syndrome (TSS). In early 1980, state health departments in Minnesota and Wisconsin reported nine women with TSS.[12] Most had become ill during their menstrual period. In May, CDC reported 55 cases;[13] 95% were women and only a month later, the *MMWR* posted the results of three case-control studies (Wisconsin, CDC-I, and Utah) each of which had found an association with tampon use.[14] The Utah study also found an increased risk associated with one tampon brand, Rely. To confirm the risk, CDC conducted another case-control study and again found increased use of Rely-brand tampons. Later studies showed increased risk with other higher absorbance tampons. CDC reported the findings to the FDA and Proctor and Gamble voluntarily removed the tampons from the market in September 1980.

Only four months had passed between the first report of a link with the tampon and the manufacturer's action. In 1980, 38 women with menstrual TSS had died.[15] The same year 234 children with Reye's syndrome (of 555 cases) reported to CDC had died.[16] The design and results of the TSS studies were strikingly like those of the Reye's syndrome studies. In both, three independent case-control studies had found a link between an agent and an illness. The similarities, however, stopped there. The reactions of the CDC, the FDA, and the manufacturers were inexplicably different.

Aspirin for heart disease

Meanwhile, Sterling Drug was looking toward a large new market for aspirin—prevention of coronary artery disease. During the 1940s, an English physician had suggested aspirin as treatment for a heart attack.[17] In 1950, Lawrence Craven, an ear, nose, and throat physician from Glendale, California, after seeing his tonsillectomy patients bleed, thought aspirin might be useful in preventing the clots (thrombi) thought to precipitate heart attacks. He advised some 400 patients to take two to six tablets a day and later reported that not one had suffered a coronary thrombosis (clot).[18]

The idea was resurrected in 1961 when two pathologists suggested that platelets might play a role in clot formation.[19] Platelets are tiny disc-shaped wafers that float in the blood and initiate the formation of clots in both bleeding sites (good) and coronary arteries (not good). Ten years later, the discovery that aspirin inhibits platelet function won English pharmacologist John Vane and his colleagues a Nobel Prize.[20] Only a fraction of the amount used for everyday aches and pains was thought to inhibit platelets—81 to 325 mg per day or about 1–5 mg/kg/day for a 60-kg adult. Peter Elwood, a physician and epidemiologist at the Medical Research Council in Britain, performed a study of prevention of heart disease with aspirin, however, it was not large enough to produce a statistically convincing conclusion.[21] Undeterred, Elwood conducted two more studies that also proved to be inconclusive. In 1975, encouraged by Elwood's work, the US National Heart, Lung, and Blood Institute began a much larger trial with more than 4500 participants called Aspirin in Myocardial Infarction (AMIS). The AMIS study and the Reye's syndrome studies would soon converge on the FDA.

In 1979 R. William (Bill) Soller had joined Sterling as Medical Director and had become the leader behind Sterling's FDA application for permission to market aspirin for the prevention of heart attacks.[22] Soller, with a doctorate in Medical Sciences from Cornell University in 1975 and a stint as associate professor of pharmacology at the University of Pennsylvania, was well trained for the task.[23] All he needed were data. Soller also became one of Sterling's main voices concerning the Reye's syndrome studies. His work would soon involve two very different research methods: prospective methods which are generally required for FDA drug approval and retrospective methods which are employed when prospective research is difficult, unfeasible, or unethical (as it would be for a fatal illness in children). Case-control studies are retrospective.

When I spoke with pediatrician Ralph Kauffman in 2009, he recalled that before the case-control studies, the "reports" suggesting aspirin was involved in causing or exacerbating Reye's syndrome didn't carry much weight despite the passion of Ted Mortimer "who really believed aspirin played a role." Kauffman mused, "[A]spirin had been heavily marketed and had been accepted for 100 plus years. So, it was really hard to overcome that." I was soon to learn, the aspirin industry would appear to be confident that the Arizona, Michigan, and Ohio studies were deeply flawed and that the very idea of informing parents that aspirin could be at the root of Reye's syndrome was nothing less than preposterous.

PART V

BUT WAIT—WHO TELLS? WHO DECIDES WHO TELLS? 1980–1982

Chapter 19

Warnings—with Caveats, Late 1980

We are all afraid—for our confidence, for the future, for the world.
That is the nature of the human imagination.
Yet every man, every civilization has gone forward
because of its engagement with what it has set itself to do.
Jacob Bronowski, *The Ascent of Man*, 1973

In October 1980, five months after the Arizona study had been previewed in the *MMWR*, flu season was approaching. The full Arizona findings were to be published in *Pediatrics* in December, and Halpin was planning to present the Ohio data at the Ohio foundation's meeting in Detroit on 6 November.[1] CDC was struggling with the results and their potential impact. Absolute proof was elusive, yet three studies had identified a link with aspirin. The situation lacked a randomized, double-blind, placebo-controlled clinical trial (which would be unethical), and a mountain of case-control studies could not remediate this.

To add urgency, Fay Luscombe, Arnold Monto, and Joseph Baublis at the University of Michigan had just bolstered physicians' perception that Reye's syndrome was one of the more common causes of death in childhood in the United States.[2] After studying Michigan death certificates, the researchers had estimated the average death rate of Reye's syndrome for the years 1969–1976 was between 0.43 (for certificates coded as Reye's syndrome) and 1.03 (for certificates that could be Reye's syndrome) per 100,000 < 19 years of age.[3] If these rates are applied to the United States population less than 18 years of age, a staggering number of mostly perfectly healthy children—between 274 and 656—would have died of Reye's syndrome in 1980 alone. (Appendix 2) By contrast, measles was averaging about 35 deaths per year[4] and the previously terrifying illnesses diphtheria and polio were on the way to extinction.

Further, Sullivan-Bolyai had just reported that the rate of death in those with Reye's syndrome was decreasing in Ohio.[5] The implication was sobering. Whereas Reye's initial cases were almost all fatal, the death rates reported in 1974 and 1975 were 23%, in 1976 13%, and in 1977 only 3%. At first this seemed to be good news, but it likely meant that more and more non-fatal cases were being uncovered, a result of the foundations' efforts to encourage early diagnosis. As Reye's syndrome was not uniformly reportable to public health systems, and had not always been coded on death certificates, the 2244 cases that had been reported to CDC since 1950 was surely a marked underestimate. The actual number of cases could have been tens of thousands more. (Appendix 3)

CDC decided to hold the meeting that Lyle Conrad had suggested on 28 October. Although I had finished my two-year commitment with the Public Health Service in September, I was invited along with the investigators from Michigan and Ohio. The three studies would be reviewed. (Appendix 5) Ohio, the largest, and therefore the most robust and impactful, would be particularly scrutinized. The objective of the meeting was to determine if any additional studies were indicated. First, Diane Rowley, EIS Officer in the Viral Disease Division, reviewed early studies. I followed with a summary of the Arizona findings, then Ron Waldman presented the Michigan study.

The Michigan results were striking and in line with those in Arizona. Waldman and colleagues had decided to study only children registered in day care or school so that controls could be easily obtained. Controls (two for each case) were matched on age, sex, and type of prodromal illness (flu-like or upper respiratory infection vs. chickenpox). Only cases above Stage 1 were included and 68 potential exposure factors were examined. 96% of the 25 cases and only 73% of the controls recalled the use of aspirin (prior to protracted vomiting for cases and during the entire illness for controls); this difference was estimated to occur by chance alone less than one time out of 1000. A statistically significant reverse association was found with being given acetaminophen. Children with Reye's syndrome were also more likely to be taking other regular medications and vitamins and to be drinking soft drinks. Waldman thought the main flaws in his study were that the cases and controls had not been matched for degree of fever and that considerable time had gone by prior to the interviews, possibly affecting memory of exposures.

Halpin presented the Ohio findings which were consistent with those in Arizona and Michigan and replicated the association between Reye's syndrome and aspirin. By the time the study ended on 31 March 1980, 227 cases had been reported in the state, coinciding with outbreaks of influenza A the first winter (1978–1979) and influenza B the second winter (1979–1980). Identification of mild cases continued. Of the 227 cases, 160 were in Stage 1 or higher, 16% refused to participate, and 24% could not be matched with a control. Included in the study were 98 cases and 160 controls. The control children were selected from the classrooms of the cases or neighborhood and matched on several characteristics including age, gender, race, and the occurrence of a similar antecedent illness (respiratory, varicella, or gastrointestinal) within one week of the case's illness. The second year of the study included a detailed day-by-day accounting of dosing for all medications and identification of the time of onset of severe vomiting.

The use of only two medicines differed between cases and controls: (1) a salicylate-containing medication was used by 97% of 98 cases versus 71% of 160 controls, and (2) a reverse association with acetaminophen was found again. The estimated increased odds of use of a salicylate was 11-fold, a level unusually high for any epidemiologic study. The results were almost identical to Waldman's. Halpin also reported a significant decrease in fluid intake in the case group, possibly indicating dehydration. An additional statistical analysis indicated that differences in fever, headache, or sore throat between cases and controls did not explain the results. Importantly, the majority of children with Reye's syndrome had not taken more than the recommended dose of aspirin.

All three studies—Arizona, Michigan, and Ohio—had found the same patterns supporting the reliability of the observation. *Only two possibilities existed—all three studies were flawed or there was a causal relationship between Reye's syndrome and being given recommended doses of aspirin.* The chance of a statistical fluke was negligible.

As expected in a scientific setting, various angles were examined. The discussion however quickly focused on the possibility that a flaw in the study design or conduct of the studies accounted for the results. The fact that case-control studies are both observational and retrospective raised many concerns, ones that would be mainly negated with an experimental study design (prospective, randomized, double-blind, placebo controlled). Were all the cases truly cases of Reye's syndrome? Was the medication taken before the onset of the syndrome? Did differential recall affect the results? Were the cases representative of the illness? Did parents confuse drugs? Was there interviewer bias or confounding, i.e., an unknown factor unrelated to causation that caused the differences? An experimental design, however, would not only be impractical (because thousands of children would be needed) but randomizing children to identify a poison would obviously be unethical. A case-control study was one of the few ways to get at the problem. As the meeting wound down, renowned aspirin authority Gerhardt Levy discussed salicylate metabolism and electron microscopy expert Jacqueline Partin discussed pathology. No conclusions were reached.

On 29 October 1980, FDA staff on detail to the CDC for toxic shock syndrome notified physician Judith Jones, Director of the FDA Division of Drug Experience, Bureau of Drugs,[6] that CDC was planning to publish a report on aspirin in the *MMWR*. Jones called Michael Gregg and a four-way call with Hurwitz and Schonberger ensued. Jones wrote that CDC was concerned that the data in Halpin's upcoming presentation in Detroit "would be released and cause a problem with the media" and that CDC was considering a report of its own. Things were now moving fast. They told her that Hurwitz was going to Ohio to convince the investigators to complete a careful analysis before the presentation and that CDC would simultaneously prepare a summary article for potential publication in the *MMWR* for November. They also told Jones that a Bayer representative had told them that aspirin use based on [parental] recall was totally unreliable. The same day, an EIS officer in Tennessee called Schonberger about an outbreak of chickenpox. CDC sent an officer to investigate antipyretic (fever reducers) use.[7] Faulty parental recall became a theme of industry's response to the studies.

Jones then called physician Eileen Barker of the FDA's Division of Neuropharmacology Drug Products to obtain information on prior FDA actions. Barker told her about the two advisory committee meetings that had "warned against all pharmacotherapy in sick children, especially those suspected of potential Reye's syndrome." Barker also relayed that the "American Association of Pediatrics" [unclear to whom she was referring] considered the relationship with aspirin "not impressive," and that recently published articles had "not emphasized drug relatedness."[8] Jones called a doctor at the NIH, learned of an upcoming conference in March on Reye's syndrome, and told him that the FDA was concerned about the role of drugs in the etiology of the syndrome.[9]

During the last two days of October, Jones and Hurwitz had several discussions by phone. The Ohio researchers had conducted some additional analyses. Hurwitz told Jones that most subjects had taken recommended doses of aspirin and that a scatterplot of peak days of intake of aspirin showed a peak after two to three days during the prodromal period "suggesting the time being in support of a causative association."[10] (A time analysis had been critical in Schonberger's analysis of Guillain-Barré syndrome after swine flu vaccination.) Hurwitz suggested that an expert committee might be helpful, and Jones agreed and expressed concern about a publication "based not on examining the data" and the need for FDA to examine the data.[11]

Nineteen months, which seems a long time given the dire nature of the illness, would pass before FDA reported its examination of the data in May 1982. It is unknown if anyone at FDA reviewed the statements in the 1977 FDA monograph panel which came very close to the heart of the matter when they described concerns about the unusual pharmacokinetics of aspirin and duration of dosing.

CDC was facing the realities that aspirin was an iconic medication, CDC had not directly analyzed the data (Ohio had), and the manufacturers indicated that medication histories were unreliable. Nevertheless, Phil Brachman, Director, Bureau of Epidemiology, approved the *MMWR* article drafted by Schonberger's group. The group would continue to play a pivotal role informing health professionals and the media via *MMWR* articles. On 5 November 1980, CDC reported to Jones that CDC would be publishing the article on 7 November, even though CDC did not yet have the raw data.[12]

On 6 November 1980 at the Detroit Plaza Hotel, Tom Halpin presented the Ohio findings to the attendees of the Third International Reye's Syndrome Symposium, including the NRSF Ohio Scientific Advisory Board members, June Aprille of Tufts University, John Crocker of Dalhousie University, Darryl De Vivo of Columbia University, Ellen Kang of the University of Tennessee, John Partin of Cincinnati's Children's Research Foundation who was moving to State University of New York at Stony Brook, Bennett Shaywitz of Yale University, and J. Dennis Pollack of Ohio State University.

Halpin informed the group that the Ohio study had found aspirin to be a risk factor for Reye's syndrome. Unfortunately, in contrast to three other Reye's symposia (1974, 1978, and 1984), the proceedings of this meeting were not published. Nevertheless, parent-advocate John Freudenberger, in his "Presidential Notes" for the winter issue of the NRSF [Ohio] newsletter, explained to the membership that the preliminary data in three state studies suggested "aspirin is a 'risk' factor in the viral illness or the chickenpox" and that "Officials stress that caution be used if administering aspirin to children."[13, 14]

On 7 November 1980, preliminary results of the Ohio and Michigan studies appeared in the *MMWR*.[15, 16] The report noted that children with the syndrome in Ohio had generally taken no more than recommended doses of aspirin. The scatterplot of doses, however, was not included. The editorial note by CDC staff focused on an academic description of potential biases with case-control studies. In the end, however, the article referred readers to the 1976 FDA bulletin and advised "caution when administering salicylate to treat children with viral illnesses, particularly chickenpox and influenza-like illnesses."

The anticipated media attention followed. On 8 November 1980, the *Chicago Tribune* headlined "Aspirin Link to Reye's Syndrome Revealed."[17] The *New York Times* announced, "Studies Warn Parents about Link of Aspirin to Childhood Disease." Gregg equivocated. He told the *Times* that CDC officials were "not saying don't use aspirin" but that parents and physicians should be aware and "act prudently and wisely with this information under their belt."[18] Advising prudent action—while better than silence—was hardly definitive guidance.

The aspirin companies were the first to question the study results. Sterling was "surprised" that CDC had not considered a study by the FDA (in collaboration with investigators from the Children's Hospital Medical Center in Washington, D.C. and Wayne State University) presented at the Detroit meeting that reported acetaminophen-induced Reye's-like syndrome in mice with influenza.[19] Representatives of the industry, particularly H. Stander of Sterling-Winthrop Research Institute (Biometrics) and R. William Soller of Sterling's Glenbrook Laboratories, immediately sought more details about the studies.[20] In late November, Sterling representatives met with the Michigan investigators in Lansing and then with the Ohio investigators in Columbus. Pediatrician and aspirin expert Alan Done, who was now at Wayne State, served as a consultant to Plough at the Lansing meeting. Hurwitz attended both meetings. According to Sterling, the meetings were "cordial."[21] Yet Ohio's Holtzhauer recalled that frustrated Ohio State statistician Richard Lanese had pulled his chair to the head of the table, sat upon its back, and gave the aspirin companies "a lecture about statistical rigor and academic rigor ... and how ... you can ... pick, pick, pick ... any case-control study."

At this point the health departments had provided only summary tables to the companies.[22] Sterling wrote its own critique of the data focusing on flaws in the study design and the data analysis "in an attempt to place in doubt the putative association between aspirin and Reye's syndrome."[23] In late November Jones suggested to the

FDA Associate Director for New Drug Evaluation some type of public announcement [about Reye's] "but only after we have obtained the actual data." Halpin told FDA he was sending the material.[24] In December, Jones reported a conversation between Hurwitz, aspirin expert Alan Done, and two drug company representatives questioning the possibility of a dye contaminant in the medication,[25] while Sterling Drug applied for permission to market aspirin for prevention of second heart attacks, a new, large, and lucrative market.[26]

Our baby boy was born on 8 December. His brother was now an active toddler. The Arizona study had just been published in *Pediatrics*.[27] Coming on the heels of the *MMWR* reports, I hoped the *Pediatrics* paper would result in prompt preventive action. In addition to suggesting that aspirin was the cause of Reye's syndrome, I pointed out that the doses received by the children with Reye's syndrome were within the range of the doses being used every day, that low blood levels can be present during salicylate poisoning, and that mitochondria are involved in both Reye's syndrome and salicylate toxicity. Aspirin experts from several universities and the Rocky Mountain Poison Control Center would soon summarize data on salicylate accumulation in *Clinical Toxicology*.[28] The *Pediatrics* report closed, "It is postulated that salicylate, operating in a dose-dependent manner, possibly potentiated by fever, represents a primary causative agent in Reye's syndrome."

I sent a letter of thanks to the families who had participated in the Arizona study. I was happy the results were out and naively believed that soon no child would ever get Reye's syndrome again.

Chapter 20

Smackdown, Early 1981

Because aspirin's so commonly used, it's hard to tie it to anything.
It's like blaming cancer on our drinking water.

Physician, *Medical World News*, March 1981

Physicians, toxicologists, AAP, and industry weigh in

On Sunday 4 January 1981, the *Chicago Tribune's* page one headline read: "Reye's Disease Linked to Aspirin." [1] "Mild fevers do not require aspirin," the article explained, "no one knows the amount of aspirin needed to foster the development of Reye's syndrome." Well, this was not exactly true. Most of the children in the studies had taken recommended doses. I told the *Tribune*, "People have to seriously consider aspirin as a possible cause." Ron Waldman added, "We are advising parents to not give aspirin to the children when they have mild flu or chickenpox ... some degree of prevention is possible by avoiding aspirin."

Any further action concerning warnings about the link between aspirin and Reye's syndrome seemed now to stall.

Only three days later aspirin was again front-and-center, this time as the time-tested treatment for influenza. A *New York Times* headline read: "PLS USE; Remedies for Influenza Stress Rest and Aspirin." [2] Health writer Jane Brody echoed the longstanding recommendation for treatment with aspirin. [3] After all, aspirin had been the treatment of choice for influenza since Surgeon General Rupert Blue recommended it during the 1918 pandemic. [4] During the 1957 Asian flu pandemic, [5] Sterling's sales soared to a record high of $55 million; [6] and Plough had reported a sales record of $16 million for the first half of 1958. [7] During the Hong Kong flu pandemic of 1968, a buyer for a drug store chain in the Midwest reported that sales of remedies had been "stupendous and fantastic."[8] Again, in 1978, aspirin was standard treatment during the Russian flu outbreak.[9] During the winter of 1979–1980, its primacy as the home remedy of choice during the flu remained.[10] Aspirin for influenza seemed to be a mantra firmly entrenched in the minds of all.

In late January Montana Senator John Melcher introduced the Reye's Syndrome Act of 1981. A previous Bill had died in committee. He reported that the NIH had received 13 applications for Reye's research during the year preceding January 1980 yet, as of April 1980, only two had been funded. The new bill provided for nearly $5 million over a 3-year period, including $4.5 million for research grants and $450,000 for new mobile teams. Curiously, no mention was made of the CDC-state studies implicating aspirin. John Freudenberger informed NRSF members of the Act on 11 February 1981.

In response to the *MMWR* article, industry began to conduct its own evaluations and present its views. Plough made several requests for data in early 1981.[11,12] In February, Dr M. Trout, Sterling's Senior Vice President and Director of Scientific and Medical Affairs, met with CDC Director William Foege and elaborated on the methodological problems he perceived.[13] Schonberger later recalled that industry representatives had indicated that, based on data from a survey, the ratio of aspirin to acetaminophen usage among children was 13 to 1—"a far cry from what our data was showing among control children." Schonberger was "extremely skeptical, but the representative did indicate that he would be willing to share the data with us." As far as Schonberger knew, he never did.

Once again, adjectives, reflecting perceptions, reigned. The results of the three studies, rather than being "important" or "groundbreaking" became "controversial." Organizations including the American Academy of Pediatrics (AAP), the National Institutes of Health (NIH), *Medical World News*, the widely read pharmacology journal the *Medical Letter*, rival company McNeil Consumer Products Company makers of Tylenol, and the NRSF [Ohio] became involved. Industry would meet with most. Its approach would soon resemble whack-a-mole.

Physicians in practice were among the first to join the controversy in print. Within weeks of the publication of the Arizona study (the only study published in full), several doctors shot letters to *Pediatrics* editor Jerold Lucey criticizing it. Simply put, the data made no sense to those who had been recommending aspirin for years. As one physician in Fayetteville, Tennessee, put it, "If this study proves more than the fact that the sicker the child is the more salicylates his parents give him, it is certainly well hidden." [14,15] Gastroenterology specialist-pediatricians, Joseph H. Clark and Joseph F. Fitzgerald of Indiana University School of Medicine,[16] and doctors in Canada[17] wrote that the salicylate levels (the average level for Reye's patients in Indiana was 8.01 mg/dL) did not support salicylate as a cause. They also noted possible flaws in the Arizona study, claimed liver pathology of salicylate poisoning differed, and expressed concern with the potential danger of increased use of acetaminophen, a drug considered potentially more toxic. (Fitzgerald would later become a consultant to Plough.) A Toledo, Ohio, physician pointed out that the Arizona study fulfilled only one of Yale epidemiologist Alvin Feinstein's five "fundamental criteria for validity in case-control research" and recommended a cohort study in which aspirin users and non-users would be followed to measure rates of Reye's syndrome over time (an impractical and unethical solution that would require thousands of participants and take years).[18] Lucey waited until the fall of 1981, just before flu season, to publish these letters along with our reply.

On 23 February, aspirin rival McNeil sponsored a symposium at Georgetown University.[19] Preeminent scientists and clinician experts on aspirin and acetaminophen attended and their work was published in the *Archives of Internal Medicine*. Salicylate toxicity was described by the guest editor as "salicylate overdosage (often a result of therapeutic misadventure [another vague term] in the pediatric age group)." [20] Notwithstanding the colorful and unhelpful term "therapeutic misadventure," aspirin expert Anthony Temple, who had begun to work at McNeil, raised a concern—that prolonged use of therapeutic doses of salicylate could cause intoxication.[21]

Mortimer was now Chairman of the Committee on Infectious Diseases, known by most as the AAP Redbook Committee. The committee drafted an AAP Policy Statement entitled "Reye's Syndrome and Aspirin" and sent it to the Academy's leadership for approval. It was no slam-dunk. In January 1981 at AAP headquarters in Evanston, Illinois, the AAP Board decided to return the draft for a revision.[22] On 2 March, Mortimer told the *Medical World News* (*MWN*) that any warning about aspirin "cannot be regarded as the official position of the academy until—and if—it's approved by the group's governors." The flu season was almost over by the time the Board approved the statement as a major AAP policy statement for the March issue of *News and Comment*. The statement, signed by both the Redbook Committee and the Committee on Drugs, appraised the membership of the association between aspirin use and Reye's Syndrome but offered no recommendation.[23] *MWN* noted that the "health department studies" had been challenged by Soller, Sterling's Director of Scientific Affairs. Indeed, Soller had provided the AAP with material that questioned the validity of the studies.[24]

In a March 1981 article entitled "Salicylate Toxicity Following Therapeutic Doses in Young Children" in *Clinical Toxicology*, academics explained how therapeutic doses of aspirin could be dangerous— at least to those who read the toxicology literature.[25] While not mentioning Reye's syndrome specifically, Wayne Snodgrass and Barry H. Rumack of the University of Colorado and the Rocky Mountain Poison Center, and colleagues from Colorado and the University of Louisville School of Medicine, wrote aspirin should not be used in young children as accumulation was a problem: "Because of the cumulative kinetics of salicylates and the risk of chronic [treatment for more than 12 hours] toxicity from therapeutic doses, we recommend that salicylates not be used in young children" to reduce fever and, if salicylates were used, physicians should limit use to 24 hours. They proposed that "Labels of children's aspirin should reflect this risk clearly to consumers." These recommendations likely sent chills over the industry.

The response was swift. Wayne State's Alan Done, who had recently served as a consultant to Plough, shot a letter to the editor objecting to Snodgrass and colleagues' "unwarranted conclusion that therapeutic doses of aspirin pose sufficient risk that salicylate should not be used in the young child for antipyresis."[26] Done was a heavyweight. A graduate of the University of Utah School of Medicine, he had developed the famous Done diagram for single aspirin ingestions, had been the first director of the Salt Lake City Poison Control Center and an early president of the American Association of Poison Control Centers, and had served on the editorial board of *Clinical Toxicology* since 1968.[27] His comment, however, seemed to contradict his own philosophy. He had recently lamented the fact that 78% of drugs on the market had not been "proved" safe and effective for children.[28] Now he claimed aspirin was just as safe as other fever-reducers but offered no proof.

No immediate action resulted from Snodgrass' recommendation for a warning on labels. In fact, in keeping with the frosty weather, anything that smacked of government regulation was slowly being frozen. In his Inaugural Address, the newly elected president of the United States Ronald Reagan declared "government is the problem."[29] According to author Philip J. Hilts, the administration's plans to "solve the crisis of overregulation" included "stopping the creation of new regulation, cutting the budgets of regulatory agencies, and infiltrating the agencies with conservatives."[30] "Nine days after Reagan's inauguration, he ordered a sixty-day freeze on all new regulations."[31] A warning label requirement would require a new FDA regulation. Within weeks, Reagan signed Executive order 12291 which gave the president the power to control all regulations. Agencies wanting a new regulation would be required to apply to the Office of Management and Budget (OMB). OMB immediately made a list of the 20 regulations to be eliminated, including former FDA Commissioner Jere Goyan's plan to require information about drugs on patient package inserts (PPI).[32]

Government-mandated package inserts (also called the "label" for prescribing physicians) had long generated controversy. In 1967, Neil Chayet of the Law Medicine Institute at Boston University had written an article in the *New England Journal of Medicine*. Entitled "the Power of the Package Insert," it had described a potential liability problem for physicians if a package insert was considered the exclusive authority. He argued that other publications and reports should "stand on equal footing." [33]

The first *patient* package insert (PPI) required by the FDA had saved lives. When inhalers for asthma were first introduced, the rate of asthma deaths curiously began to rise. A bronchodilator inhaler contained the drug isoproterenol. [34] In 1968, experts concluded that inappropriate use of the inhaler was actually "*causing* the condition it was intended to treat." Each inhaler was then required to "bear a two-sentence warning on the container advising of an association between repeated and excessive use and severe paradoxical bronchoconstriction." [35] In 1970, the government required another PPI—for oral contraceptives. Goyan's planned regulations, announced in September 1980, involved 10 categories of drugs based on the importance of precise use, widespread use, potential for serious side effects, the likelihood of severe problems if directions were not followed, and whether use of the drug was largely a matter of patient choice. Goyan later called the PPI effort the "single issue that occupied more of my personal time." [36] By May 1981, the PPI program was stopped providing a tangible indication of the administration's view of informing consumers of information on medicines.

Reagan appointed Arthur Hayes, Jr, a Cornell medical graduate, as commissioner of the FDA. Hayes was director of clinical pharmacology at the Pennsylvania State University Medical School when he was called to serve. [37] He had been "a regular consultant for many drug companies" and "continued to receive industry money ... after he was in office, which was not illegal at the time." [38] His philosophy was "the industry should be regulated with its voluntary consent and cooperation." [39]

In March 1981, the NIH held a Consensus Development Conference on the diagnosis and treatment of Reye's syndrome. [40] Seven specialty associations (CDC was not listed) were represented. The conference chairman, appointed an "Aspirin Subcommittee" to write a section for the final statement.[41] Sterling accepted an invitation to present its position.[42] The final statement published in *JAMA* in November 1981 punted the Reye's syndrome issue, calling the link an "apparent" association and stating the cause of Reye's syndrome "remains unknown"—but curiously accepted as "well-established" the connection between Reye's and influenza B and chickenpox, associations established only by coincidental occurrence and not by the more rigorous case-control study method. The statement—a harbinger of things to come—recommended "carefully designed" studies before recommending changes in antipyretic therapy."

Were more studies really needed or was it time for action on par with the tampon-toxic shock syndrome link? Sterling Drug straddled the issue by agreeing more studies were needed and urging doctors and parents to heed cautionary statements, because *all* medications can have deleterious effects.[43] Plough, however, was resolute that no meaningful scientific evidence existed regarding the link.[44] The Canadian publication *Forefronts in Neurology* contacted me. I said, "We need to broadcast the notion of caution in giving children salicylate or medications containing them for viral infections, especially when there is fever. There is no evidence that salicylate plays a role in recovery from such infections."[45]

In early June Mark Abramowicz, editor of the *Medical Letter,* a respected and widely read publication on therapeutics, asked for my comments on a draft article.[46] The article reported that an unnamed researcher suggested "that higher salicylate levels in patients with Reye's syndrome are secondary to reduced metabolism of salicylate by an injured liver and are not the cause of the disease." I suggested the author provide evidence to back up this statement and expressed "hope that the potential significance of the epidemiological association between aspirin use and Reye's syndrome is clear to your readership."[47] Hope didn't work. On 24 July, the *Medical Letter* ignored my suggestion and published the statement. The author was J.C. Partin, et al.[48] During the 1970s Partin, a member of the Cincinnati group, had suggested that the liver pathology of salicylate intoxication and Reye's syndrome differed. The Partin data did show that children with Reye's syndrome had more salicylate—*ten times more*—in their serum than did control subjects. The levels, like the doses, were not in the so-called toxic range. Surprisingly, no evidence supporting Partin's speculation was offered.[49]

Charlie Haley, physician at the University of Virginia and former fellow EIS officer, became livid when he read the *Medical Letter* and asked if I wanted to co-author a rebuttal. Of course, I did! As the *Medical Letter* had no format for this, we wrote to the *New England Journal of Medicine* explaining that we believed the *Letter* had published misleading statements and we wanted to set the record straight.[50] Criticizing one journal in another was admittedly unusual. Our letter was not published. I wondered why the *Medical Letter* printed Partin's speculation but did not mention the case-control studies? Things were getting "curiouser and curiouser" to quote Alice from Lewis Carroll's famous Wonderland story.

Industry funds research

On 5 June 1981, the *MMWR* published a landmark investigation by a group of Los Angeles physicians and the local EIS officer Wayne Shandera. Five previously healthy young men had developed a rare type of pneumonia—*Pneumocystis carinii*. All were homosexual.[51] Soon more cases were identified in New York, San Francisco, and other cities. Within 18 months, epidemiologists had identified major risk factors for the new illness, acquired immunodeficiency syndrome—AIDS.[52] On 16 June, my husband, physician Donald Francis, an expert on retroviruses, speculated to his mentor Myron Essex at Harvard that a retrovirus might be involved.[53] Francis was one of the few CDC staff with expertise in retroviruses, viruses that become incorporated in their host's DNA. Not long before, NIH researcher Robert Gallo had found that just such a virus caused a type of human leukemia in Japan.[54] Francis began travelling regularly to Atlanta.

While I was taking time off to be with our children before starting a new position at the Maricopa County Health Department, I continued working with Floribel Mullick at the AFIP on our analysis of the liver samples from children with salicylate intoxication. The liver cells as seen with a light microscope, and the brain, as seen with the naked eye, appeared to be indistinguishable from those of children with Reye's syndrome. [55] To publicize the data, I asked CDC for permission to present our findings at an upcoming Reye's syndrome meeting in Vail, Colorado. While the request was granted, CDC could not pay for the trip. Conrad wrote that he hoped I could go on my own dollar.[56] So I did.

The meeting, held 19–20 June 1981, was a joint meeting of the National Reye's Syndrome Foundation [Ohio] and a new foundation based in Denver called the American Reye's Syndrome Foundation.[57] I presented the AFIP data showing fatty degeneration in children with salicylate poisoning and to my surprise was questioned quite aggressively. I felt like a student who had not studied rather than a guest scientist. The harsh criticism made it clear that something was terribly wrong. The meeting proceedings published in the *Journal of the National Reye's Syndrome Foundation* (Ohio) did not include the abstract of my presentation.[58] Soon, industry would send a critique of my Vail presentation to the FDA stating that there was "apparent confusion" on my part. (In 1983, Tim Miller wrote in *The Nation* that the American Reye's Syndrome Foundation had received money from the makers of Bayer aspirin.[59])

Someone must have had enough of the deniers, the distracters, and the cautious. In August 1981, an anonymous editorial entitled "Aspirin or Paracetamol?" in *The Lancet* boldly reiterated Snodgrass' warning that with aspirin therapy there is "great danger of accumulation and toxicity especially in young children." It went further, expressing "particular concern" with evidence that salicylate may be a primary causal agent in Reye's syndrome, "a condition which has many features in common with sub-acute salicylate intoxication in children."[60] That month the NRSF [Ohio] and Ohio State University College of Medicine opened a new NRSF Research Laboratory at the university. Brian Andreson, the laboratory director who specialized in chemicals, focused on the idea that the "disease was first identified in the 1960s" and speculated that a new chemical or virus could be involved. When he talked to the AP press, he discussed early diagnosis and did not mention the aspirin studies.[61]

In September 1981, as I began my new position at the Bureau of Communicable Diseases at the Maricopa County Health Department in Phoenix, the editor of *Pediatrics* published the letters critiquing the Arizona study and a rebuttal George Ray and I had written. We called for caution in using any medication for fever, quoting 17th-century English physician Thomas Sydenham's famous line: "Fever is Nature's engine which she brings into the field to remove her enemy."[62]

By late 1981, makers of both aspirin and acetaminophen were providing funds to interested parties, which was common practice. For example, Sterling's subsidiary Glenbrook Laboratories funded research by Pollack, Chairman of the Scientific Advisory Board of the NRSF of Ohio. In 2015 Pollack told me that he had received an unsolicited and unrestricted grant from Glenbrook Laboratories around "1981–1982." Sterling reported to the FDA that it had funded an "outstanding proposal" for basic research by Pollack in December 1981.[63,64] While Pollack had no recollection of submitting a formal proposal, he did recall sending a letter "inquiring of their interest in whatever idea I wrote about" and that about $7500 appeared. All went into the Ohio State Research Fund marked for Reye's syndrome research. Pollack later explained that he had no money to finance the Reye's meetings "and felt compelled" to accept all gifts, an acceptable practice among researchers at the time. He learned many years later that Glenbrook was a subsidiary of Sterling Drug. His primary goal at the time was to connect experts and keep them "informed, contributory, and hopefully active" through the congresses, the proceedings, and the *Journal of the NRSF of Ohio*. Sterling also funded NRSF [Ohio] Scientific Board member John Crocker of Dalhousie University who was studying the role of pesticides in Reye's.[65] Meanwhile, the Johnson & Johnson (J&J) unit McNeil Consumer Products Company, makers of aspirin's rival Tylenol, provided support to the NRSF [Ohio] for their 1980 brochure.[66] Plough supported John Wilson, professor of pharmacology and pediatrics at Louisiana State University Medical Center. Wilson asked me for the Arizona data, indicating he wanted to prepare a letter to the editor.[67] Pleased by his interest, I sent him the data from the cases and controls and suggested that work be done on drug metabolism in children.[68] Later, in 1982, Wilson and his co-author wrote a detailed critique of case-control methods, with no mention of pharmacology. Their work, the report noted, was in part supported by Schering-Plough, makers of St Joseph Aspirin for Children.[69]

Accelerating decline in aspirin use

Quietly, a major shift in the use of aspirin was occurring. At the time few knew that several months after the case-control studies were published in late 1980, the already ongoing slow decline in physicians' recommendations for aspirin for children accelerated.[70] In the United States, this decline had begun in 1976 when J&J launched a campaign to boost sales of Tylenol, which then represented only 4% of the pain-relief market.[71] By 1979, however, sales of aspirin and acetaminophen for children were neck and neck.[72] By 1981, Tylenol's overall market share had risen to 35.4%.[73] This trend had occurred at least a decade earlier in Australia as consumers there more quickly embraced acetaminophen products. (Appendix 4)

Sadly, parents, for whom the aspirin data carried critical importance, were the least likely to be involved in discussions about aspirin use. If they didn't hear from their physician or read about the link with Reye's syndrome in the newspaper, they were in the dark. Children continued to die of Reye's syndrome.

Chapter 21

Would You Give This? Late 1981

How wonderful to think that nobody need wait a single moment,
we can start now, start slowly changing the world.

Anne Frank, *Tales from the Secret Annex*, 1949

During the fall of 1981, with the annual flu season once again approaching, a fourth study, another by Ron Waldman in Michigan, showed the same link with aspirin. In a move that would mark the opening shot of an epic five-year battle over if and how parents and other consumers should be informed of the link between aspirin and Reye's syndrome, CDC called in outside expert consultants. Schonberger later explained that to speed up the process, instead of going through the red tape required to organize an official advisory committee, the CDC hired each expert individually and asked them to attend a meeting at CDC in Atlanta on 13–14 October 1981. I travelled to Atlanta a third time to present the Arizona study.

Pediatrician E. Russell Alexander MD of the University of Arizona would lead the group. The members included well-known experts in the fields of pediatrics, epidemiology, statistics, Reye's syndrome, infectious diseases, drug regulation, pathology, and pharmacology. The FDA sent Franz Rosa MD. Statistical expert Stuart Hartz SCD from Tufts University in Boston attended as did Jacqueline Partin MS. AAP members included Alexander, Mortimer, Rosa, Wayne State pediatrician Ralph Kauffman MD, and David J. Lang MD of Baltimore. Brian Strom MD MPH, a faculty member at the University of Pennsylvania, was the youngest member. These were no lightweights. Strom, for example, was a graduate of the Johns Hopkins School of Medicine and his credentials were impressive. He had been a Fellow in Clinical Pharmacology at the University of California, San Francisco, while simultaneously earning a Master of Public Health in epidemiology. Penn was one of only three academic programs in the country devoted to the new field of pharmaco-epidemiology. The stated purpose of the meeting was to evaluate the studies and determine recommendations, if any, regarding treatment and further studies.[1] In 2006, reflecting on CDC's angst, Strom put it another way. As he recalled, CDC had received heat for the studies and wanted to know if it had "gone too far." The consultants were tasked with preparing individual statements and, as a group, a final summary.[2]

Opening remarks by CDC staff and Hurwitz, moderator of the workshop, were followed by Diane Rowley's literature review and presentations by Tom Halpin, Ohio biostatistician Richard Lanese, Ron Waldman, and me. Waldman had sought to improve his first study by questioning cases and controls more promptly and matching the cases and controls by year in school, race, febrile response, and type of prodromal illness. Amazingly the interviews occurred on average 5.5 days after the child came to medical care. The results revealed that all 12 children with Reye's syndrome had used an aspirin-containing medication during the presumed viral illness prior to the protracted vomiting that signaled Reye's syndrome, whereas only 41% of the controls had used it. The average dose for cases was 25 mg/kg/day—an amount clearly in the generally recommended range.

Now, at the interface between scientific purity and public health action, where intellect and common sense must come together, the experts met long into the night. Each had been trained to analyze data based on research principles. They methodically discussed possible study flaws. They struggled with these and with the bottom line. How would they put academic concerns in context with the real world? There were critical questions to answer. Could four separate studies with essentially the same results all be wrong? Could they all have some common unidentified flaw? Was any flaw severe enough to invalidate the conclusions? What should be done?

Strom recalled asking the group, sometime after midnight, "Would any of us give aspirin to our own kids after hearing these data?" The answer was unequivocal. The conclusion of the draft report, which they completed the next day, was now clearly focused. The panel stated the results of the four studies were strong and consistent and could not be explained away.

On 12 November 1981, Alexander mailed the group's final edited summary statement to Walter Dowdle, Director, Center for Infectious Diseases at CDC.[3] It indicated that the CDC had not gone far enough. "Until the nature of the association between salicylates and Reye syndrome is clarified, the use of salicylates should be *avoided*, [emphasis added] when possible, for children with varicella infections and during presumed influenza outbreaks." It also made recommendations regarding labeling of salicylate and other antipyretics in combination products and questioned the usefulness of antipyretics in such products. Essentially, the experts had shot down decades of physician practice and consumer habit.

In a letter to the editor in the November issue of *Pediatrics*, former EIS Officer Calvin Linnemann of the University of Cincinnati suggested that a decline in Reye's syndrome commensurate with a decline in aspirin use would provide additional evidence of a link.[4] At the same time University of Chicago physicians were doubting the link as the blood or urine was completely negative for salicylate in 15 of 43 consecutive Reye's cases seen at their hospital since 1975.[5]

A year had passed since CDC and FDA first had discussions about the link. On 4 December 1981, CDC Director William Foege forwarded the consultant report to FDA Commissioner Hayes "because most of our consultants' recommendation normally come under the aegis of the Food and Drug Administration."[6,7] CDC made plans to publish a fourth article on Reye's syndrome and the link with aspirin in the *MMWR*. The article would contain the consultants' recommendations.

What happened next can best be described as a free-for-all with the CDC, the FDA, industry, and various academic researchers each advancing a point of view. In 2009 Foege recalled the aspirin manufacturers went directly to his office and even phoned him at home when he was visiting his parents in Portland, Oregon, during the 1981 Christmas holiday. Six-foot-seven-inch-tall Foege was no pushover. The son of a Lutheran minister, he had grown up in the state of Washington and as a teenager had wanted to work in Africa after reading about Albert Schweitzer. He earned a medical degree from the University of Washington and volunteered for a church mission in Nigeria where the CDC was launching its smallpox eradication program. In 1966 Foege played a pivotal role in the eradication of smallpox in West and Central Africa by developing a system of vaccinating around cases rather than using blanket vaccination. Foege was known for his brilliant insightfulness, sense of fairness, down-to-earth speaking ability, and love of practical jokes.

A myriad of public health issues was pressing when the aspirin manufacturers knocked on Foege's door. According to Foege, as he later recalled, they kept making the point that no single study was statistically significant on its own. While each of the studies, if analyzed simply by comparing use between the case and control groups, was "statistically significant," the manufacturers focused on a statistical concept whereby if many factors are evaluated, there should be an adjustment to the probability calculations. Their strategy was clear, though. They were trying to punch holes in the studies. According to the *San Francisco Chronicle*, two aspirin manufacturers "directly urged the CDC not to publish any statement linking aspirin to Reye's syndrome without consulting the FDA, or before 'more reliable' studies could be undertaken."[8] In research terms reliable is a synonym for reproducible. The Arizona study had been reproduced three times.

The eyes of epidemiologists are trained on three things—the reproducibility of the findings, the magnitude of the association, and biologic plausibility. The Arizona results had been replicated three times and the magnitude was rarely seen. The FDA had the facts on biologic plausibility laid out in the 1977 draft monograph as well as in the publication in *Clinical Toxicology* and *The Lancet* editorial. Yet, as Foege recalled,

They [the manufacturers] repeatedly came back and said CDC doesn't have anything ... they would come with new information ... to be reanalyzed ... that was always the same things rewritten ... you could not ignore it until you had gone through it ... I had been saying we are going to publish this [the consultant's report] whether it is statistically significant or not. We are going to let everyone know what we know, and they were trying to abort that. Here was their big argument: The reputation of CDC is so good it would be a shame if you ruined it on the basis of a publication that is not statistically significant.

On 19 January 1982, Sterling met with CDC. Sterling's statistical consultants from the School of Public Health at the University of North Carolina, and Rensselaer Polytechnic Institute had concluded that problems in the design, execution, and analysis were of sufficient magnitude to question support of a warning statement. According to Sterling, the meeting terminated with CDC stating it would not publish the entire consultant group report, would notify Sterling of the content of any summary it published (before publication), and would approach the FDA.[9]

When Foege and FDA communicated on 20 January 1982, the FDA agreed to put its name on the MMWR article, if appropriate, according to a handwritten note on file at the FDA dated 11 February.[10] The memo also noted its first contact with industry on the topic had been the previous week. On 1 February, the Director, Bureau of Drugs, FDA, sent a memo to the FDA's Executive Communication Staff with the subject line "Bureau of Drugs' Hot Items" stating that some observers consider Reye's syndrome to be among the top 10 causes of death in children ages one to 10 years.[11] The memo indicated that FDA was working with CDC on the MMWR article.

Chapter 22

Misbranded, Early 1982

> *You cannot reason people out of a position that they*
> *did not reason themselves into.*
>
> Ben Goldacre, *Bad Science*, 2010

Cincinnati produces fifth case-control study

In any field beside the conservative field of medicine the report published in *The Lancet* in January 1982 would have been called a bombshell.[1] It was a fifth case-control study pointing at aspirin. The authors, Cincinnati researchers (some had moved to the State University of New York at Stonybrook) led by Jacqueline Partin, were careful not to overstate their findings, yet the numbers spoke for themselves. They introduced their study with a description of a child on chronic salicylate therapy, a very high serum salicylate level, and Reye's syndrome. Altogether they studied 130 children with confirmed Reye's syndrome and controls. The children with Reye's syndrome had taken two to three times more salicylate than controls. The amounts were at or close to the typically recommended amounts. The total average amount of salicylate taken by cases and controls in Cincinnati was almost identical to that of the Arizona children as shown in Table 22.1, around 5000 mg.

At hospital admission, the children with Reye's syndrome had higher serum salicylate levels than several different control groups. The difference was stark. For 27 children with Reye's syndrome, the average initial salicylate level was 9.6 mg/dL. For 79 healthy controls, 37 with upper respiratory infections, and 17 with varicella, the levels were 0.8, 1.0, and 1.5 respectively. Because many of the children had vomited for 33 to 55 hours before admission, the authors concluded: "It seems

Table 22.1 Salicylate reported to have been taken before vomiting by children in Arizona and Cincinnati, Ohio

	Average amount of salicylate (mg) (Number who took aspirin/total studied)	
Children with	Arizona Study, 1980	Cincinnati Study, 1982
Reye's syndrome	5164 (7/7)	5434 (61/64)
Upper respiratory infection controls	2607 (8/16)	2220 (29/35)
Chickenpox controls	Not done	3114 (12/13)

likely that serum salicylate concentrations entered the toxic range in many patients with Reye's disease before they presented for treatment." Twenty-one patients who died or had serious neurologic deficits had significantly higher average levels (15 mg/dL) than the 103 patients who survived without neurologic consequences (10 mg/dL). The authors wrote: "Salicylates are mitochondrial toxins and mitochondria are known to be significantly injured in Reye's disease." They concluded, "it seems wise to avoid the use of aspirin [emphasis added] in children during outbreaks of Reye's disease."

This stunning research spawned a tit-for-tat string of letters in *The Lancet*. Researchers from Louisville and Syracuse agreed the levels must have been previously higher.[2] In contrast, Brian Andresen of the NRSF [Ohio] Research Laboratory at Ohio State and Ohio State colleagues suggested serum salicylate levels were not sufficiently accurate.[3] Later that year Andresen and colleagues wrote about the "folly" of wrongly accusing a drug.[4] The same month another editorial in *The Lancet* stated, "[t]he cause" of Reye's syndrome remains "unknown" pointing out that more genetic disorders related to altered metabolism were being discovered.[5]

Aspirin visits the AAP

The AAP Redbook Committee with the CDC consultants' report in hand drafted another statement for publication, this time for the January 1982 issue of AAP *News and Comment*.[6] By early February, the

AAP Committee on Drugs had unanimously endorsed (with a minor edit) the statement that the Redbook Committee had written. The statement was definitive: children with febrile illnesses resembling influenza or varicella should not be given aspirin.[7]

Then, Plough "got wind" of it.[8] According to AAP Executive Director pediatrician M. Harry Jennison who in 2008 reflected on the events of early 1982, Plough's representatives travelled to the AAP headquarters in Evanston, Illinois and met with him. Jennison's position was a non-voting but influential one. Jennison recalled that Plough had sent three men. "Flew up in their private jet, three of these suits, looked pretty impressive," he said. "The guy who may have flown the plane, he was a take-charge guy ... and he just looked ominous. I remember that well. He had a scowl on his face, and they quickly got to the point that ... if you publish that statement 'We are going to sue you all the way to the Supreme [Court].' I was in no position to respond for the academy. I said, 'I hear you and I will take your message to the Executive Board.'"[9, 10] Plough denied threatening a lawsuit, but according to a report in the *San Francisco Chronicle*, "warned the academy that publishing the paragraph without further scientific review would be 'precipitous.'"[11]

Ralph Kauffman recalled that on the day that *News and Comment* was to be mailed out to the membership an AAP staffer made a frantic call to him. He was Professor of Pediatrics and Pharmacology at Wayne State University, a member of the CDC consultant group, and chairman of the AAP Section Committee on Clinical Pharmacology and Therapeutics. The staffer asked if he could hop on a plane and come down that morning because lawyers representing the aspirin industry were meeting with the Executive Board and were threatening all kinds of things. The Board needed technical support. Kauffman flew to Chicago but was not allowed into the meeting.

After the meeting, the AAP withheld the controversial issue of *News and Comment*, all 30, 000 copies,[12] and printed a revised issue.[13] Along with news of the promotion of pediatrics as a medical specialty, marketing of breast milk substitutes, and Board approval to move their headquarters to a new location, the new issue contained a memo from the Executive Board to its members at large entitled "Reye Syndrome and Aspirin." *The memo summarized the CDC consultant group statement but made no direct statement of the Academy's position on aspirin use in children.*[14]

CDC publishes recommendations—without the FDA

On 9 February, Soller called Marion Finkle, Associate Director, New Drug Evaluation, Bureau of Drugs, indicating he was aware that FDA "would be included in the forthcoming *MMWR* of CDC as an endorser of CDC's position of a possible association between ASA and Reye's syndrome." He said Glenbrook had obtained access to the data from Ohio and its position was there were serious flaws with the conclusions. According to Finkle, Soller asked the FDA to keep an open mind until a meeting on 11 February and suggested the FDA ask CDC to remove its name from the *MMWR*.[15] On 11 February at 3 pm, the day before the *MMWR* was to be released, nine representatives from Sterling Drug, Bristol Myer Products, and Schering-Plough met with 13 FDA staff.[16] After the meeting, an FDA deputy director urgently called Foege and told him the aspirin manufacturers had new information and, therefore, CDC could not publish the next day.

Foege later recalled wrestling with the problem that entire evening. In the morning, he got into his car, drove to the CDC, climbed the stairs to his office, greeted his co-workers, and did not say a word about the call. "So, no one else was on the hook except me." The *MMWR* was published as planned. The 12 February issue of the *MMWR* first reported that CDC had received half as many reports of Reye's syndrome—221 cases—than it had during the previous year when 555 cases had been logged. Of these, 77% had been hospitalized between 5 December 1980 and 27 March 1981, coincident with reports of influenza A and while the three state study reports were first being publicized. It noted that another Michigan study confirmed the first three.[17] The editorial note contained the consultants' recommendation, which stated, "the use of salicylates should be *avoided*, when possible, for children with varicella infections and during presumed influenza outbreaks."

Foege later recalled that

The aspirin manufacturers just went ballistic. The first thing they did was they went to Ed Brandt, my boss, [Edward N. Brandt, Jr was the Assistant Secretary of the Department of Health and Human Services (DHHS) and acting Surgeon General of the Public Health Service] and, believe it or not, he stood up for what I had done. And he would not back down. They then went to [DHHS] Secretary Richard Schweicker and he backed me, unbelievably, when you think about this ... and they then went to the White House and the next thing we [CDC] got was to cease and desist ... and to do another study. My reaction to that was fine. We will do that because the word is already out. You can't pull that back. So, the whole world knows what we know even if we do not know what it means.

Now the FDA, facing both its legal responsibilities and the Reagan administration's hands-off philosophy, issued a "Talk Paper" summarizing the *MMWR* article.[18]

Sidney Wolfe and the FDA

The four CDC-state studies, the Partin study, the independent consultants' analysis, and the explanations of biologic plausibility by both Snodgrass and colleagues and the anonymous editorial in *The Lancet* had created a growing belief in the validity of the aspirin–Reye's link, and its implication for prevention. In terms of action, however, it was physician Sidney Wolfe, Director of Public Citizen's Health Research Group (HRG), who turned up the heat. Wolfe had co-founded the HRG with consumer advocate Ralph Nader in 1971. According to the *New York Times*, Wolfe had become "incensed" when he had learned that, while patients were dying from contaminated intravenous drugs made by Abbott Laboratories, the FDA had allowed continued sale of the products and instructed hospitals to disconnect the fluids at the first sign of infection. Wolfe and Nader wrote a letter to the agency "insisting the FDA force the drug's withdrawal" and "gave it to every major news organization." Abbott announced a recall. This event cemented Wolfe's passion for health-related consumer activism. Unconcerned with formality or style, his entire persona contrasted sharply with the demeanor and reserve of the corporate executives and lawyers with whom he battled. "Dr Wolfe agrees that he has trouble being polite with adversaries. He almost never speaks with drug company executives, and he avoids lobbying on Capitol Hill because his tendency to speak his mind hurts his cause."[19] He considered his work to be that of the people's advocate.

Wolfe learned of industry's attempts to stop the publication of the consultant's report. In a four-page press release he stated "the Reagan Administration, yielding to pressure from drug companies, has delayed for more than two months a major public health warning that could have prevented the injuries and deaths of many children" and that according to its sources and a memo, "two manufacturers have urged that CDC make no premature statements until FDA takes action."[20] On 12 February, CDC's Public Affairs Director Don Berreth explained to the *Atlanta Journal* that, unlike the FDA which does issue warnings, CDC is not a regulatory agency and can only issue advice.[21] On 27 February, Wolfe called FDA's Frank Rosa recommending the FDA add a warning to the drug label and issue an "immediate statement to avoid any further deaths." He accused the CDC, the FDA, and the Executive Board of the American Academy of Pediatrics of being stalled by the aspirin companies.[22]

Wolfe's proposal to inform both consumers and physicians would become the blueprint for solving the problem of Reye's syndrome. A warning on the label seemed to be the only practical way to ensure that everyone had an equal opportunity to know about the potential danger. Yet, vastly different resources funded the various positions on a warning label. The pain-reliever market in the United States was worth more than $1 billion. Wolfe quoted an estimate of the 1980 market for aspirin-containing products of $671 million with children's aspirin contributing about $50 million.[23] In 1982, an article in the *Wall Street Journal* estimated the market for children's aspirin to be $85 to

$100 million.[24] (Industry reported that about 49 million packages of children's aspirin were sold annually from 1971–1981.[25]) Most children with Reye's syndrome in the Arizona study however had taken adult-size aspirin. In 1982, the FDA and CDC budget were similar at about $675 million each (in fiscal year 2000 dollars) with NIH funding being about sevenfold greater.[26] In real-time dollars, the CDC budget was about $105 million.[27] Wolfe's Public Citizen was non-profit.

Skeptics

Industry had already approached the CDC, FDA, NIH, AAP, and others with attempts to control the narrative. Now it set it eyes on no less than the entire US federal government—all three branches. But first it needed skeptical scientists and physicians aligned with its position. A skeptic could present an opinion of the situation and oppose a label. Industry would tout the experts in memos to the FDA, to the media, and in Congressional testimony.

The skeptics fell into several groups. The first were basic science researchers. Skeptical by profession and accustomed to the definitive answers of laboratory experiments, they found the epidemiologic studies, which used data from humans in real-life situations and gave answers in probabilities, messy, complex, and potentially biased. Industry relied heavily on the words of researchers including members of the Scientific Advisory Board of the NRSF [Ohio], Ohio State University colleagues, and Ohio State researcher Brian Andresen.

On 17 February, Sterling provided the FDA with a summary of studies refuting the biology of the link.[28] One by Board member June Aprille showing that high blood salicylate levels were needed to inhibit mitochondria in the lab implied these levels were not reached in children with Reye's syndrome.[29] Another, by Board member F.J.S. Crocker, suggested an environmental toxin,[30] and two by Ohio State University researchers summarized (in numbers too small to be definitive) chemical differences between Reye's syndrome and salicylism.[31, 32] The summary also refuted my talk at the Vail conference in June 1981 stating there was "apparent confusion on the part of one study investigator (Dr K. Starko at the Vail Conference) … as to the distinction between the liver pathology of salicylism and that of Reye's Syndrome."[33] This "apparent confusion" was all there would be during 1982 because despite submissions to three journals Mullick and I could not get the liver pathology paper published.

Senior academic and practicing physicians comprised a second group of skeptics. Some physicians generally believed that a warning would hurt the practice of pediatrics by inhibiting aspirin use or possibly engendering lawsuits. Therefore, they reasoned more certainty was necessary. Doctors caring for children with arthritis and George Johnson the EIS officer who claimed to have investigated the first outbreak in the United States fell in this group, as did academic pediatricians at Wayne State University School of Medicine, who simply believed the studies were not good enough. The Wayne State doctors included Alan Done the aspirin expert who had been a Special Assistant to the Director of Pediatric Pharmacology at the FDA from 1972 to 1975 and was now a consultant to Plough, Sanford Cohen, and Henry Nadler. Both Cohen and Nadler were influential with the AAP. Cohen was Professor of Pediatrics, Associate in the Department of Pharmacology, and Associate Dean and had served six years on the AAP Committee on Drugs.[34] Nadler, known for his work in genetics, was Dean of the School of Medicine.[35] Nadler would submit comments for an upcoming FDA meeting and Cohen would speak.[36]

In addition, a new group was spawned by academic pediatricians Sydney Gellis at Tufts (who had been sparring with Mortimer over the role aspirin played in Reye's for years) and Heinz Eichenwald, Professor of Pediatrics at the University of Texas Southwestern Medical School in Dallas. Eichenwald, the group's first leader, was a graduate of Harvard University and Cornell University Medical College and known as a man of high integrity. In 1969, he had told Senate investigators that "… 'misleading advertising' had lured 'the gullible physician' into prescribing useless and sometime dangerous drug combinations."[37] Eichenwald told me in 2008 that he had first discussed the issue casually with Gellis and Gellis had suggested the names of most of the invitees for a meeting at the American Pediatric Society in May 1982. The men agreed the link remained unproven. Gellis had then introduced him to Neil Chayet, in a phone conversation, "I believe, as a public interest lawyer, whom he knew personally and held in high regard ... He [Chayet] assured me that any necessary funding would be from private donors that he had access to, so Gellis and I got busy recruiting [interested parties]."

Chayet had previously studied potential abuse of package inserts. As an attorney with a Boston firm, chairman of the Health and Disability Law Committee of the Massachusetts Bar Association, and founder of Doctor's Protective, he had recently written an article for *The Internist* encouraging doctors to get involved in drug issues lest they become victims of lawsuits.[38] Eichenwald recalled that he himself had contacted four experts, two Yale professors, a World Health Organization statistician, and a Johns Hopkins statistician who, according to Eichenwald, agreed the CDC-state studies "should never have been published."

As Eichenwald later recalled, the group first decided to review the data. He said, "It is possible that a pharmaceutical company, hearing about these activities, also asked us to review the data, but I frankly don't remember that ... I personally had no contact with the aspirin industry ... Among our activities was to enlist the AAP to call for a definitive study as well as other professional organizations such as the Infectious Disease Society ... etc."

Indiana University pediatrician Joseph Fitzgerald recalled attending the first committee meeting. A straight shooter who cared deeply for children, Fitzgerald had founded pediatric gastroenterology at the Riley Hospital for Children in 1969. The members of the group, he remembered, were "all reasonable, and were going to try to just make people really look at this data ... How do you explain the other 45% [who used aspirin and didn't get Reye's]?" It is unclear where he got that number. Years later, after he had accepted the link, he recalled his early impression: "[M]y career was always skeptical of statistics. You know—statistics are needed ... but I was always skeptical naturally as

a guy that spends hours and hours at the bedside of these patients …
I probably had an inherent prejudice." Fitzgerald had trained during a
time when statistics classes were rare in medical school curricula.

Chayet soon would help the fledgling group formalize under the
name the Committee on the Care of Children (CCC). (Much later, the
San Francisco Chronicle reported Chayet had organized a similar group
earlier, the Committee on the Care of Diabetics, which "successfully
delayed efforts to inform diabetics" that diet and exercise might control
their illness.[39])

Another source of skepticism was the new Colorado Foundation,
which received funds from Sterling.[40] Executive Director Paul Hinson
voiced the opinion of the foundation, which generally seemed to echo
that of the manufacturers.

Finally, industry hired professional statisticians. Sterling hired
a private statistical organization called Biometric Resource Institute
(BRI) and Plough sought the help of physicians John Wilson and R.
Don Brown at Louisiana State University Health Sciences Center.
Wilson was influential because of his lifelong interest in pediatric
pharmacology and advocacy for the study of drugs used for children.[41]
According to Wilson who spoke with me in 2009, Brown, a colleague,
had recently taken a class in statistics and used his new knowledge to
write an article critiquing the CDC-state studies. On 16 February 1982,
a Plough representative indicated he would send a copy of Wilson and
Brown's analysis to the FDA and request a meeting between FDA staff
and Plough's consultants.[42]

At the same time, medical advisors of the Michigan foundation
were feeling compassion for parents, many of whom must have by now
been realizing that they had given aspirin to their children. Empathic
physician Wallace Berman, chairman of the NRSF of Michigan
treatment study group, spoke of it to me later. "We were all pretty
much on the same page, it was interesting; there was no causal link. We
were concerned about it … we were afraid that families were not going
to deal well with it … unless we could really nail it down and prove

it." The Michigan advisors, whose natural interest was to find a way to treat the critically ill children, were busy with a major campaign to get a treatment trial up-and-running.

This powerful mix of alleged study flaws and influential skeptics created a swirl of controversy. Industry would soon use the purported flaws and skeptics to lobby the powerful bodies of Congress, the executive branch of the Federal Government, the US court system, and, in a final coup de grace, the American Academy of Pediatrics.

Wolfe, the FDA, and the AAP

I was now overseeing immunization programs and managing the sexually transmitted disease clinics at the Maricopa County Health Department in Phoenix. The boys were growing. *Goodnight Moon.* Yellow trucks. Nursery school. Walks to the Circle K. Dusty summer desert storms. I monitored the situation from afar and obsessed over the evidence. Everything lined up, the epidemiology, the pharmacology, and the pathology. But could it be wrong? The counter narratives were unnerving. The criticisms by industry and the negative reviews of the liver paper weighed heavily upon me. It was obvious that most children did not need aspirin for colds, flu, or chickenpox. The label was a good idea. What better way to let everyone know? Parents should have this information. My goal now was to get the AFIP liver data published. Between January and July 1982, three US medical journals declined publication[43, 44, 45]

Although summaries of the Ohio and Michigan data had been provided to industry, it had not been able to review the "raw" data. And what it had seen it did not agree with. In March 1982 the FDA finally convened a Reye's Syndrome Working Group tasked with reviewing the state studies, performing site visits to Ohio and Michigan, conducting audits/analyses, meeting with industry, and preparing reports. The work was to be completed by May 1982. [46] Wolfe found this delay unacceptable. On 9 March, Wolfe's HRG formally petitioned the FDA "to immediately change the labeling on all aspirin-containing products."[47] HRG supplemented its petition on 8 April by letter, citing the Food Drug and Cosmetic Act, 21 US, prohibiting the sale in interstate commerce of any "misbranded" drug. The Act read:

> A drug or device shall be deemed misbranded ...
>
> Unless its labeling bears (1) adequate directions for use; and (2) such adequate warning against use in those pathological conditions or by children where its use may be dangerous to health, or against unsafe dosage or methods or duration of administration or application ...[48]
>
> 1938 Food Drug and Cosmetic Act, 21 US

According to the HRG, aspirin products were "misbranded" within the meaning of law and a warning label was therefore required. If the FDA did not respond by 30 April 1982, HRG would consider its petition denied.[49]

Plough went directly to doctors to set the record straight. In early March, John M. Clayton, PhD, Vice President of Clinical Research at Plough, sent a letter to US pediatricians claiming, "in view of a just-completed in-depth analysis at the Medical Center of a major [unnamed] University ... Aspirin is a safe and highly effective medication for the reduction of fever in children." The letter noted that the analysis had found the reports linking aspirin and Reye's syndrome were "misleading and unjustified." Clayton's letter exuded certainty: "Therefore, you should feel confident in continuing to recommend aspirin for the reduction of fever in children."[50]

On 5 and 6 March, AAP Executive Director Jennison briefed the AAP Committee on Drugs meeting in Alexandria, Virginia. First, a new statement from the Redbook Committee [the Committee on Drugs would not be a co-signer as it had been in 1981] would be published in the June issue of *Pediatrics*. Also, during the spring AAP meeting in Hawaii, the aspirin industry was planning to hold a non-Academy session with a presentation by John Wilson. And, finally, *Medical World News* was going to carry a story.[51] When the Board met in Maui in mid-March, AAP Vice President James Strain reported that "the Academy acted responsibly in publishing the summary of the CDC panel in the February *News and Comment*." He noted, "At the same time, the Academy wasn't exposed to the legal action that would have occurred if we had published the *original statement* of the Committee on Infectious Disease [Redbook Committee]."[52] (No record of the original statement can be found, even though 30,000 copies had been printed before being withdrawn and possibly destroyed.) Strain noted that the new statement the Redbook Committee had drafted would be published in *Pediatrics* if "approved by the Executive Board." He explained that in the future the AAP Executive Committee would make all final decisions on publication of committee statements.[53] It was becoming clear that the Executive Board and its Executive Committee intended to maintain tight control of messaging.

Meanwhile, Sterling's Soller widely shared the industry's doubt. According to Jennison, Soller lobbied the Academy with academic reasoning. In 2008, Jennison told me that he was "really very impressed" with him. He and Soller had become "good friends." Jennisen felt Soller "was really obliged to say that he didn't see the clarity or legitimate connection between aspirin and Reye's syndrome." The Freudenbergers recalled that Soller visited McDonald's with them and called at their home in Bryan. Michigan EIS officer Waldman told me Soller frequently stopped by the Health Department in Michigan. Doubt played right into Michigan politics. Waldman recalled, "Parents' meetings were happening all the time. They were very emotional ... so sad. All those parents had lost their kids. And they were just angry. I mean it was just awful. And, you know the state ... a lot of antigovernment feeling. The interpretation was that we were telling them that it was their fault. And they wanted it to be somebody else's fault."

Epidemiology studies define probabilities. To anyone without training (at the time few physicians had epidemiology training), the studies must have seemed full of pitfalls and biases, and Soller persuasively pointed out each one.

In April, the FDA met with Sterling, Bristol Meyers, Dow, and Monsanto. They apparently thought the outcome was to their liking as the companies' summary of the meeting concluded, "publication of further cautionary statements by FDA on salicylate usage and Reye's Syndrome is not warranted at this time." Calling the CDC-state studies "preliminary surveys," they recommended "the development of studies based on sound scientific principles, early recognition of Reye's Syndrome, and prudent use of all medications in children."[54]

On 23 April, the FDA provided an "interim response" to Wolfe's petition. Under their regulations, the agency had 180 days to respond to citizen petitions like Wolfe's, and its final response would not be completed until the special working group reviewed and analyzed the data. Undeterred, on 17 May 1982, Wolfe sought an order in the District Court to either direct the FDA to require an appropriate warning label or require the FDA to respond to the merits of HRG's petition within 30 days.[55] The American Public Health Association also petitioned the FDA to require warning labels and threatened legal action.[56]

FDA steps up

On 10 May, the AAP Redbook Committee met in Washington, D.C., and reviewed the "sad saga" of Reye's syndrome. An FDA representative reported that the FDA had reviewed the full data tapes from the Ohio study and had scheduled an open review meeting on 24 May. The big news, however, was that the Committee's new statement, set to appear in the June issue of *Pediatrics, had not been approved by the Board and would be issued only as a committee statement.* Also, several members were upset by the fact that *Pediatrics* had given equal status to an editorial by John Wilson and his associate "on behalf of Plough" rather than printing it as a subsequent letter to the editor. Members voiced concern over "preemptory decisions by the Board or the Executive Committee without consultation with expert committees."[57]

A public review of the FDA working group analysis of the Ohio and Michigan studies was held on 24 May in Wilson Hall on the NIH campus in Bethesda. The full reports of the studies were slated to be published over the summer in the *Journal of the American Medical Association (JAMA).* CDC invited me to Bethesda. I arrived from

Phoenix the night before and checked into the nearby Holiday Inn. I had prepared a statement in the event I was given the opportunity to speak.

In 2011, Joseph Fitzgerald reminded me that he had attended the meeting on behalf of Plough. The relationship had developed through his professional relationship with colleague Sanford Cohen at Wayne State. Both were oral examiners for the American Board of Pediatrics. Cohen, a former member of the AAP Committee on Drugs, would also be testifying. When Fitzgerald arrived, however, he became uncomfortable. "We met all night, but the person who led the meeting was a lawyer by the name of [Robert A.] Altman ... a lot of money was being spent on us ... a lawyer is actually kind of guiding what's going to be the testimony." In the morning, Fitzgerald was driven to Wilson Hall in a limousine. "Just the whole aspect of it was something that, when I got back home, I was not very comfortable with," he recalled. Emotions were running high. Fitzgerald later recalled, "Sidney Wolfe is standing in the hallway hollering—Children are dying while we're talking about this, you know. And I'm trying to give, you know, a rational discussion of the clinical data and the pathology."

It rained that day. The wake-up call I had requested never came. Fortunately, Russ Alexander, who had been chairman of CDC's consultant group, called when I failed to show up for our taxi. We arrived at Wilson Hall at the last minute. The large meeting room was full. Someone led me to the long table that ran down the center of the room. I looked around at my tablemates, a panel of outstanding epidemiologists and physicians. The chairperson of the morning session was Reuel Stallones, Dean of the School of Public Health at the University of Texas, Houston. The chair of the afternoon session was virologist Richard Johnson, Eisenhower Professor of Neurology at the Johns Hopkins University School of Medicine. Others included Walter Dowdle of the CDC; Harry Meyer of the FDA; William S. Jordan of the NIH; and academics Ralph Kauffman, Ted Mortimer, Albert Pruitt, David Lang, Russ Alexander, Neal Nathanson, Jacqueline Partin, Richard Lanese, and Stuart Hartz. Although I had not been scheduled to speak, I sent a message to the chairperson that I would like the opportunity to do so.

Harry Meyer, Director of the Bureau of Biologics at the FDA, opened the meeting by stating that its purpose was a scientific discussion of the FDA's working group audit of the larger studies.[58] The morning session consisted of presentations by the CDC, investigators from Michigan and Ohio, and the members of the FDA working group. The working group's analysis was long and complicated, but the bottom line was that they had not identified any methodological flaw or statistical mistake accounting for the association between aspirin and Reye's syndrome.

The children in the Michigan studies ranged from five to 17 years old. The first study was completed in April 1980; the second study in April 1981. The first showed that 96% of 25 cases took aspirin and the second showed that 100% of 12 cases took aspirin. In both, aspirin use occurred statistically more often than in controls. A reverse and statistically significant association was found with acetaminophen use. No specific brand of aspirin was implicated. The second study revealed that each child had used aspirin previously and even when fever was considered, aspirin was still used more often by cases than controls. [59] (Appendix 5)

The Ohio study enrollment had ended two years earlier on 31 March 1980. The children's initial illness was an upper respiratory tract infection in 85% of cases, chickenpox in 10%, and other illnesses in 5% of subjects. Aspirin was the only drug used by significantly more cases than controls. In a statistical model that considered multiple factors, both aspirin and decreased fluid intake were significantly associated with Reye's syndrome. The maximum and mean daily doses were significantly greater in cases than in controls although for 46 cases (where both body weight and aspirin dose were obtained) the average dose was 47 mg/kg/day. Only 7% received a maximum daily dose greater than 80 mg/kg. In the upcoming publication, the authors would conclude, "This study shows that aspirin at normal doses is associated with Reye's syndrome."[60] (Appendix 5)

Johnson introduced the afternoon speakers. Except for Sidney Wolfe and me, all spoke on behalf of the manufacturers.* Pediatricians from Boston University, State University of New York at Stony Brook, and Wayne State University submitted letters recommending additional studies. The industry presenters discussed inadequacies of the data and called for more study.

In complete opposition, Sidney Wolfe called for "immediate action by the FDA to order warning labels." Failure to do so, he said, not only violated drug laws, but also would "guarantee the continued deaths and injuries." The last speaker, I presented new data from Arizona. All 22 of the children with Reye's syndrome in Arizona since December 1978, including eight who had died, gave a history of salicylate use (in one more usage was unknown). Doctors had measured salicylate levels at hospital admission for 13. All had salicylate present. Six had levels over 20 mg/dL and the doses the children received were in the range normally recommended. Finally, after summarizing a few aspects of epidemiology, I pointed out that aspirin can be toxic to the liver and affect mitochondria and that data on metabolism in children were sparse.

Johnson asked for a reading of the panel's "feeling on summary." Individual comments are paraphrased as follows:

- I came to listen. The FDA will have to decide risk benefit.
- Regulatory decision will have to be based on risk benefit.
- It's a difficult call. I'm not on one side or the other. Let's be

---

* Joseph White, President, represented the Aspirin Foundation. Speakers for Sterling Drug included William Soller, Vice President and Director of Scientific Affairs; Robert Klein of Dartmouth Medical Center; Larry Kupper, Professor of Biostatistics at the University of North Carolina; and Albert Palson, Professor and Chairman of Management Operations, Research and Statistics at Rensselaer Polytechnic Institute. Speakers for Plough included: attorney Robert Altman; internationally recognized biostatistician and developer of the Mantel-Haenszel test Nathan Mantel; Joseph F. Fitzgerald, pediatric gastroenterologist from the James Whitcomb Riley Hospital for Children, Indiana University; Sanford Cohen, Professor of Pediatrics, Associate in the Department of Pharmacology, and Associate Dean at the Wayne State University School of Medicine in Detroit; John Wilson, Professor of Pediatrics and Pharmacology at LSU Medical Center in Shreveport, Louisiana; and John Clayton, Vice President of Clinical Research for Plough, Inc.

careful about what one advises pediatricians.

- Pediatricians should be kept informed, and they should be concerned about prescribing aspirin for their patient with influenza and varicella.
- A note of caution is still justified.
- Aspirin is obviously not the cause of Reye's syndrome. Labeling changes would be inappropriate.
- Caution should be shared with our colleagues and the public.
- It's appropriate for the FDA to advise and caution parents and physicians to manage the symptoms associated with varicella and flu like illnesses ... without antipyretics and with a minimum of pharmacologic preparations altogether. More than that is not warranted.
- I came here to listen; it's appropriate and prudent not to administer any medications including salicylates to children with influenza-like illness or varicella in the absence of other medical indications for their use. How you get the message across is the responsibility of the FDA or the Academy of Pediatrics.
- Inappropriate for me to comment.

As the meeting wound down, I realized that the FDA's 1977 aspirin monograph addressing aspirin pharmacology and concerns with the dose schedule had not been mentioned. The FDA task force consisted of infectious disease internists, pediatricians, epidemiologists, biostatisticians, and a pathologist and had been focused on the epidemiologic studies and certainty.[61] Yet epidemiology studies alone *never* provide certainty. Other information—history, biology, pharmacology, etc.—is needed to shore up certainty.

The meeting ended quietly leaving the FDA to decide if the public should be informed. When I returned to Arizona, I wrote to Harry Meyer stating my belief that the association between Reye's and salicylate use warranted inclusion in the label.[62] The last pillar—FDA oversight—was on the line.

PART VI

POLITICS DECIDES
1982–1986

Chapter 23

Stand Don't Walk, Late 1982

What we want you to do is stand instead of walk.

Representative James H. Scheuer,
Reye's syndrome Hearings
US House of Representatives, 97th Congress
17 and 29 September 1982

During its June meeting, the AAP Executive Board undertook a full agenda including consideration of a major relocation from Evanston to Elk Grove Village, Itasca, or Schaumberg, three sites near Chicago International O'Hare airport. AAP President Glenn Austin reported the Academy's involvement with Washington, including "open discourse with the White House policy advisors and with many HHS luminaries," work with the CDC on the "Aspirin/Reyes Issue," and DHHS Assistant Secretary Edward Brandt, Jr's request for advice. The stark reality was, however, that the Board was distancing itself from the recommendations of its own committee. As AAP Executive Director Jennisen later recalled,

> Bill Soller from Sterling and others ... were very effective lobbyists ... and there was seemingly enough uncertainty and, I don't remember the exact moment, but I can certainly remember the tenor of the discussion of the full Board ... And there was enough uncertainty that they said, "Well, let's just lay it on the committee. Let the committee take the responsibility." But they did authorize its publication in our journal *Pediatrics*. So, that was a tacit endorsement.

AAP member James Cherry put it more bluntly. His recollection was that "[T]hey were afraid of getting sued by St Joseph." The Academy, however, was not yet off the hook.

The Special Report by the AAP Redbook Committee appeared in the June issue of *Pediatrics*. The report concluded there was "a high probability that the administration of aspirin contributes to the causation of Reye's syndrome … and it is the opinion of the Committee that aspirin should *not* [emphasis added] be prescribed under usual circumstances for children with varicella or those suspected of having influenza on the basis of clinical or epidemiological evidence." As for action, the government should "undertake … necessary action to inform the public at large."[2] The AAP Board had not endorsed it. (Curiously a summary of the Bethesda meeting presented to the AAP Board in June, under the title "Reye's and Aspirin Controversy," stated: "The FDA concluded that no warning label for package inserts was necessary, but influenza should be deleted from the list of diseases for which aspirin is indicated."[3])

The Special Report was followed by Wilson and Brown's counterbalancing statement, which was supported in part by Schering-Plough.[4] Wilson and Brown concluded the link was a result of the cases being more ill during the prodromal phase, even though the FDA working group had just disproved that. Wilson and Brown, pharmacology experts, did not mention pharmacology. Yet when it came to a recommendation, they hedged their bets saying their report "should not be construed as our approval or disapproval of aspirin use in children." The same month, in a detailed 34-page article replete with charts and figures in the specialty journal *Therapeutic Drug Monitoring*, Wilson and colleagues predicted that aspirin (80 mg/kg/day) resulted in peak plasma salicylate levels of about 37 milligrams per deciliter as shown in Figure 23.1.[5] These were simulated by computer and not tests of actual children, but the authors concluded such levels could be reached and "associated with salicylate toxicity in the young children." Their work was supported by a grant from Glenbrook Laboratories, Schering-Plough Corporation, and by a Clinical Pharmacology Development grant from the Pharmaceutical Manufacturers Association Foundation. Like the AAP, Wilson and colleagues seemed to be walking a fine line.

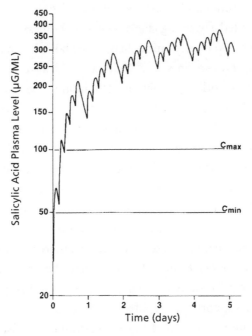

Figure 23.1 Predicted average plasma levels for current (1981) aspirin dose recommendations. The average ASA dose was 13.3 mg/kg (as ASA) or 10.2 mg/kg (as SA) and the dosing interval was 4 h in accordance with that calculated from the package label instructions. One dose was deleted each night.[6]
Wilson, J.T., Brown, R.D., Bocchini, J.A., & Kearns, G.L. (June 1982). Efficacy, disposition and pharmacodynamics of aspirin, acetaminophen and choline salicylate in young febrile children. *Therapeutic Drug Monitoring,* 4(2), 147–180.
Copyright © 1982, Reproduced with permission from Wolters Kluwer Health, Inc.

On 4 June 1982, DHHS Secretary Richard Schweiker, with scientific backing from the CDC, the FDA, and the AAP Redbook Committee, issued a major press release stating that DHSS would launch three actions—a Surgeon General's Advisory, an educational campaign, and a new regulation requiring a Reye's syndrome warning on the label of salicylate-containing medications. The medicine, it said, "has been sufficiently associated with Reye's syndrome to warrant warning physicians and parents."[7] If only it could be that simple.

Aspirin was now under attack on two fronts. Public health professionals wanted a warning label about a fatal illness on the product and the Tylenol brand of acetaminophen, with about 35% market share, was encroaching on aspirin sales.[8] Neither could have been welcome while Sterling was working to obtain FDA approval to market aspirin for prevention of second heart attacks.[9] A warning on aspirin had been successfully thwarted in 1966 when inclusion in the Child Safety Act was abandoned. Now, 16 years later, efforts to avoid a warning label were renewed and escalated like blitzkrieg, the tactic used during World War II, during which "doubt, confusion and rumour were sure to paralyse both the government and the defending military." [10]

On 5 June 1982, a spokesperson for Sterling called Schweiker's proposed warning "inappropriate," and claimed there was "no scientific basis for a causal association." [11] The same day the head of the NRSF [Ohio] laboratory Brian Andresen reported that his preliminary findings did not support the "rapidly growing view" of a relationship between salicylate products and Reye's syndrome. He also expressed concern that parents might think "they may have poisoned their child." [12] The "trouble," he said was that "most of the findings have been based on epidemiologic 'surveys,' not sophisticated chemical research." Andresen's group later called the link "flimsy." [13] In early June, actor Bill Cosby announced he would donate his time to film commercials to be used as public service announcements about Reye's.[14] He began working with the Ohio foundation.

On 6 June, Joseph White, president of the Aspirin Foundation, a nonprofit educational foundation that had been established in January, ignored the fact that industry had just commented at the large meeting in May, accused the Federal Government of acting "hastily and without sound scientific basis," and complained he had asked to present the industry's views to the FDA before they took action.[15] White, a long-time champion of self-medication and consumer access to over-the-counter medicines, had, during the 1960s, served as medical advisor to Miles Laboratories in an important legal case. This case had established that the FDA couldn't limit a "safe OTC drug to prescription use merely because there may be some underlying condition that goes undetected."[16] It was a precarious argument as almost all "side effects" occur only in *some* people, presumably because of their underlying physiology, yet the court had bought it. Members of the Aspirin Foundation would come to include Bristol-Myers Company, Burroughs Wellcome Company, Sterling Drug, Inc., Whitehall Laboratories, Miles Laboratories, Inc., Squibb Corporation, and Proctor & Gamble Company.[17] Schering-Plough remained independent. Soller, now Sterling's Vice President of Scientific Affairs, echoed White.[18]

On 22 June, in a memorandum to DHHS, attorneys for Sterling and Schering-Plough stated there was "no factual or legal basis for the proposed measures." They characterized the case-control studies as "surveys" and "defective" and concluded that a warning label would be unlawful and against the public interest.[19] They had four arguments. First, "there is no reliable record evidence." They backed this up with Ohio State researcher Milo Hilty's comment that the Ohio study "does not in any way establish causal connection," which, of course, is true of all epidemiologic studies. Second, "neither the Department nor interested members of the public have yet had an opportunity—as is customary in public health matters—to conduct a thorough review of all the raw data that underlie the proffered conclusions of the state surveys." It was true the companies had been blocked from access to the raw data (individual records). For reasons of individual patient confidentiality, only summaries had been shared. (In early June, Schering-Plough filed lawsuits in Ohio and Michigan for the data. The Ohio State Attorney General's office agreed to release them. However, Michigan officials continued to block access and a hearing was set.) Their third and fourth arguments were that regulatory action would be unlawful and against the public interest. The memo concluded: "For these reasons, the Department cannot lawfully issue a warning for aspirin products. The Department must instead undertake a full and careful review of all the available data, with an opportunity for proper scientific review."

In July, six FDA medical staff and attorneys met with Joseph White of the Aspirin Foundation, John Clayton of Plough, Kenneth Weiner and William Soller of Sterling, Frank Hurley of Biometrics Research Institute (BRI), and a lawyer named Bruce Dixon. Clayton told the group the case report forms (the forms on which the raw data for each subject are recorded) had been released by the State of Ohio but not by Michigan. BRI would perform a review for industry. It would take eight to 10 weeks.[20]

The NRSF [Ohio] now comprised 106 chapters.[21] It had recently received an anonymous award of $100,000 by an unnamed DC firm to hire an executive director and establish an office a few blocks from the US Senate Building in Washington.[22] A director was hired in May.[23] In its spring 1982 newsletter the foundation published the CDC statement regarding the aspirin–Reye's link in its entirety and summarized the government's plan to require the warning label in its fall newsletter. It now moved toward a vigorous campaign focusing on early diagnosis. Wallace Berman, chairman of the NRSF (Michigan) study group later told me that he had been concerned about blaming parents for killing their kids. Just as Fitzgerald had described Wolfe, Berman talked about a "crazy guy with some of the private agencies who was screaming about labeling" On the issue of the warning label, the new Denver-based American Reye's Syndrome Foundation became the most public voice of parents during most of 1982.

On 25 and 26 June, in Tampa, Florida, at the NRSF (Ohio) annual meeting, keynote speaker Betty Mathias expressed the view that more research was needed on Reye's syndrome.[24] Mathias, a spokesperson for Consolidated Capital Companies of Emeryville, California, discussed recent news articles on salicylates, building up to her punchline: "The implication is pretty clear. What reader, with little or no proper knowledge of Reye's, would not get the impression that aspirin is the culprit responsible for the deaths and injuries of children afflicted with Reye's?" After more examples of "misinformation" and "erroneous material," Mathias read the Foundation's statement indicating that it merited widespread circulation.

> The evidence linking salicylates with Reye's syndrome is epidemiological ...
> A statistical correlation like this one does not indicate cause and effect ...
> In fact, researchers have documented that 25% of all the children who had
> Reye's Syndrome were not given aspirin [it is unclear where this number
> came from because the CDC/state studies found that 95% or greater had
> taken aspirin] ... The Foundation believes that ... further research on the
> cause of Reye's Syndrome is necessary. The Foundation will continue to
> substantively support and encourage research and attention to the diagnosis,
> etiology, and therapy and management of Reye's Syndrome.[25]

Mathias, with a nod to programs such as breast self-examination, indicated that the correct action was *early diagnosis* when the prognosis is most favorable. She said, "Most of the volunteers ... want the answers to this medical mystery."[26] Mathias' plan aligned solidly with that of the Aspirin Foundation of America, Inc. who had recently written: "The only responsible statements that can be made in relation to Reye's syndrome at this time are those that pertain to early recognition of RS and to prudent use of all medications."[27] No one would argue against early diagnosis but this tack seemed to be a distractor. On 19 July, *The Times* of Bryan, Ohio, reported on the Foundation's Florida meeting. It mentioned four studies "on the controversial issue of salicylate use and Reye's syndrome."[28]

The United States House of Representatives soon became involved. In July the House Subcommittee on Natural Resources chaired by Representative James Scheuer, Democrat of New York, "launched an inquiry into government warnings ... after learning there was 'considerable doubt.' ... among some quarters."[29] Nevertheless, the FDA stood by its assessment. On 22 July it estimated "[c]ases of Reye's Syndrome are approximately three to five times more likely to have used salicylate than their matched controls."[30] Yet a visible sign that the government might be backtracking on its stated intention to require a warning label emerged on 25 July during an interview between *New York Times* reporter Michael de Courcy Hinds and FDA Commissioner Arthur Hull Hayes Jr:

Q. What about labeling the risks associated with aspirin? As many as 300 children have died in one year from Reye's syndrome, which medical experts have linked to aspirin used to treat influenza or chickenpox.

A. We've got to decide what that label will say.

Q. Previous warnings to doctors and parents simply noted the statistical association between Reye's syndrome and aspirin. Couldn't labels do the same?

A. There is no data that children who take aspirin for generic flu-like symptoms, as against true viral flu, are at risk for Reye's. Therefore, we must be careful and rather specific about the label, so its wording can be defended in court and so we do not underwarn or overwarn people. Just telling people not to use aspirin is no answer, since for many aspirin is a valuable drug.[31]

On the spot Hayes had invented a new diagnostic paradigm pitting "generic flu-like symptoms" against "true viral flu." Was this distinction part of a strategy to decrease the number of conditions that would appear on any subsequent label? Or was it a step toward eliminating the requirement altogether? Soon after the interview, adjectives describing the upcoming FDA action on the warning label began to change. The August issue of FDA's *Drug Bulletin* stated the "FDA is evaluating *possible* [emphasis added] change in the labeling of products containing aspirin or other salicylates."[32]

Industry analysis versus FDA analysis

On 20 August, the BRI on behalf of Sterling's Glenbrook Laboratory and Schering-Plough completed its report.[33] It asserted that Ohio's second-year data did not "provide sound statistical evidence that the use of aspirin increases the risk of Reye's syndrome." On 31 August, an attorney for Sterling sent to a DHSS General Council a protocol for a new case-control study prepared by Soller and his associates stating this was the type of study they believed should be undertaken.[34]

Sterling Drug asked me for a copy of the CDC-AFIP liver pathology manuscript, which had been sent to *Pediatrics* on 7 July and was under review. I sent a copy.[35] In September, lawyers for Schering-Plough requested the original case forms from the Arizona Department of Health Services which, citing privacy issues, it declined.

In early September, Bruce Gelb, President of the Consumer Products Group of Bristol-Myers, brought up a new concern with HHS Secretary Schweiker. Gelb was worried that a "massive switch" to acetaminophen [mainly Tylenol] based on "seriously flawed studies" could be dangerous. He said the Aspirin Foundation was providing a grant to "the National Foundation on Reye's Syndrome" (not clarifying which one) for a symposium gathering its distinguished "Scientific Advisory Council" to generate ideas for research.[36] Around this time Sterling's Monroe Trout communicated with James Orlowski, Assistant Director of the pediatric ICU at the Cleveland Clinic, who was concerned his patients had not been properly enrolled in the Ohio study.[37] In mid-September, FDA's Gerald Quinnan concluded there was no evidence of Orlowski's claim.[38]

On 17 September, editor Jerold Lucey informed me the CDC-AFIP liver pathology paper would not be accepted by *Pediatrics* based on the assessment of two reviewers.[39] One felt it was an "important paper" and should be "featured prominently" and the other provided a five-page, single-spaced negative review. Frustrated by the divergent assessments, I called Ted Mortimer who wrote to Lucey imploring him to offer me the opportunity to resubmit the paper.[40] Lucey agreed.[41] By then though I had sent the manuscript to *The Lancet* for consideration.

The American Academy of Pediatrics had not yet weighed in on the label and seemed to be off the hook. However, a series of chess-like movements was about to place the Academy in a pivotal position—one that could checkmate the warning label requirement. But first there was still time to air more negative assessments of the studies.

Congress hears testimony on a warning label

In mid-September 1982, Jonah Shacknai, a young lawyer and chief aide to the US House of Representatives, organized a Congressional hearing on the advisability of labeling aspirin. Shacknai, with a bachelor's degree from Colgate and a law degree from Georgetown, would later develop a successful career in the pharmaceutical industry. From 1982 to 1988, he worked as senior partner in the law firm Royer, Shacknai, and Mehle, a group that represented multinational pharmaceutical and medical device companies and four trade organizations. He served as an executive with Key Pharmaceuticals, a company purchased by Schering-Plough. In 1988, he founded Medicis, a wildly successful publicly traded company with products for the treatment of skin and aesthetic conditions.[42] In late 1982, however, Shacknai's job was to assist Representative James H. Scheuer of New York in bringing the issue of protecting children with a warning label on aspirin into the political arena.

On 17 September 1982, Scheuer, Chairman of the House Subcommittee on Natural Resources, Agriculture Research, and Environment, convened a hearing in the Rayburn House Office Building.[43] Scheuer opened by discussing the importance of the "public health of our children" noting that his 87-year-old mother had raised five happy and healthy kids on two nostrums, Vaseline for the outside and aspirin for the inside. "Hundreds of physicians" had called, he said, asking the committee to conduct an investigation because HHS had acted "prematurely." The subject, he noted, was "the controversy surrounding the alleged association between aspirin use and Reye's syndrome."

It was time to hear from some of the skeptics. The witness list was comprised of six persons who opposed the warning label and two who favored it. Absent were academicians from the CDC consultant list, experts on aspirin pharmacology, and representatives of the AAP. Pediatrician George Johnson of Fargo, North Dakota, the former EIS officer, testified he was worried that "the clamor over this tenuous association … would … divert practicing physicians from the urgent task of future research." Other speakers, including Heinz Eichenwald, focused on two points: more review and/or data were needed, and parents might be frightened away from a needed medication. The Director of the Dartmouth-Hitchcock Arthritis Center stressed the needs of children with rheumatic disorders, especially juvenile arthritis. Paul Hinson, executive director of the National (previously called "American") Reye's Syndrome Association of Colorado, expressed concern that if parents had not given aspirin, they would not bring their child to a doctor for early diagnosis and that the warning "laid a very heavy guilt trip with parents who had recently lost children." John Crocker, professor of epidemiology at Dalhousie University in Halifax and a member of the Ohio Scientific Advisory Board, brought methodology concerns, but concluded: "I am not as committed to an absolute clean bill of health for aspirin as many of my colleagues." Nonetheless, he added that warning the public was "a bit of an overkill." Frank Hurley, president of BRI, testified that BRI had concluded that the second year of the Ohio study did not provide "sound statistical evidence."

During the first day of the hearing, the only witness to testify in complete support of a warning for physicians and parents as "a minimal response" was Dr Reuel Stallones, Dean of the School of Public Health at University of Texas in Houston. Stallones had been the co-chairman of the FDA's 24 May meeting. Shacknai asked Stallones if he would change his view if the AAP did. Stallones replied, "If evidence is presented to indicate that there is no credible link between salicylates and Reye's syndrome, I think we should all change our minds."

In a final note, Scheuer thanked Shacknai for his "outstanding professionalism" and meticulous concern. The hearing would be continued on 29 September 1982, a day that Americans would remember for years.

On Monday 21 September, DHHS Secretary Schweiker, who presided over the FDA, NIH, and CDC, stubbornly ignored the testimony at Scheur's hearing and reiterated his plan to propose a new labeling requirement for aspirin, and to conduct a public awareness program.[44] The warning label, however, required a specific regulatory process: publication of the proposed rule in the Federal Register followed by a 90-day period to allow for comments, after which the warning would become mandatory if no compelling argument was made to indicate otherwise. Schweiker's proposed label for OTC aspirin would read:

Warning: This product contains a salicylate. Do not use in persons under 16 years of age with flu or chickenpox unless directed by your doctor. The use of salicylates to treat these conditions has been reported to be associated with a rare but serious childhood disease called Reye's syndrome.[45]

The label for prescription aspirin would be similar.[46]

An educational campaign by FDA did not require a regulation. Thus, Schweiker also planned to roll out a public service campaign through newspapers and broadcast outlets and a brochure that would consist of mailings to 150,000 pharmacists and 100,000 other healthcare professionals.[47]

Each time Schweiker spoke, however, industry responded. Joseph White immediately advised that efforts should be directed toward early diagnosis and treatment.[48] Sterling said a warning would be "inappropriate and scientifically unjustified," and the data were "fatally flawed."[49] Yet Al Gore of Tennessee, member of the House of Representatives, complained, "It won't be done in time for the flu season, will it?"[50] Schweiker responded that he believed the public service campaign would alert the public in time for the peak months of winter flu. Exasperated, Gore noted that Schweiker had started the process on 4 June, "and it takes so much time that we'll go through another flu season without labels on the product." "Well, you won't go through another flu season without the warning," Schweiker snapped back.[51]

The educational campaign might have to do. Another roadblock to the regulation was in place—approval by the Office of Management and Budget (OMB).

On 21 September, I received a letter from Vincent A. Fulginiti, Chairman of the AAP Redbook Committee and founder of the Department of Pediatrics at the University of Arizona, School of Medicine. Lucey had asked him to respond to a new letter sent to *Pediatrics* from Louisiana State researchers Brown and Wilson.[52] Fulginiti asked if I would write the reply. Of course. I submitted a response in October, but it would not be published until February, too late to have any effect on what would happen next.[53]

On 28 September the NIH held a Workshop on Disease Mechanisms and Prospects for Prevention of Reye's Syndrome.[54] In attendance were representatives of the Ohio and Michigan foundations, staff from CDC, NIH, the FDA, and others. A summary (published in November 1983) concluded that identification of risk factors was "clearly the most important area of investigation" and current poorly defined risk factors included: viral infection, age <18 years, suburban habitat, and "possibly" salicylate use during the prodromal illness. *The Wall Street Journal* even dubbed the link "theoretical." After citing the conclusion of the AAP Redbook Committee that the data were sufficient for a warning and the concept that a decline in Reye's syndrome after a decline in aspirin use would be evidence strengthening the link, the *Journal* presented counter arguments. For example, Sanford Cohen of Wayne State described a "climate of hysteria" at the FDA meeting and Soller suggested rural cases may be due to a flame retardant and complained of a "railroad mentality."[55]

That evening, Congressman Scheuer consulted AAP President Glenn Austin as to the Academy's position on the warning label. Austin dodged the issue and informed Scheuer that the full membership of the AAP and its governing body had not yet weighed in.[56] In other words, the AAP did not yet have a position.

September 29 began like any other day in Washington, D.C. Scheuer summarized his view of the testimony to date saying that the evidence "is far too tentative and far too flawed for any type of regulatory action to be contemplated." He also stated that the actions being considered by DHSS "could actually do great injury to the 150,000 juvenile arthritics in our country for whom aspirin is by far the best drug of choice." Scheuer expressed particular concern with Secretary Schweiker's announcement.

Scheuer then assured the first witness, DHHS Assistant Secretary Edward Brandt, Jr, that "[t]he only thing that will be questioned are the judgmental factors involved in making this decision." Brandt was accompanied by Walter Dowdle, Director of CDC's Center for Infectious Diseases; Harry Meyer, Director of the National Center for

Drugs and Biologics; and Jerry Quinnan, Director of the FDA's Division of Virology of the National Center for Drugs and Biologics.

Brandt reviewed the long history that culminated in the conclusions of both the outside CDC consultant group and the FDA Working Group. He summarized the DHSS action plan, noting that physicians and other health-care professionals had already been alerted to the link in a June 1982 Surgeon General's Advisory in the *MMWR*, and in the August *FDA Bulletin*. Brandt concluded: "We believe … that we are obliged to inform the public." He quoted the testimony of Reuel Stallones: "Taking action on evidence that is incomplete or inconclusive is commonly required and the decision to do so is usually uncomfortable and sometimes agonizing. However, in this instance we have sufficient information that salicylates may pose a hazard that to do nothing appears to me to be irresponsible."

Vigorous questioning ensued as Scheuer probed various areas including malpractice litigation, the objectivity of participants at the May meeting, the qualifications of the Ohio investigators, the complaint by Ohio clinician Orlowski that his cases were not included, and a statement that the parent foundations (American and National) had not been consulted before Schweiker's label announcement.

Scheuer complained that HSS had gone over the heads of physicians to speak directly to (ironically) mothers, and that in the "fuzzy business of communicating," parents … might get an "inchoate fear that aspirin is bad and leads to all kinds of horrible diseases, and therefore don't give your kid aspirin." Brandt replied the message was not that aspirin was bad, but that "if your child has either chickenpox or a flu-like syndrome, you should not give aspirin without consulting your physician. Now, I do not find that this is bad advice to tell them to do that. That is advice that is shared in by the American Academy of Pediatrics."

Scheuer was prepared. He interrupted and informed Brandt that he had talked with the AAP president the previous night, "I understand that that was their infectious disease committee and that the full membership and governing body have not acted yet." Brandt was caught off guard. The AAP's position was unclear. This left a huge void, one that was unanticipated, at least by Brandt. Scheuer then clarified that a targeted physician advisory would be acceptable: "We know that physicians are capable of coping intelligently with the information that you have to give them." Informing the public at large was the problem.

Scheuer then commented that recent studies had failed to show a link with pesticides and perhaps the same would be true of aspirin "and it all goes to underline the need in this extraordinarily difficult area, for all parties concerned to tread very carefully in, as I said before, what is proving to be a minefield." To this, Brandt replied "let me assure you, Mr. Chairman, that we do intend to walk cautiously through that minefield. As one who had been standing in it for a while, I can assure you that we will be as careful as we can be."

Scheuer then made his position crystal clear: "What we want you to do is stand instead of walk."

As the hearing ended, Scheuer said he understood how the public could be confused about the difference between association and causation and pointed out that Brandt may have added to the confusion in that he had "interlarded" his testimony by using softened language, like "tended" to indicate an association. Scheuer wondered if Brandt himself was not even sure of an association, let alone possible causation between aspirin and Reye's syndrome.

Extra Strength Tylenol capsules laced with cyanide

As the hearing proceeded in Washington, a horrific tragedy was unfolding in Chicago.[57, 58] That morning, 12-year-old Mary Kellerman of Elk Grove Village, Illinois, collapsed after taking cyanide-laced Extra Strength Tylenol for a cold. By evening six others, including three members of a single family, the Janus family, had suddenly and unexpectedly fallen gravely ill after taking the same medication. All would soon be dead. The cause was not in doubt—cyanide poisoning.

The bottles of cyanide-laced Extra Strength Tylenol capsules had likely been purchased from Chicago area stores, most near O'Hare Airport. The police were "reasonably certain the killer delivered the packages of death in a single day probably Tuesday September 28th." [59] The perpetrator left no firm clue as to his or her identity or motive.

Death by cyanide follows a progression like that of salicylate intoxication, only faster. Both disrupt the formation of ATP by insertion, like a proverbial monkey wrench, into the critical ATP production pathway. It is a matter of dose. Minuscule and safe amounts of cyanide can be found naturally in foods such as almonds, soy, and spinach. In high enough quantities, what happens next is horrifying. The victim starts to breathe rapidly and deeply. The body abruptly shifts from its usual aerobic (oxygen-derived) metabolism to an anaerobic state, which is much less efficient. Extreme anxiety and agitation precede faintness and a sense of impending doom. Coma and death are not far behind. When a large amount is taken at one time, this sequence of events occurs within seconds to minutes, a result of a profound decline in cellular energy.

Chicago toxicologist Michael Shaffer smelled the characteristic bitter almond odor of cyanide as soon as he opened the bottles retrieved from the Kellerman and the Janus households. [60] Quickly Cook County's medical examiner publicized the news of contaminated bottles of Tylenol and warned that use of the product stop, at least temporarily. [61] The makers of Tylenol Johnson & Johnson (J&J) immediately recalled suspect lots and, as an even more conservative measure, FDA officials advised customers not to take *any* Extra Strength Tylenol capsules, regardless of the lot number, until more information became available. [62]

Investigators quickly concluded that the tampering must have taken place in the retail stores in the Chicago area, likely the evening before. Chicago police and health authorities warned area residents by cruising neighborhoods with bullhorns; Boy Scouts went door to door; church groups initiated telephone drives; schools notified parents; police visited taverns; and cyanide antidote kits were added to area paramedic units. The list of suspects was long—a disgruntled employee or a murderer covering his or her tracks by committing multiple murders. *Newsweek* suggested that "aspirin manufacturers, bloodied by Tylenol in the battle for market share and lately stung by the government studies suggesting a link to Reye's syndrome, seemed to have the most to gain from the Tylenol scare." [63]

Sterling itself had experienced a tampering episode during the summer. Two bottles of its Milk of Magnesia had been spiked with lye and bleach at two stores in Los Angeles. [64]

The Tylenol murders were never solved. The total annual OTC pain-relief market remained at about $1.2 billion. [65] Tylenol suffered only in the short term. The previous year, Tylenol had brought J&J about $425 million in revenue. [66] However, by late October 1982, Tylenol's market share had plummeted from 35.4% in 1981 to 7%. [67] As reported in the *Chicago Tribune*, " 'It appears that regular aspirin products picked up most of Tylenol's share loss,' said the president of Information Resources." [68] However, the effect of the Chicago incident was temporary. J&J quickly restored public confidence by conducting what was later touted as a textbook response to the tragedy. As for the children's pain-relief market, acetaminophen—mainly Tylenol—never again lost the lead it had taken from aspirin in 1981.

Chapter 24

Keep Parents in the Dark, Late 1982

In every battle there comes a time when both sides
consider themselves beaten,
then he who continues the attack wins.

Widely attributed to Ulysses S. Grant,
President of the United States

Warning, now or later?

In the weeks following the Tylenol murders, the manufacturers pressed
the government, the AAP, and others to delay the proposed labeling
rule on aspirin. For those who thought five separate studies (the four
CDC studies and the Partin study) with the same result as well as the
recommendation from aspirin experts that, because of accumulation,
"Labels of children's aspirin should reflect this risk clearly to
consumers," were sufficient, any delay was unconscionable.

DHHS Secretary Schweiker was still hell bent on pursuing the
regulation. However, the Office of Management and Budget (OMB),
pursuant to Executive Order 12291, had to complete a review before
any new rule could be published in the *Federal Register*.[1] Aspirin
Foundation President Joseph White had "consulted with his attorneys
and learned of the OMB's veto power" over rules "whose costs would
exceed the benefits they were intended to bring about."[2] While the size
of the children's aspirin market was estimated at $50 million,[3] avoiding
a blemish on aspirin's image could be priceless. No analysis of the
benefit and cost to children appeared.

As the regulation was making its way through this new layer of
review, DHSS blanketed the country with print and radio warnings
about the link.[4] Although FDA had already published an advisory
article in the August *FDA Bulletin* for over a million health-care
professionals, Surgeon General Koop now issued advisories to the

public which included a newspaper column to 8000 news outlets and recorded public service announcements for 8000 radio stations. FDA included an article in the October issue of *FDA Consumer* and soon made available upon request about 673,000 question and answer brochures. The brochure stated that the AAP "has independently recommended against using aspirin products in such situations."[5]

Meanwhile a *School Awareness Bulletin* sent home with children in St Paul, Minnesota, stressed the need for early diagnosis, but did not mention the link to aspirin or the recommendations to prevent it. More information though, the bulletin said, could be obtained from the NRSF of Bryan, Ohio.[6]

In early October I received another request from editor Mark Abramowicz to review a draft for the *Medical Letter*.[7] This article stated the studies had "many flaws" and concluded they were "unconvincing." I wrote a strongly worded reply.[8] Upon seeing the draft, Waldman reached the end of his tether. In a cover note to me with a copy of the letter he had sent to Abramowicz, Waldman wrote: "I just can't take this Sh—anymore." His three-page letter to Abramowicz concluded:

> Does the author of the draft think that the independent panels convoked by the CDC and the FDA were composed of a random selection of imbeciles? He or she seems to have about the same regard for the readership of the *Medical Letter*. The conclusion as written, I am afraid to say is ludicrous … I strongly believe that publication of this draft in anything resembling its present form would be a major disservice not only to the medical community but to the public as well.

On 15 October, Shacknai bolstered the industry's position in a take-no-prisoners op-ed in the *Wall Street Journal*. He asserted the data were "significantly flawed," the Ohio study was too small to be significant, and the others were "discredited." He quoted Cleveland pediatrician James Orlowski, who thought cases "may have been systematically excluded" and the conclusion "biased." Further, Shacknai claimed the "Reye's Syndrome Association" (without clarifying which one) opposed the HHS efforts, arguing that doctors and parents would treat Reye's "as a preventable disease" and "be less alert to its symptoms." He went further in stating that most "strident advocates admitted that Reye's syndrome would not disappear even with complete cessation of aspirin use in children with flu and chickenpox," and doctors treating arthritic children with aspirin were experiencing "tremendous resistance." [9] Subsequent events would show that Shacknai was wrong on almost every point.

On 21 October, I penned my response to Wilson and Brown's letter to the editor of *Pediatrics*. Emboldened by the escalating print war, I wrote: "The attempts of Brown and Wilson to obfuscate the findings of the Arizona, Michigan, and Ohio studies by reiterating arguments that have been deemed unlikely … do not serve to enhance knowledge in this area. The Arizona, Michigan, and Ohio investigators have noted that the observed association between salicylate use and Reye's syndrome does not prove causality. Causality, however, must be considered given the lack of evidence to the contrary." [10] Brown and Wilson's letter and my reply did not appear in *Pediatrics* until February 1983. [11,12]

The AAP Executive Board seemed to be hoping the June Redbook committee statement would suffice. However, skeptics were organizing. Six academic pediatricians wrote in the October issue of *Hospital Practice* that a "warning might be a premature act." In addition to Eichenwald and Gellis who had first met in May around the time of the FDA meeting, the academics included Henry Nadler, Dean of the Wayne State University School of Medicine, and Philip Lanzkowsky Chairman of the Department of Pediatrics at Long Island Jewish/ Hillside Medical Center, both of whom had written letters prior to the May FDA meeting, Robert Hoekelmann, Professor of Pediatrics at the University of Rochester School of Medicine, and Irving Schulman Chairman of the Department of Medicine of Stanford University. The academics indicated that at the suggestion of Sterling's Glenbrook Laboratories, they had reviewed the studies and were "disturbed to learn that the raw data … were never analyzed by independent agencies until very recently." They cited the BRI analysis that questioned the validity of the studies. [13] The pediatricians suggested the HHS Secretary and the FDA name a panel of "distinguished objective scientists," (implying the scientists who had already reviewed the data were neither distinguished nor objective) to review the data and to delay labeling. Finally, they noted that aspirin had been used by "hundreds of millions" of children over the past 80 years and its widespread use was one of the largest clinical trials ever conducted. "A short term solution," they said, "should not set the stage for removal of a time-honored and useful drug."[14]

In October Colorado pediatrician James Strain took the reins as the president of the AAP and updated the AAP Board.[15] He clarified that the Redbook Committee's publication in *Pediatrics* was "not an official Academy policy, but rather a committee statement." But the AAP had inadvertently backed itself into a corner and now seemed to be leaning on delay. The Board decided it "needed more information to come up with a position on any new labeling for aspirin." The minutes stated: "MOTION was made and carried that this issue be referred to the Executive Committee for appropriate consultation and that it be finalized after a conference call with the entire Board within one month."[16]

The 11 board members who hailed from Alabama, California, Colorado, Georgia, New York, New Jersey, Michigan, Minnesota, and Vermont were now the voice of the AAP on the issue of a warning label on aspirin products.[17]

On 10 November, after three medical journals based in the United States had rejected the CDC-AFIP liver manuscript, I wrote to *The Lancet*.

> In the United States there is considerable controversy surrounding the epidemiological association between salicylates and Reye's syndrome. Scientists, the aspirin industry, and the government have been deeply and at times bitterly, embroiled in the public health action which should (or should not) result from these studies. For this reason I request that you select reviewers which are not involved in this controversy ... this may be an important avenue to further define the aspirin-Reye's syndrome link. [18]

The Lancet promptly accepted the AFIP paper.[19]

I still had a slim hope that even if the liver finding was brought to light, it would make a difference.

At the same time, OMB's Christopher Clay DeMuth, who could single-handedly quash the warning label rule, consulted with several analysts who supported the warning label. Plucked from the Kennedy School of Government at Harvard in 1981, DeMuth was now Executive Director of the Presidential Task Force on Regulatory Relief, as well as Administrator of the Office of Information and Regulatory Affairs of the OMB.[20] DeMuth's own OMB statisticians had rejected industry's BRI's analysis [21] as did Denis J. Prager, an electrical engineer with a PhD from Stanford University who was Associate Director of the White House Office of Science and Technology Policy (OSTP).[22] Prager found "the [labeling] decision to be a prudent public health action and would only support negotiations with HHS to make the warning label less unequivocal."[23]

However, these two analyses soon took a backseat. Five Aspirin Foundation representatives met with James Tozzi, deputy administrator of the Office of Information and Regulatory Affairs and gave him the name of a physician who opposed the label. Tozzi spoke with the physician and then summarized his findings in a memorandum to DeMuth.[24] In early November, "DeMuth telephoned Schweiker and suggested that he withdraw the rule."

Later DeMuth told Tim Miller, writer for *The Nation*, "his decision was based on conversations with his wife, a pediatrician, on arguments in Shacknai's article, and on the Congressional testimony [organized by Shacknai] in late September." Put another way, DeMuth seemed to be balancing the four studies as well as "carefully weighted decisions" by the AAP Redbook Committee, the scientific staff of the CDC, the external review committee of the CDC, the analysis of the FDA, and the analysis by OSTP against the opinion of his wife, Shacknai, and the Shacknai's selected Congressional testimonials. The Aspirin Foundation's president told a *WSJ* reporter, "It is a wonderful thing that the government finally has a system to review these recommendations."[25] The OMB was now poised to shoot down the regulation if Schweiker did not withdraw it. Yet the OMB would not have to act. The AAP took the OMB off the hook.

As the Redbook Committee reaffirmed its recommendation concerning the treatment of fever with antipyretics, especially salicylate, in the November issue of *Pediatrics*,[26] Brandt called AAP President Jim Strain and asked for the AAP's position on the label. Strain told Brandt that the AAP still did not have one.[27] The Academy could delay no longer.

The Executive Board held a hastily arranged teleconference. Strain, who like many of the board members was a practicing pediatrician, led the discussion. He clearly remembered the call and shared his recollection with me. The Board, he recalled, discussed the pros and cons of a warning label on aspirin. No single person influenced the discussion. Some focused on the fact they had used aspirin for 30 years and had never seen a case of Reye's syndrome. Others felt a warning label was a serious step. Before the call, Strain had talked with members of the AAP Redbook Committee and the Committee on Drugs. The board members had also listened carefully to others in the Academy. He recalled there may have been a discussion of legal issues, but Strain said that was not an overriding concern. The Board then made its decision. The AAP would support more studies and not the warning label. Strain recalled the vote was unanimous or nearly so. (In 2021, the AAP archivist reported that no minutes of the meeting were preserved in the archive.)[28] According to Strain, the number-one reason for the decision was that "we were getting a lot of information from people we respected in the academy that didn't think there was an association." One whose name he could not recall "really bugged us about refuting any connection."

The AAP had chosen a position. Strain called Brandt and told him the Board did not endorse the warning label. Brandt now had no choice but to relay the absence of AAP support to Schweiker. On 10 November 1982, Jennisen, on behalf of Strain, sent a letter to the FDA which included in part:

at the present time, we do not feel that labeling aspirin-containing preparations as being contraindicated in these illnesses is in the best interest of children or the practice of pediatrics. We believe labeling should be delayed until more conclusive evidence of the association of aspirin administration and Reye's Syndrome is shown by further investigation …

Approved by the Executive Board, November 8, 1982[29,30]

The AAP explained its decision to its membership: "The AAP Board had objected to the mandatory warning label because it might cause widespread undue alarm and avoidance of aspirin use by children, some with conditions needing aspirin therapy. An increasing number of physicians were questioning the validity of the scientific studies on which the Academy based this warning of an association earlier in the year. The AAP asked HHS to delay the labeling until more conclusive evidence of an association is shown and urged support of more research."[31]

The same day, according to a court filing, the now formalized physician group called the Committee on the Care of Children (CCC), took credit for influencing the AAP and strongly urged the FDA to abandon the proposed aspirin-labeling rule via a letter addressed to the President and Vice President of the United States, the Vice President's counsel in charge of the Task Force on Regulatory Affairs, the Director of OMB, the Secretary of HHS, the Commissioner of FDA, and other government officials. It suggested the AAP had changed its position at the urging of the CCC whose members "worked with members of the Academy."[32]

Now the CCC attacked Schweiker's education campaign. On 16 November, the CCC of Boston, Massachusetts issued a press release stating that the committee planned to seek a court order that would impose a moratorium on the Health and Human Services Secretary's campaign to stop the use of aspirin to treat children with influenza or chickenpox for fear of causing Reye's syndrome pending further investigation."[33,34] Several members of the original physician group writing in *Hospital Practice* (Lanzkowsky, Nadler, and Schulman) had not joined the CCC and were replaced by others. Heinz Eichenwald, the chairman, was quoted as saying, "The government is behaving like it has found the mass murderer ... In reality, we do not yet have even a fingerprint of the villain that causes Reye's." He continued that the NRSF (Denver), the NRSF (Ohio),* and the American Academy of Pediatrics "agree that there is insufficient evidence justifying a relabeling of aspirin at this time." The NRSF of Michigan was notably absent from the list. NRSF (Michigan) founder Jim Crawford told me in 2011 that his recollection was that "we joined the group that wanted the label on ... We never took a position of let's wait and see."

Furious over the AAP Board's decision, Ted Mortimer and Vince Fulginiti resigned their seats on the Redbook Committee. According to Mortimer, the reversal came in response to "heavy pressure from certain members of the Academy who were recruited by the aspirin industry."[35] He said the Reagan administration had been "looking for a face-saving way out [of requiring warning labels] and the Academy gave them one." He told the AAP that if industry pressure could compromise such organizations, their statements on anything would be worth little.[36]

Wolfe complained that the HHS retrenchment was "political" and the Reagan administration under the influence of the aspirin industry had "taken a giant step backward."[37] According to a court filing, Mortimer sent a letter of resignation to Strain on 17 November stating as one ground for his resignation the following: "I feel that the Academy has now set a most unfortunate and potentially dangerous precedent for itself and for other public or quasi-public advisory bodies in terms of responding to outside pressures. I find this to be unacceptable." He added, "I, as one who has spent literally hundreds of hours studying this matter, feel that the Board made this decision in cursory fashion without adequate examination of the facts or permitting its technical advisory committee to have an adequate hearing in this matter."[38]

---

* I was unable to verify Eichenwald's statement concerning the opinion of the NRSF [Ohio] during this time.

But the warning label was dead in the water, at least for now. On 18 November, Schweiker announced that "following a recent statement by the American Academy of Pediatrics Executive Board" new government studies would be conducted to resolve the scientific dispute over the reported link."[39,40] He explained: "This is the first time concerns have been raised by an independent scientific body, and it is critical that they be resolved."[41] In order to protect the public, he stated, the department would continue educating parents and professionals on the need for caution and pursue resolution of the dispute.

The Academy apparently had second thoughts. On the day of Schweiker's announcement, the Academy sent Schweiker an additional statement noting that although they reaffirmed their earlier opposition to warning labels on aspirin at this time, they recommended that treatment of "flu" be deleted from children's aspirin-containing preparations.[42]

The blitz to delay a warning on the label of aspirin had worked.

Stick-on labels and FDA's vast public information campaign

Now a coalition unleashed red stick-on warning labels. The CCC and others may have convinced the AAP Board, but others were tired of waiting. By early November, a coalition (which included the American Pharmaceutical Association, the American Public Health Association, the National Wholesale Druggists Association, a major trade group, the National Association of Chain Drug Stores representing 150 corporations, and Pharmex, a Connecticut manufacturer of labels) announced a voluntary labeling program to warn consumers of the association.[43] Their plan was to ask retailers to place red warning stickers on every product containing aspirin sold over-the-counter. The stickers would cost less than a penny and state: "WARNING: Do not give this product to children under age 18 with chicken pox or flu. It contains an ingredient associated with Reye' syndrome, an often fatal disease."

As expected, the stick-on labels generated strong commentary, as noted by *New York Times* journalist Michael DeCourcy Hinds.[44]

Aspirin Foundation president Joseph White said the coalition's plan was "novel," but possibly "illegal and impractical." "This is just a group of people getting together and taking the law over," he said. Grigg, spokesman for the FDA, countered, "in general, I welcome the idea."

The FDA continued blanketing the United States with educational messages. In a "Talk Paper," the FDA cleared up eight misconceptions about the studies and noted the FDA's recommendation for new labeling of aspirin and its program for public and professional education.[45] On 17 November, FDA's W.Y. Cobb, Associate Director for Federal and State Relationships, pushed the button on his fax machine and transmitted the "Talk Paper" to State Health Officers, State Boards of Pharmacy, and State Drug Officials as well as a staggering 673,000 pharmacies and primary-care physicians. With that transmission, information about the link between Reye's syndrome and aspirin continued its spread throughout the United States.[46]

On 23 November, the FDA Working Group reported that it "continues to strongly support the interpretation that there is an association between salicylate and Reye syndrome ... we disagree with a number of points raised by BRI on the grounds of scientific merit. BRI's analyses and interpretation of the data do not change our scientific judgment."[47] The same day Eileen Barker, Acting Group Leader of the FDA's Neurology/Analgesic Group, pointed out that page one of the BRI report stated it had performed an "independent" audit and that "... in a technical sense the report cannot be considered independent as it was paid for by commercial manufacturers of the products under discussion."[48]

Nevertheless, the stark reality was there would be no warning on aspirin labels in the foreseeable future because the government was now going to perform more studies.

Lawsuits over informing the public

Then the lawsuits began. With the warning label on hold—seemingly along with the 1977 draft aspirin monograph—the CCC requested a temporary restraining order to stop the FDA's campaign in Federal

District Court in Boston.[49,50,51] On 25 November, a Federal District Judge in Boston denied the request.

In December, *Pediatrics* published CDC's report of a cluster of New Mexico children with Reye's syndrome studied in 1980. All five children had taken aspirin, yet the CDC investigators wrote, "Continued investigations are needed in an effort to identify and study suspected risk factors."[52]

On 7 December 1982, I wrote to Mortimer.[53] The first case of Reye's syndrome for the winter season had just been reported in Arizona. The mother had given her baby children's aspirin.

That month, John Vane, a scientist at the Wellcome Research Laboratories in Beckenham, United Kingdom, won the Nobel Prize for figuring out one of the ways aspirin works. Among its many effects, aspirin inhibits prostaglandins, substances in the body that cause inflammation, fever, and blood clots. A world of opportunity was awaiting, especially in the fight against the leading cause of death in the United States, vascular disease. Only a small fraction of the usual recommended dose for pain and fever was necessary to powerfully inhibit the formation of a blood clot. Curiously, no such fanfare had accompanied Brody's amazing 1955 discovery that salicylate, the most popular drug in the world, inhibits the production of ATP, the life-sustaining energy in cells. Researchers now had to prove that aspirin by inhibiting a clot could translate into help for patients with heart disease.

On 28 December 1982, the FDA, rather than publishing a "proposed rule," issued an "advance notice of proposed rulemaking" in the *Federal Register*. It stated that FDA was "considering proposing" a rule requiring aspirin warning labels and was proceeding by way of an advance notice "so that the agency would have the benefit of a broad range of views early in the rulemaking process."[54] Brandt appointed a new group, the US Public Health Service (PHS) Reye's Syndrome Task Force, consisting of members from the CDC, FDA, NIH, and the Office of the Assistant Secretary of Health to develop research protocols. He estimated the studies would take three or four years. The *Medical*

Letter never ran the article on Reye's syndrome. The FDA continued its massive education campaign under pressure from both the CCC on the one side and Wolfe's Public Citizen group on the other.

While the new studies were being planned, conducted, and analyzed, parents could still buy a bottle of aspirin, read the label, and have no idea that giving it to their child might be dangerous.

The new studies would, indeed, take several years.

Chapter 25

Delay, Delay, Delay, 1983–1986

*Industry has learned that debating the science is
much easier and more effective than debating policy.*

David Michaels, *Doubt is Their Product:
How Industry's Assault on Science Threatens Your Health*, 2008

Science and legal limbo

Failing to quash the government's education campaign in court, the
CCC began an education campaign of its own. In late February 1983,
a letter from the CCC to pediatricians across the country claimed,
"40% of those questioned believe that aspirin causes Reye syndrome—
leading to almost unprecedented panic." In it, Eichenwald noted he had
personally reviewed the study data, and the conclusions of the studies
were not supported.[1]

In March 1983, Mary Margaret Heckler, an attorney and longtime
Republican congresswoman from Massachusetts, took the reins
from Richard Schweiker as Secretary of the Department of Health
and Human Services.[2] AIDS would be her most visible and pressing
problem. More than 1000 persons had already contracted the
disease and the nation's blood supply was in jeopardy.[3] Heckler also
inherited the FDA's seemingly opposing goals on aspirin—educating
the country on the aspirin–Reye's link while delaying the warning
label requirement until new studies were completed. Public health
professionals were clearly supporting warnings. For example, the
Commissioner of the New York City Department of Consumer Affairs
told the *New York Times*, "There should be strong warning with respect
to aspirin use when children have the flu."[4]

Heckler's agency was also still fighting legal action initiated in May
1982 by Sidney Wolfe's Public Citizen Health Research Group (HRG),

which had asked the court to compel the FDA to require an appropriate warning. In March 1983, the US Court of Appeals for the District of Columbia Circuit issued a summary judgment for the FDA stating it was reluctant to interfere with FDA decision-making. HRG appealed the case. On 7 December 1983, the HRG argued its case against the FDA and the Aspirin Foundation to the US Court of Appeals.[5] On 7 July 1984, the Court of Appeals affirmed that such decisions belonged with experts at the FDA, not the courts, and returned the decision to the lower court, asking the lower court to decide if the FDA's process in making a final ruling was being unreasonably delayed.[6,7] The HRG pressed for a summary judgment.[8]

The mandatory warning label was now tied up in both scientific and legal limbo. Shacknai, now working as counsel for the American Foundation (which had been called the National Reye's Syndrome Foundation, Denver, Colorado, during the hearings in September 1982), said the Foundation had "great concern" over the proposed warning label and wanted additional research aimed at finding the causes of Reye's syndrome.[9]

On 22 March 1983, healthy, athletic 11-year-old Dana Ivy Wigutoff of Seacliff, Long Island, got the sniffles and ran a temperature of 101 °F.[10] Her parents, Edwin and Sharon, reached for Bayer aspirin. The label said nothing about Reye's syndrome. The Wigutoffs kept Dana home from school on Wednesday and gave her aspirin again. That evening she seemed better, but the following evening she complained of a stomachache. On Friday, she vomited. Her doctor suggested it might be premenstrual discomfort or a stomach virus. At 6 am Saturday morning, however, Dana awakened her parents. She was walking into walls, delirious. They wrapped her in a blanket and took her to the hospital, where the doctors immediately suspected spinal meningitis or Reye's. They inserted an IV with glucose and transferred her by ambulance to a larger hospital. The doctors there told the Wigutoffs they were 95% certain Dana had Reye's syndrome. By Monday morning, Dana was dead. In 1985 Edwin Wigutoff would submit a letter to a congressional hearing on Reye's syndrome explaining, "We, as parents are also struggling with the guilt of having given aspirin to our child which may have contributed to her death. If warning labels had been on the aspirin in 1982 our daughter might still be alive!"

CCC activism

Over the next several years, the CCC focused an intense public information campaign discrediting the link and intermingling doctors' concerns over autonomy with the question of the warning label. The AAP made it clear it was not associated with the CCC,[11] and the FDA voiced outrage over the CCC announcements.[12]

According to an Associated Press report on 19 November 1982, aspirin companies were financing the CCC.[13] In 1983, a court record stated the "CCC is funded by Schering-Plough and Sterling Drug ..."[14] By late 1983, public communications from the CCC seemed to be coming mainly from Chayet himself. Chairman Eichenwald recalled when I talked with him in 2008 that when the FDA asked for new studies in 1983, the CCC had voted to disband. In other words, according to Eichenwald, the physician arm of the CCC's leadership had ceased to exist, at least formally. In 1984, the *Washington Post* reported that an administrator at one of Chayet's organizations, the International Science Exchange, acknowledged the CCC had been launched with pharmaceutical funds.[15] The source of funding of the CCC however was apparently unclear to its members. In 2008 Eichenwald told me that his understanding of Chayet's role was that "he provided secretarial and similar support, and advice about regulatory matters which we knew little about, and about the workings of the FDA which were rather opaque." In November 1984, CCC member Robert Hoekelmann, chair of the Department of Pediatrics at the University of Rochester, reported that he had been assured the aspirin industry was not behind the CCC. "If it is, then I think I would get out [of the CCC]," he said. When asked who funded the group, Hoekelmann said, "some benefactor, but I'm not sure who they are."[16] Several months later, Chayet wrote that the CCC "does not represent industry and is not part of industry."[17] However in 1985 before a congressional committee, he would testify, "From its inception, the CCC indicated that its work in areas which relate to industry would be funded primarily by industry ... by arm's length efforts to seek the truth with regard to matters of controversy."[18]

Regardless of the miasma surrounding the members' view of the source of funding, the CCC remained ever-present. The CCC aggressively sought to stop the DHHS and others from distributing information about the link. In the fall of 1983, "due in part to strong lobbying and threatened lawsuits by the CCC," the secretary of DHHS banned distribution of half-a-million pamphlets for supermarkets.[19] Nevertheless the government had already distributed public service announcements (PSAs) by the likes of Star Trek's Leonard Nemoy.[20] According to Stephen Soumerai and colleagues at Harvard Medical School:

> An October 1983 letter from the CCC's attorney outlined the industry's charge that the supermarket pamphlet was misleading in implicating aspirin and salicylates as causes of RS, and specifically called for a halt to the publicity campaign and recalls of distributed materials (Chayet, 1983). Distribution of a 30-second radio announcement to 5000 radio stations was also canceled. Television PSAs, however, had already been sent to approximately 800 commercial television stations in fall 1983. During this time, a newspaper column prepared by the FDA was distributed to approximately 1500 newspapers, as well as a new 60-second PSA to 200 television stations.[21]

In response, the CCC sent letters to television stations across the country arguing that equal-time doctrines applied and to supermarkets claiming that by displaying the FDA brochure, the stores were violating labeling requirements. A CCC press release stated that experts felt the FDA's information was deceptive and misleading.[22]

Again, on schedule before flu season, in October 1984, the CCC countered government warnings with PSAs to radio and television stations, including one featuring a physician who said he represented 1200 pediatricians across the country: "We do know that no medication has been proven to cause Reye's." Incensed, Wolfe and

HRG brought the announcement to the attention of the FDA and wrote to over a thousand radio and television stations asking them not to broadcast the CCC's announcement and to broadcast the FDA ads instead.[23,24] According to the *New York Times*, the CCC and the FDA had a "stormy meeting" during which the CCC declined to withdraw their announcements saying they were fair, accurate, and informative. Chayet said the studies had been "completely discredited."[25] An FDA spokesperson reported the CCC had threatened legal action against stations broadcasting FDA public service announcements and drug stores using voluntary warning labels.[26]

In 1984, the NRSF [Ohio] conducted its largest school awareness campaign to date sending copies of the *School Awareness Bulletin* to 16,000 school superintendents. Later, it estimated that approximately six million homes had received the information.[27] Its bulletin contained the recommendations of the Surgeon General, the FDA, and the CDC "that aspirin and combination products not be given to children 18 years of age and under during episodes of these illnesses [influenza-like illnesses, chickenpox, and colds]." The foundation's medical director, Cincinnati pediatrician William Schubert, approved the Foundation's updated brochure "Because You Need to Know."[28]

New research

As the media battle continued, studies further supported the link. First, the CDC-AFIP liver pathology study was published by *The Lancet* in February 1983.[29] Mullick and I reported 13 children logged into the AFIP data base with fatal accidental or therapeutically induced salicylate intoxication. Each had, at some point, a salicylate level of 30 mg/dL or higher—which was probably why they had been identified at all. Liver tissue from 12 of the children had been stained in the standard way for light microscopy; microvesicles were observed in 10 samples. Six of the samples had also been stained with a special fat stain, and microvesicular fat was observed in all six. Information on brain pathology was available for 12 cases. Nine showed brain swelling. Essentially, they had Reye's syndrome.

Second, Duke University researcher Kwan-sa You published a laboratory study in *Science*.[30] He had dropped salicylate onto rat liver mitochondria and within minutes watched them swell. Swelling was first noticeable at a concentration of 1.6 mM and maximal swelling at 32 mM. Levels inside of cells of children were unknown but blood levels attained during treatment, he noted, are 7 to 40 mg/dL (0.5 to 3 mM). The mitochondria, he observed, "resembled those from patients with Reye's syndrome."

Third, a surprising study negated decades of dogma about treatment of influenza. Scott Younkin and colleagues at the University of Rochester School of Medicine reported that aspirin provided little benefit.[31] In addition, many of the young adults he studied could not tolerate it. The researchers had set out to study a drug called amantadine and decided to compare it to aspirin at a dose of 46 mg/kg/day. Forty-eight college students with influenza A were randomly assigned to receive one or the other treatment. By the third day, most of the students felt well enough to return to class. Amantadine was generally superior to aspirin in reducing symptoms (except fever which was reduced more quickly in the aspirin group). But the most surprising result was that a whopping 35% of the students treated with aspirin (compared with only 3% treated with amantadine) discontinued therapy because of bothersome side effects. This study suggested that aspirin, the darling of influenza treatment since 1918, might have been making some influenza sufferers feel worse.

Reports expressing skepticism about the link also surfaced. The *Medical Tribune*, for example, reported on two presentations from the Ninth Annual Meeting of the NRSF (Ohio) in St Louis in June 1983. One found that only 9% of 54 cases of Reye's in Japan had used aspirin. The other by NIH researcher Anita Chu noted that five Reye's survivors, compared with their unaffected family members, had no trouble "handling salicylate." Chu reported that aspirin doses of 10 to 30 mg/kg/day had "built up" over six days but produced no abnormalities.[32] In other words, these children with Reye's syndrome and their families under these conditions metabolized salicylate normally. While this finding was interpreted as failing to implicate aspirin in Reye's syndrome, it also found no metabolic defect, and left unanswered the question of the safety of the recommended doses.

Findings from these studies had no apparent impact on the regulatory actions of the FDA, which was, as planned, waiting for results of the new government case-control studies.

PHS Task Force embarks on new case-control studies

The PHS Reye's Syndrome Task Force designed the new studies in consultation with the aspirin companies. An independent body, the Institute of Medicine (IOM) of the National Academy of Sciences, provided oversight and served as an advisory board, evaluating the proposed protocol, monitoring the studies' progress, and reviewing the data and results. The goal was to produce a near perfect case-control study. According to CDC's Schonberger, industry representatives at first balked at having a control group as they wanted to test the accuracy of parental recall. But without a control group, there would be no possibility of evaluating the link, so the task force insisted on having one and proposed that every type of control thought to be reasonable be included. According to Schonberger, the IOM also came up with a plan that made neither side particularly happy. The first study would be a "pilot," to determine feasibility and establish the methods. A main study would then follow.

The PHS pilot study finally got underway in February 1984, exactly two years after the CDC consultants' strong recommendation to avoid aspirin was published in the MMWR. By May 1984, 30 children and teenagers and 145 controls at 16 pediatric centers in 11 states were enrolled. The incidence of Reye's syndrome was decreasing. CDC's Martha Rogers observed that chickenpox had not decreased yet Reye's cases after chickenpox had. This suggested that a decrease in aspirin use might be the reason.[33] Indeed, the once ubiquitous children's aspirin ads were becoming hard to find.

As enrollment in the pilot study closed in the spring of 1984, scientists gathered in Columbus for the Fourth International

Conference on Reye's Syndrome, sponsored in part by the Upjohn company of Kalamazoo, Michigan, makers of the new fever and pain reliever ibuprofen, along with the Children's Hospital of Columbus, the Departments of Pediatrics at the Ohio State University and the University of Cincinnati, and the NSRF of Ohio. Ibuprofen would compete directly with aspirin and acetaminophen. During the conference, scientist and clinician George Rodgers, Director of the Division of Pediatric Pharmacology and Toxicology of the Kosair Children's Hospital in Louisville, Kentucky, stated, "I must conclude that the data strongly suggest a role for aspirin or salicylate in conjunction with virus, in the etiology of Reye's syndrome." [34] The author of the foreword of the conference proceedings, however, still seemed flummoxed by the aspirin–Reye's link: "Since then [the first meeting 10 years earlier] we have shed little light on the most important questions concerning the disease. We still do not know its [Reye's syndrome] etiology, nor the exact location of the pathology and metabolic insults that result in the metabolic cascade leading to the clinical picture, nor specific therapy." [35]

The PHS pilot study data were ready for the IOM review on 13 December 1984. Two days earlier, on 11 December, the FDA's Cardiovascular and Renal Drugs Advisory Committee had reviewed the new data on aspirin's ability to prevent second heart attacks. For Sterling the gates to a huge new market rested on the committee decision. At the time, 20% of men died within a year of first heart attack and, of those who survived, the risk of death over the next five years was 25%. [36] Thus, hundreds of thousands of Americans suffered second heart attacks. A medicine that could help prevent these would instantly claim a lucrative place in the pharmacopeia. In the face of the increasing popularity of acetaminophen and ibuprofen, this was a much-needed opportunity. In 1980, the FDA reviewed an NIH-sponsored study showing no benefit. But now the results of a large Veterans Administration study, as well as a summary analysis, favored the preventive efficacy of aspirin treatment. [37,38] This time the FDA review committee voted unanimously to recommend new labeling for the use of aspirin to prevent recurrent heart attacks.[39]

That night, the founder and president of the NRSF of Michigan, John Dieckman, disappeared. In 2011, I spoke with Dieckman's widow about the incident. As she recalled, her husband had been driving home to Benzonia from a meeting he attended regularly in Lansing. The study he and Wallace Berman's medical team had worked so hard to create was limping along, given the decreasing number of Reye's cases. Dieckman did not arrive home. On 17 December, Dieckman's car was found on its nose in a creek in the highway median. She said that the autopsy indicated he had died immediately.

Foundation co-founder Crawford knew that whatever had happened, alcohol wasn't involved. He recalled that he had never seen Dieckman drink but that he did tend to become remote when thinking about his deceased son. Maybe, Crawford speculated, Dieckman was in one of those states. Sadly, John Dieckman, who had worked so hard for Reye's syndrome, would not hear the results of the pilot PHS Reye's syndrome study, which were unveiled to the IOM oversight committee two days after his death.

The IOM committee reviewed the results of the PHS pilot study in a closed session and found that the results replicated those of the Arizona, Ohio, and Michigan studies.[40] Because of the declining use of aspirin in the general population, the data were more statistically persuasive.[41] Yet the IOM members faced a dilemma. The pilot study had been planned as a feasibility study, not for public release. Nevertheless, with the results so clear, the IOM members determined that ethically the data should be published while awaiting results of the main study. Sidney Wolfe was not going to wait. He obtained the pilot data through the efforts of Michigan Representative John Dingell and released them in early 1985. Wolfe observed that the risk assessment was "one of the largest risk ratios found in any recent epidemiological study."[42] It showed 96% of children with Reye's had used aspirin compared with only 45% of 145 controls. The findings indicated that children with Reye's were *16 times* more likely to have taken aspirin.[43] (Appendix 5)

When he saw the pilot results, Ohio researcher Frank Holtzhauer, now Chief of the Division of Epidemiology of the Ohio Department of Health, was outraged and called for a code of ethics for epidemiologists.[44] During the previous four years, he felt he and his colleagues had been the victims of a "witch-hunt" that had served only one purpose—to discredit their data. They had been subjected to hours of depositions by pharmaceutical company attorneys, and their data had been inappropriately used by "epidemiologists for hire" who analyzed subsets of subsets, "cherry-picking" groups within the case and control groups (a practice useful for exploration but not for conclusions) that "tortured the data to the point that it did confess to whatever charge they wanted to prove." Ted Mortimer, now Elisabeth Severance Prentiss Professor Emeritus, Case Western Reserve University, later wrote that the manufacturers had "subpoenaed me, asked for "everything [in his office] related to Reye's Syndrome and worked me over in a deposition for six hours, trying to prove I had a financial interest, or other relationship with Tylenol."[45]

On 8 January, the *MMWR* posted the results of the pilot study and that "The [IOM] committee recommends that steps should be taken to protect the public health before the full study is completed."[46]

On 10 January 1985, as if using an old industry playbook from the 1960s for accidental ingestions, Heckler requested that aspirin makers *voluntarily* warn consumers of a possible association with Reye's syndrome via warning labels and immediately remove recommendations to use aspirin to treat flu and chickenpox in children and teenagers.[47] Schering-Plough was the first to respond and "members of the Aspirin Foundation (Sterling, Bristol-Myers, Miles, Burroughs-Wellcome, Merrill-Dow, and Proctor & Gamble) followed."[48] Voluntary warnings were not good enough for Wolfe. He demanded the warnings be strengthened, that all children's aspirin be seized, or new warning stickers affixed, and a new regulation state that all persons 19 and younger should not use aspirin for flu or chickenpox. Of course, CCC attorney Neil Chayet disagreed, claiming the new results were premature and unreliable. A spokesperson for DHHS politically admitted that while the pilot study strengthened the "possible link," the findings "do not at this time warrant stronger action than we have taken."[49] Wolfe also asked the Federal Trade Commission, which oversees advertisements across public airwaves, to require the warning.[50]

That weekend, the front page of *USA Today* headlined: "Flu Season—Aspirin Warnings Out."[51] The manufacturer's position began to soften. By 24 January, the Aspirin Foundation agreed to labeling changes in a "spirit of cooperation." Without admitting to the veracity of the link, it nevertheless agreed to remove the suggestion that aspirin be used for flu and add a warning: "Consult a physician before giving this medicine to children, including teenagers, with chickenpox or flu."[52]

After five studies, six including the Partin study, with the same results, FDA was still dragging its heels and touting corporate volunteerism. Congress was not happy.

Chapter 26

In the Best Interest of Children, 1986

Children cannot protect themselves.
Parents cannot protect their children from dangers they know nothing about.

Representative Henry A. Waxman,
Emergency Reye's Syndrome Prevention Act of 1985; Hearing
US House of Representatives, 99th Congress
15 March 1985

California Representative Henry Waxman was astounded that Ronald Reagan's administration under DHHS Secretary Margaret Heckler had decided upon a voluntary approach. Public health experts had been advising the government to place a warning on the label of aspirin products since 1982 and an NIH notice entitled "What to do About Flu" did not even mention Reye's syndrome and was still recommending aspirin therapy.[1]

Waxman and Senator Howard Metzenbaum of Ohio co-authored the "Emergency Reye's Syndrome Prevention Act of 1985" and introduced it in both the House (HR 1381) and Senate (S. 538).[2] On passage, it would require a warning on labels of any salicylate-containing drug: "WARNING: This product should not be given to individuals under the age of 21 years who have chickenpox, influenza, or flu symptoms. This product contains aspirin or another salicylate, which has been strongly associated with the development of Reye's Syndrome, a serious and often fatal childhood disease."[3]

On 15 March 1985, Waxman, Chairman of the House of Representatives Subcommittee on Health and the Environment, held a hearing.[4] He had asked Heckler to report on the progress of the voluntary labeling efforts. DHHS Assistant Secretary Edward

Brandt, Jr had reported that labels were variously vague, did not even mention Reye's syndrome, and were lacking in prominence. Indeed, most changes in the label would not appear until after the flu season. Waxman declared, "If the Department of Health and Human Services can identify risks but then is unwilling or unable to take strong enough measures, the Congress must act." [5]

Metzenbaum put it in real terms. He described the situation of a child crying in the middle of the night and parents reaching for the aspirin bottle that merely says, "Consult your physician first." The parents don't want to bother the doctor, so they think: It won't hurt. I'll just give him (or her) two aspirins. "That is begging the question because if the doctor says what the doctor should say, the doctor is going to say, 'Don't give the child aspirin.' So why not put it on the label?" Metzenbaum went on, "Children of America are exposed to enough risks at the present time without exposing them to something that we know is dangerous ... and if it is a known problem why don't we do something about it and why do we have to use our efforts to pass legislation to force them [the aspirin manufacturers] to do something that they should be doing on their own?"[6] James Scheuer, who had chaired the September 1982 hearing deriding the warning label requirement, appeared to have a change of heart. He thanked Metzenbaum for coming [to the Committee hearing] and for his "sheer unadulterated guts."[7]

Waxman called several groups to testify. The first were parents, including Joel Taubin, a physician and vice president of the NRSF (Ohio). Taubin described the loss of his 11-year-old son Greg in 1978 after receiving aspirin for chickenpox. NRSF (Ohio) President John Freudenberger explained, "That little bottle of aspirin may be the reason our daughter Tifinni died in 1973. I have been fighting Reye's Syndrome for the past twelve years by building the National Reye's Syndrome Foundation ... one hundred thirty chapters in forty states." He explained the mistakes that had been made as he saw them—the NIH refusing to fund research in 1974 and the FDA yielding to the manufacturers and reversing its decision to label aspirin in 1982. He put it simply: "All that needs to be decided is whether you want a clear, strong statement or whether you want to trust the judgment and motives of the aspirin companies."[8] When asked about the American Reye's Syndrome Foundation in Colorado, Freudenberger responded it was a small group and "has always yielded to the Aspirin Foundation." He concluded, "[I]gnorance is no way to solve the problem."[9]

Sidney Wolfe and pediatrician Albert Pruit, Chairman of the AAP Committee on Drugs, accompanied by AAP Executive Director Harry Jennison testified next. Wolfe, with characteristic definitiveness, spoke first: "It is classic preventive medicine, yet we have got a really unethical, illegal, and immoral response by the Federal Government and its partner, the aspirin industry."[10] Heckler, he said, had asked the manufacturers to voluntarily remove flu from the label and add a warning. He said there was rampant non-compliance and hundreds (this would turn out to be a low estimate) of children had died or suffered brain damage after the Reagan administration yielded to pressure from the drug industry two-and-a—half years earlier and canceled the mandatory label.[11]

Pruitt, speaking on behalf of the AAP's 27,000 pediatricians, explained the Academy now supports labeling.

FDA Commissioner Frank Young had the unenviable job of trying to explain how data on the link could be strong enough for the FDA to conduct a vigorous educational campaign, yet not strong enough for a label warning. He defended voluntary action yet also reported that HHS had stepped up its awareness campaign and the major manufacturers had agreed to revise their labeling by the next season.[12] Waxman challenged him:

> You have got two values here, doing things voluntarily and doing what is necessary to protect the public health ... Why do you think volunteerism is so important? Aren't you entrusted not with doing things voluntarily with the industry, but doing what is helpful to protect the public from dangers? [13]

Young replied that the information was "not completely definitive." Waxman, seemingly frustrated, responded, "I know, but you are throwing away one of the most important ways to reach people at the time when they are about to use the product that might kill their kids. It seems to me you are throwing away an effective vehicle to communicate, because you don't want to offend the aspirin industry, and I am just astounded by that." Young held his ground, saying the FDA had studied the pilot data and concluded there was not enough there to go with mandatory labeling.[14]

Finally, witnesses from industry included Joseph White with counsel and James Cope, president of the Proprietary Association. Chayet was also called upon, and pointed out that the CCC, although funded by the industry, was independent.[15] White reported the Aspirin Foundation was willing to undertake voluntary labeling, but it was not "accepting that there is a connection [between aspirin and Reye's syndrome]." Regarding his grandson, White announced he had not informed his own son of the link.[16] Cope, whose association represented all OTC medicines, relayed that his organization felt congressional action was "premature, because there is disagreement among scientists."[17] Chayet launched into his criticism of the studies. A letter from Chayet on behalf of the CCC requested "action on H.R.1381 be delayed pending further analysis of the conclusions of the pilot study." He reiterated that "the CCC does not represent and is not part of industry; it never has been and it never will be."[18] It seemed he was drawing a distinction between funding and representation.

Other organizations, many involved with the marketing and distribution of aspirin products, submitted objections to the proposed labeling law. The American Advertising Federation, for example, said, "we cannot agree that lawful product advertising is an appropriate or effective vehicle for the dissemination of warnings of this kind."[19] The American Pharmaceutical Association was "concerned that this vehicle for action may have an inhibitive effect on voluntary efforts in this and future situations."[20] The American Reye's Syndrome Association stated it "opposes H.R.1381 ... because it would require manufacturers to misinform consumers that an association has been established between the use of salicylates and

Reye's syndrome." And "could mislead consumers into thinking that by avoiding salicylates they would eliminate the risk of Reye's syndrome."[21]

With the American Academy of Pediatrics in support of a warning label, the government and the aspirin manufacturers were left to solve the problem. Another year would go by before a mandatory warning label became a reality. For many months, the Emergency Reye's Syndrome Act of 1985 circulated in Senate and House committees while the industry made substantial voluntary efforts to educate the public. The Aspirin Foundation reported that under its auspices 800,000 warning posters were distributed and television public service announcements had been prepared.[22]

Although fewer, deaths from Reye's syndrome continued, proving the voluntary approach ineffective. The AAP discovered that only 35% of aspirin bottles carried the warning (68% of children's aspirin containers). Wallace Berman, who had been leading the NRSF of Michigan's treatment trial, complained about the lack of warnings on aspirin bottles on store shelves.[23] In September 1985, the district court heard oral arguments for a new motion for summary judgment filed by the HRG.[24] While the HRG's motion was undecided, the pilot study data were published in the prestigious *New England Journal of Medicine* in October.[25] In December 1985, the FDA proposed a warning label requirement.[26]

A mandatory warning label was now inevitable. Republican Senator Orrin Hatch from Utah and Democrat Howard Metzenbaum from Ohio "hammered out in negotiations" the wording of the new labeling rule. White said the agreement "headed off pending legislation."[27] The result was a label that pertained only to aspirin—not all salicylates. This made little sense; however, the parties agreed. (In 2003, the FDA would issue a final regulation requiring the warning be added to non-aspirin salicylates, including bismuth subsalicylate.[28])

On 7 March 1986, the FDA published the final rule in the *Federal Register*. The rule would become effective on 5 June 1986.[29] The required warning read:

Children or teenagers should not use this medication

for chickenpox or flu symptoms

before a doctor is consulted about Reye's syndrome,

a rare but serious illness reported to be associated with aspirin.

The UK followed suit, but its labeling was even broader.[30] Donald Aheson, Chief Medical Officer of the Department of Health, advised all doctors, dentists, and pharmacists not to give aspirin to children except on medical advice. Producers agreed to print a warning on aspirin packages stating that aspirin-based products "not be given to children under 12 unless your doctor tells you to." The aspirin brands in the UK included Reckitt and Colman's Junior Disprin, Bristol Myers's Junior Angiers, and Boots' soluble aspirin for children. The market for children's aspirin was approximately £3 million of the £40-million total market for nonprescription analgesics. Reckitt's expected no change in their financial performance as they had recently launched a paracetamol-based children's analgesic.[31] In 2002, the UK government extended the aspirin "ban" to include its use in all those younger than 16 years of age.[32]

Meanwhile, the main PHS study, which had begun in January 1985, proceeded under full steam. However, even with 70 pediatric centers participating, the study organizers were challenged to find children with Reye's syndrome to enroll. When the interim data were reviewed, the IOM once again found the results overwhelming. It recommended the study be stopped. Enrollment ended in May 1986. The final data showed that 96% of 27 cases and only 38% of 140 controls had taken aspirin. (Appendix 5) This difference indicated that greater than 90% of cases of Reye's syndrome were attributable to aspirin therapy.[33]

Nevertheless, American Home Products, Bristol-Myers, Sterling Drug, Miles Laboratories, and Proctor and Gamble planned another study.[34] They sponsored Yale University and McGill University researchers to conduct an eighth case-control study. The study, which began in 1986 and involved 108 hospitals in the United States and Canada, was specifically designed to address purported flaws in the previous studies. In 1987, its oversight committee determined the evidence that aspirin was associated with Reye's syndrome was so clinically impressive and statistically significant it advised stopping enrollment. The study confirmed once again the previous seven studies. (Appendix 5) Further analyses showed that five potential sources of bias—flaws the aspirin industry had complained about for years—did not exist.[35]

The gold-standard study for proving causality—exposing some children to aspirin therapy and others to placebo, in a random and blind manner, and determining rates of illness and death—is unethical and will never be done. However, the numbers in the case-control studies, the pharmacologic facts about salicylate, the parallel reduction in aspirin use and Reye's syndrome, and the historical events described herein indicate that for most children from the beginning through the mid-1980s, the mysterious illness called Reye's syndrome was, in fact, salicylate poisoning.

The FDA required a Reye's syndrome warning on labels in 1986, made it permanent in 1988, and required non-aspirin salicylates be added in 2003. By then the illness, once a top killer of children, had almost disappeared.

Afterword

Proof that a given condition always precedes or accompanies a phenomenon
does not warrant concluding with certainty
that a given condition is the immediate cause of that phenomenon.
It must still be established that when this condition is removed,
the phenomenon will no longer appear.

Claude Bernard,
An Introduction to the Study of Experimental Medicine, 1865

Salicylates, like all medicines, have unique characteristics and toxicities. From the beginning physicians recorded observations of pharmacologic effects. However, possible flags for therapeutics were minimized or ignored. Instead, trust, bolstered by salicylate's immediate effect on fever and pain, a confluence of opinion-based medicine, marketing creativity, and an absence of government protection prevailed.

Doctors warned about possible accumulation, particularly in children, as early as the 1800s. First attributed to faulty kidney function (dehydration), another factor at the beginning of treatment was suggested by Langmead in 1906. Later Coburn found it took several days to reach a steady level.

William Hoffman was so concerned about the danger of this accumulation in children that in 1953 he was among the first to alert the medical community. "With the modern tendency to give drugs every four hours ... extreme toxicity will develop in two or three days. Most pediatricians ... do not realize that this pyramiding takes place." A mechanism was identified during the mid-1960s when Gerhardt Levy and scientists at Nicholas Inc. learned that the rate of metabolism of salicylate is fixed (early in treatment). After this discovery, a second round of warnings was issued. For example, in 1966, J.O. Craig and colleagues in Glasgow warned that "repeated doses of salicylate cause a steady rise in blood salicylate level" and suggested "the surest way to eliminate therapeutic aspirin-poisoning of infants and toddlers is to withhold the drug entirely from children." Warnings about accumulation were prominent in Australia. Brisbane pediatrician Phyllis Cilento believed the consensus of medical opinion was that aspirin should not be administered for more than two days as it could "accumulate." In the United States, however, warnings languished as long-standing habits prevailed, an "overdose by mother" scenario emerged, government intervention was spurned, and images of safety, doctors' blessings, and maternal love lifted aspirin to the pinnacle of parents' and government's trust. Even as safety processes were put in place by the Kefauver amendment, no word of the danger got out to the public. The authors of the FDA's 1977 tentative monograph identified the risk of accumulation for *a third time in three decades* and recommended that, in the presence of fever, children should not be dosed beyond three days. The monograph remained in draft and the general use of the trusted product for children continued.

The case-control studies identified salicylate as a risk factor for Reye's syndrome and data from the Public Health Service Main Study provide evidence of a key role for accumulation during the first days of treatment. It revealed that 78% of the children with Reye's syndrome were still taking aspirin on day 3 compared with only 9% of controls.[1] The median daily dose during the first four days of the prodrome illness was only 25 mg/kg/day—far below the dose that had been recommended for decades.

Beside rate-limited metabolism, other factors that predispose to accumulation were identified: dose, frequency, duration, dehydration, individual variation, kidney function, protein levels, and the stress of infection. Variation in metabolic capacity may also have played a role, although one study showed that children with Reye's syndrome had normal salicylate metabolism.[2] Infection, while not necessary for the induction of Reye's syndrome,[3] may have increased risk by creating general metabolic stress.

The case-control studies spawned a broad, relentless, and

penetrating educational campaign concerning salicylate use in children, preventing many cases and saving lives, as shown in the Figure below (which shows only cases reported to CDC). The decline in the use of salicylates in children was accompanied by a decline in cases of Reye's syndrome.[4,5]

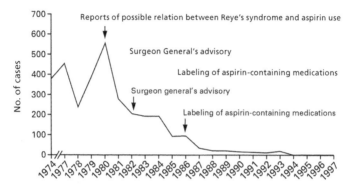

Number of Reported Cases of Reye's syndrome in relation to the Timing of Public Announcements of the Epidemiologic Association of Reye's Syndrome with Aspirin Ingestion and the Labeling of Aspirin-Containing Medications
From *New England Journal of Medicine*,
Belay, E.D., Bresee J.S., Holman R.C., Khan A.S., Shahriari A., Schonberger L.B., Reye's syndrome in the United States from 1981 through 1997, Vol. 340, p. 1389.
Copyright © 1999 Massachusetts Medical Society.
Reprinted with permission from Massachusetts Medical Society.

Cases of Reye's syndrome began to decline in 1981 after the first reports of the aspirin–Reye's syndrome link in 1980 and subsequent alerts by the CDC, the American Academy of Pediatrics, the foundations, and media giants like the *Chicago Tribune* and *New York Times*. In February 1982 CDC again put the word out and media followed. For example, the *Washington Post* headlined, "Children with chicken pox, flu should not use aspirin US says."[6] A massive FDA educational campaign soon followed and despite lawsuits necessitating careful messaging (for example: "While the cause of Reye's syndrome is *unknown, some* studies *suggest a possible association*."), the government's reach and intensity were significant.[7] By 1983, the number of reported cases dropped by about a half, even as the number of states with mandatory reporting increased (44 states had mandated reporting of Reye's syndrome by 1984). The number of tablets of children's aspirin purchased similarly decreased. By 1986, for example, 91% of pediatricians and 98% of pharmacists in Columbus, Ohio, no longer recommended aspirin for children with fever or pain.[8] The educational campaign served to alert the public until the government required a warning label in June 1986. By 1994, salicylate-associated Reye's syndrome had essentially disappeared as a clinical condition across all 50 states.[9]

Surveillance in the UK also documented a decline in Reye's syndrome[10] after the June 1986 warnings of the UK Committee on Safety of Medicines.[11] A case-control study in the UK published in 1988 demonstrated the link.[12] In 2006, John F.T. Glasgow reported knowledge of at least 13 countries globally with "some form of public health warning."[13]

Two key factors impacted recognition and resolution of the problem. First, Reye's syndrome was not reportable and neither the CDC nor the NIH had a defined program. Data from the few population-based studies available (shown in Appendices 2 and 3) indicate that the true number of cases greatly exceeded those reported, masking the likely fact that Reye's syndrome was a top killer of children. Second, the delay in implementing the warning label—the only known way to reach *all* potential users—cost lives. According to Devra Lee Davis of the National Academy of Science, and Patricia Buffler, Dean of the School of Public Health at the University of California, Berkeley, 1470 excess deaths occurred between the first proposal for the label in June 1982 and June 1986, when the label was instituted.[14] Even then, the warning did not reach everyone. On 6 April 1987, 13-year-old Jessica Van Dyke, granddaughter of television and film actor Dick Van Dyke, died of Reye's syndrome in Cincinnati, Ohio, after taking aspirin for chickenpox.[15] Nevertheless, the warning had a major impact on the illness, even though it only warns for "children and teenagers" with "flu symptoms or chicken pox" and does not address accumulation, adults, or other or no infections.

The internal analgesic monograph remains tentative except for piecemeal final rules such as, in addition to the Reye's syndrome warning, an alcohol warning (1998),[16] a stomach bleeding warning (2009), and a rule for professional labeling for vascular and rheumatic use (1998). Aspirin is not alone. In 1997, FDA's J.R. Crout explained, "Actually, to this day a lot of drugs have never made it to the final monograph."[17] In 2020, the Coronavirus Aid, Relief, and Economic Safety Act (Cares Act) addressed the delay by including statutory provisions that reform and modernize the way OTC monograph drugs are regulated. The rulemaking process was replaced with an administrative order process for issuing, revising, and amending OTC monographs.[18] This will be interesting to follow.

Some children diagnosed with Reye's syndrome during the mid-20th century may have had another illness, such as a genetically based disorder, however, the proportion appears to have been low.[19] Naturally, as aspirin use and "classic" Reye's syndrome (as the illness of the mid-20th century is often called) declined, advances in genetic testing identified more children with inborn errors of metabolism, particularly in the younger age groups.[20, 21]

Hindsight is of course 20:20. For many years, clinicians attending to the mysterious cases did not diagnose salicylate poisoning because they thought that either the child had not taken any, the aspirin dosing regimen was safe, the government was monitoring safety, poisoning could not be present at low levels, or the liver pathology differed. Years later, Jim Baral recalled his time as a trainee with Reye, "When the child [with Reye's syndrome] came to the hospital, they usually died within 27 hours of admission. The last thing on our minds would have been to ask them if they took aspirin." Nevertheless, many of the charts Baral and Morgan examined did document aspirin use.[22] Baral told conferees at the 35th Anniversary of the National Reye's Syndrome Foundation in 2009, "Ladies and gentlemen, we had the evidence. We were blinded. We didn't see it."[23] What Reye, Morgan, and Baral did see was the starkly similar pattern of illness and pathology that propelled them to alert the world and raise awareness of the deadly condition.

The parents' foundations played a key role. Beginning in 1973, as a young couple, John and Terri Freudenberger never lost sight of their goal of raising awareness. They supported hundreds if not thousands of grieving parents through their tireless efforts and assisted Ohio with the critical study. The founders of the Michigan foundation also devoted many years to the cause. Sadly, its president and driving force John Dieckman died just days before the results of the PHS pilot study were released. The National Reye's Syndrome Foundation of Ohio eventually incorporated the Michigan and American foundations. In 2011, the Freudenbergers, concerned that marketing of low-dose aspirin for the prevention of heart disease as "baby" aspirin was confusing to parents, asked me to accompany the foundation to ask the FDA to institute a moratorium on the use of the term "baby" for this use.[24] Packages marked "baby" aspirin are rarely seen today.

A few mysteries remain. The spectrum of the illness in those with Reye's syndrome is not fully understood. Since salicylate poisoning can occur without liver abnormalities and in adults, many more cases may have occurred. One report suggests just that. In 1975, Fred Hochberg of the CDC and physicians at the University of Illinois reported an outbreak of 48 grade-school children living in western Chicago hospitalized with "influenza B-related encephalopathy."[25] Fourteen of them met the standard criteria for Reye's syndrome. Could other encephalitis-like illnesses have been Reye's syndrome/ salicylate poisoning, too? How many other encephalopathies, such as the measles, rubella, and mumps encephalopathy, were in fact salicylate poisoning? Solomons and colleagues in Providence, Rhode Island, for example, observed a striking increase in the incidence of measles encephalitis from 1 per 3010 cases in 1937–1946 to 1 per 807 cases during the period 1947–1952 just after the introduction of children's aspirin.[26]

Other questions remain. Did treatment affect outcome? Many treatments for salicylate poisoning and Reye's syndrome were identical, but a few differed. Phenobarbital, for example, was shown to exacerbate salicylate intoxication, yet for a time was routinely administered to treat Reye's syndrome. Could children have had better outcomes with different therapy? Also, why, decades later, does confusion remain? Schonberger revised *Wikipedia* in 2006 as it had slanted away from the relationship with aspirin. Why did it take until 2009 for the NIH, after a letter from me, to remove from their public summary that the cause of Reye's syndrome is "a mystery"? Words matter. Finally, as aspirin has been marketed around the world for decades and Reye's syndrome was reported in many countries, how many children and adults had "Reye's syndrome"?

The introduction and popularity of acetaminophen (paracetamol in Australia, UK, and elsewhere) likely had an important impact on the incidence of Reye's syndrome. (Appendix 4) If the role of aspirin had not been identified, as acetaminophen use increased, Reye's syndrome may have simply vanished, becoming a great medical mystery.

The case-control studies described in this book lit the path to the solution. As these were observational studies rather than "gold-standard-proof" experimental studies (prospective, randomized, blinded, and placebo-controlled), they were susceptible to a well-recognized list of potential flaws. Criticism is key to scientific progress, but here it seemed excessive, self-serving, and aimed at confusing those unfamiliar with valid methods. According to Professor Arthur Reingold of the School of Public Health, University of California, Berkeley in 2021:

> Students are taught that observational studies only show association [links] but do not prove "causation" yet at the same time, for ethical and practical reasons many critically important cause and effect relationships will never be examined by experimental trials. Therefore, we still need to make decisions based on observational studies, not just parrot that "association does not prove causation," allowing naysayers to hide the truth and delay action.

This book posits that, even without an ideal experiment, a question can be answered, if not to perfection, then beyond a reasonable doubt. The historical events, the case-control studies, the lack of flaws large enough to invalidate the results, the timing of the illness related to the expected rise in salicylate levels, the presence of fatty degeneration, and, finally, the parallel decrease in the use of aspirin in children and the decline of the syndrome indicate that, for most children during the mid-20th century, the illness known as Reye's syndrome and salicylate poisoning were one and the same.

**

In March 2006, as I began to write this book, I visited Ray and Betty Hime to thank them. They were living in the town of Marana about 20 miles from the Silver Bell copper mine. Rodney's sister Teresa, now married, lived nearby with children of her own. When Ray answered the door, it was clear he was ill. Tall, slim, and still handsome, he was now jaundiced from a disease of the bile system. Betty's eyes welled as he told me he was not a candidate for a liver transplant. He was as warm, kind, and caring as I remembered, as was Betty—a perfect match. After we reminisced, we hopped into Ray's pick-up and drove up to the mine. The village was gone but the massive copper pit remained. The sky was clear. The muted desert-colored mountains were mystically beautiful. During our visit, I told Ray how his meeting in Silver Bell in May 1979 had set me on the path to finish the investigation, one that eventually had an impact on thousands of children, and I thanked him. He looked at me and smiled. "Tell my son-in-law," he said with a twinkle in his eye, "he thinks I'm just an old miner." I promised I would. Ray died on 22 May 2006, and I wrote a eulogy for his funeral. His son-in-law read it.

Appendix 1

Historical Dose and Dose Frequency
Recommendations and Selected Warnings
General Use of Aspirin for Children, United States
Examples: 1923 to 1980

Date	Recommendation and selected warnings	Multidose recommendation in mg/kg/day* Specified (s) or calculated (c) for a 16-kg four-year-old given every 4 hours unless otherwise stated.
1923	One grain [60mg] for a 6-month-old and 3–5 grains for those aged 4 and 5.No frequency given.	
1930	One grain, to be given every four hours for 1-year-old.	40 (c) (Calculated for a 9-kg 1-year-old)
1950	One grain per year of age up to age 5. No frequency given.	
1953	"With the modern tendency to give drugs every four hours, a second dose of one grain to an infant will cause a pyramiding of the blood level ... If the doses are maintained at the same rate obviously extreme toxicity will develop in two or three days."	
1956	60 mg per year of age up to age 5, no oftener than every 4 hours is "probably safe for the majority." "The safe and proper dose is controversial."	90 (c)
1964	"60 mg/year of age to age 5, and single 0.3-Gm. (5 grain) doses in older children may be given every four to six hours."	90 (c)
1964	65 mg/kg/day with maximum of 3.6 Gm. in 24 hours.	65 (s)
1969	Range includes above recommendations	
1975	65 mg/kg/day, divided into 4–6 doses with a max. 3.6 mg.	65 (s)
1977	Panel recommendation for a 4-year-old, 240 mg every 4 hours not to exceed 5 doses in 24 hours.	75 (c)
1980	For fever: 10–20 mg/kg every 6 hours not to exceed 3.6 g per day. "Children with fever and dehydration are particularly prone to intoxication from relatively small doses of salicylate."	40–80 (c)

*   If range given, the larger amount was selected for the calculation.

Note. Estimate for prevention of heart disease was 2.7 mg/kg/day.

Appendix 2

Estimates of Reye's Syndrome Deaths in Persons <18 years,
based on the Michigan population study[1]
United States, 1950–1985

Period	Population <18 years (a)	Number of deaths		
		Annual deaths, lower estimate (b)	Annual deaths, upper estimate deaths (c)	Total deaths, estimated in period
1950–59	55,738,328	239	574	2390–5740
1960–69	69,730,855	300	718	3000–7180
1970–79	67,167,846	289	691	2890–6910
1980	63,685,159	274	656	274–656
1981–1985				1700 (d)[2]
1950–1985				10,254–22,186

(a) US Census Bureau. 1 July estimates for 1955, 1965, and 1975 for each decade and for 1980. Estimate files for National, State, and County Level. Accessed 22 February 2010.
(b) Annual deaths, calculated: annual rate of death certificates coded as Reye's syndrome, i.e. 0.43 per 100,000 <18 years, January 1969 to June 1976 in Michigan applied to the US population at various time periods.
(c) Annual deaths, calculated: annual rate of death certificates coded as Reye's syndrome and others possibly related to Reye's syndrome, i.e. 1.03 per 100,000 <18 years, January 1969 to June 1976 in Michigan applied to the US population at various time periods.

Appendix 3

Reye's syndrome cases, Reported and Estimated,
United States, 1950–1985

Year	US population <18 years (a)	Cases reported to CDC (b)	Cases estimated based on CDC/Ohio study case rate of 0.9 cases per 100,000 <18 years (c)(d) applied to US population <18 years	Cases estimated based on hospital catchment study case rate of 5.6 cases per 100,000 <18 years (e) applied to US population <18 years
1950–59	55,738,328	N/A	5016	31,213
1960–69	69,730,855	69	6276	39,049
1970–79	67,167,846	1620	6045	37,614
1980	63,685,150	555	573	3566
Total 1950–80		2244	17,910	111,442

Notes:

(a) US Census Bureau. 1 July estimates for 1955, 1965, and 1975 for each decade and for 1980. Estimate files for National, State, and County Level. Retrieved from the US Census on 22 February 2010.

(b) Cases reported. CDC surveillance started in 1967, no data available 1975 and 1976. Cases 1967=11, 1968=17, 1969=41, 1970=13, 1971=83, 1972=30, 1973=32, 1974=379, 1975=Not available, 1976=Not available, 1977=454, 1978=240, 1979=389.[1–9] For 1980s, 1980=555, 1981=297, 1982=213, 1983=198, 1984=204, 1985=93.[2]

(c) Rate of 0.9 cases per 100,000, 18 years.[3]

(d) Seasonal and geographic variations make estimates difficult. However, CDC estimated "the average annual incidence of Reye's syndrome in the United States between 1 and 2 cases per 100,000 children under 18 years of age.[4, 5] The range was based on states with intense surveillance and two hospital-based record reviews: Ohio[6] and Colorado[7] and the retrospective mortality-record review conducted in Michigan."[8]

(e) Case rates ranged from 3.5 for biopsy proven cases to 5.6 for clinically diagnosed cases which met CDC case definition expressed as cases per 100,000 <17 years. For this table, the 5.6 rate is applied to the population less than 18 years.[9]

Appendix 4

Notes on Acetaminophen (Paracetamol) Sales,
Aspirin Use, and Reye's Syndrome
in Australia, the United Kingdom, and the United States

The marketing of acetaminophen (known as paracetamol in much of the world) as an alternative to aspirin had a major impact on consumer use of aspirin.

Consumer uptake of paracetamol was rapid in Australia. Pediatrician D.M. Danks of the Murdoch Institute for Research into Birth Defects, Melbourne, Australia, noted that during the 1960s "aspirin fell into disrepute in Australia ... and was replaced by equally indiscriminate use of paracetamol. Reye's syndrome almost disappeared." [1] Around this time, in addition to the coroners' inquests on therapeutic aspirin poisoning and subsequent government and media attention (Chapter 9), the Australian government required a warning on aspirin products regarding its association with kidney damage.[2] Paracetamol sales in Australia surpassed those of aspirin by 1970.[3] *By 1975 sales of pediatric forms of aspirin in Australia in retail pharmacies were practically nil.*[4]

A review of 12 cases of Reye's syndrome in Perth between 1961 and 1966 was among the last case series reports of Reye's syndrome in Australia with one exception.[5] US pediatrician James P. Orlowski, a critic of the link between aspirin and Reye's syndrome, wrote several reports which are summarized by Mark Largent in his book *Keep Out of Reach of Children*[6] and the Medicines Evaluation Committee of the Australian government.[7] Orlowski asserted after studying cases in Australia that Reye's syndrome was not attributable to salicylate and in fact may never have existed. In 1987, Orlowski reported that of 20 children with Reye's syndrome between 1973 and 1985, only one had been given aspirin. This was not surprising as during the study period aspirin accounted for only 0.3% of pediatric analgesic/

antipyretic sales.[8] In 1990 he reported 8% of 49 had been given aspirin. In 1999, he reassessed 26 surviving patients from his 1990 study and found 69% had been diagnosed with inborn errors of metabolism or other illnesses. The cases he studied occurred after aspirin use fell in Australia and likely represent Reye's-like illnesses. The Australian Institute of Health and Welfare reported 8 cases between 1993 and 2001.[9]

In the UK, Sterling Drug subsidiary Frederick Stearns and Co. introduced the Panadol (acetaminophen) brand in 1956, five years before the US launch of Tylenol.[10] It first marketed Panadol as an alternative to Disprin noting that it was not as irritating to the stomach. According to journalist Diarmuid Jeffreys this approach gave aspirin a "bad name" and caused sales of aspirin (which Sterling also sold) to fall. In 1958 Sterling released a children's formulation called Panadol Elixir and, in 1963, paracetamol for children was introduced to the British pharmacopoeia.[11] *By the early 1970s, sales of the two drugs there were "almost on par."* [12]

In 2006, John F.T. Glasgow of the Royal Belfast Hospital for Sick Children traced the history of Reye's syndrome in the UK beginning with the institution of voluntary surveillance in 1981 to the active reporting system which commenced in 1986.[13] From August 1981 to July 1986 between 40 and 81 cases were reported per year. The British Risk Factor Study, a two-year study which had begun in 1984 showed a "highly significant excess of aspirin exposure in Reye's cases." In 1986, the UK Committee on Safety of Medicines deemed public health action be taken. A letter was written to doctors, a notice was posted in the *British Medical Journal*, leaflets were placed in pharmacies, and a warning label was required on aspirin products. "Moreover, the pharmaceutical industry voluntarily withdrew paediatric aspirin products." From August 1987 to April 2001 cases slowly dropped from 32 per year to zero.

In the United States, McNeil Laboratories, maker of Tylenol, launched prescription-only Tylenol Elixir for children in 1955.[14] In

1959, Johnson & Johnson acquired McNeil and began selling children's Tylenol Elixir and drops as OTC drugs. Children's chewable tablets were introduced in 1972. (OTC adult Tylenol was launched in 1961.) *Purchases of children's Tylenol by drugstores did not surpass those of aspirin until the 1980s.*[15]

Appendix 5

Case-control Studies (1980–1989)

Salicylate Use in Children with Reye's Syndrome and Controls,

United States

Study (enrollment period)	Year Data Were First Made Public (Published)	Number Cases/ Controls	Salicylate Use Among Cases (%)	Salicylate Use Among Controls (%)	Probability of a Chance Finding or Odds Ratio
Arizona (December 1978– January 1979)[1]	1980 (1980)	7/16	100	50	<5 of 100
Michigan (March–April 1980)[2]	1980 (1982)	25/46	96	73	<1 of 100
Ohio (December 1978–March 1980)[3]	1980 (1982)	97/156	97	71	<1 of 1000
Michigan No. 2 (October 1980– February 1981)[4]	1981 (1982)	12/29	100	45	<2 of 1000
Cincinnati (Partin et al.) (December 1978–May 1980)[5]	(1982)	64/48	95	85	Not reported
Public Health Service Pilot Study (February–May 1984)[6]	1985 (1985)	30/145	93	46	OR=19a
Public Health Service Main Study (January 1985–May 1986)[7]	(1987)	27/140	96	38	OR=40b
Yale McGill Study (February 1986–August 1987)[8]	(1989)	24/48	88	17	OR=35c

(a) Cases were 16 times more likely to have taken a salicylate

(b) Cases were 40 times more likely to have taken a salicylate

(c) Cases were 35 times more likely to have taken a salicylate

Note: for the methods used to calculate the odds ratio, see the study publication.

Acknowledgements

First, I am indebted to John Sullivan-Bolyai who reported the hospitalized children to me in December 1978 and to the children's parents who provided the critical information that helped unlock a decades-old mystery. I am also grateful to the staff of the Arizona Department of Health Services who despite my fledgling skills supported my investigation: State Epidemiologist Phil Hotchkiss; Director of the State Laboratory Jon Counts; Assistant Director of Disease Control Services James Sarn; disease investigator Lee Dominguez; and laboratory experts Warren Stromberg and Dora Woodall. Indeed, this history may have been entirely different were it not for the critical meeting in Silver Bell organized by parent Raymond Hime in May 1979, and the encouraging words of former and current CDC scientists J. Lyle Conrad, C. George Ray, and Lawrence Schonberger.

I thank and deeply respect all those who devoted themselves to understanding the mysterious deaths and shared their stories with me, especially: Larry Schonberger who not only supported research and national surveillance over many years but was also a valuable source of information and encouragement to me, Graeme Morgan and Jacob (Jim) Baral, who co-wrote the landmark paper with R.D.K. Reye; American Academy of Pediatrics member Ted Mortimer, who refused to let go of his prescient deduction; John and Terri Freudenberger, John Dieckman, Jim Crawford, and Louis Pettine, parents who selflessly dedicated themselves to Reye's syndrome; J. Dennis Pollack, a dedicated scientist motivated by curiosity who brought experts together; Wallace Berman, a young investigator who threw himself into finding a treatment; Nelson Irey and Floribel Mullick of the Armed Forces Institute of Pathology who helped uncover a missing piece of the puzzle; Louis Hall, Milo Hilty, and Frank Holtzhauer, Ohio researchers who stepped up for Reye's syndrome; the physicians and researchers at the Cincinnati Children's Hospital Medical Center, particularly Charles Linnemann, John Partin, Jacqueline Partin, and William Schubert, who contributed to the understanding of Reye's syndrome over many years; CDC's Ronald Waldman, who took on the directive of the Michigan legislature; pioneering pharmacoepidemiologist Brian Strom, who supported the sharing of information with the public; CDC Director William Foege, compelled by the principle of doing the right thing; pediatricians James Strain and Harry Jennisen, AAP president and executive director respectively, Heinz Eichenwald, Joseph Fitzgerald, Ralph Kauffman, and John Wilson for their lifetime commitment to children and their candor; and Raymond Hime, a parent who wanted to do something and did. For their dedication and work, I also thank those I did not meet, especially Eugene Hurwitz, a young CDC doctor who worked under immense pressure to complete the large case-control studies; Sidney Wolfe, a man unafraid of jumping into the middle of a controversy and staying there; California representative Henry Waxman, whose eloquent summary of the problem said it all: "Parents cannot protect their children from dangers they know nothing about." I extend heartfelt thanks to these and so many other epidemiologists, physicians, scientists, parents, legislators, media, librarians, and professionals at the CDC, FDA, AAP, and the state health departments especially those in Arizona, Ohio, and Michigan—whose selfless efforts helped end this tragedy.

I extend very special thanks to those providing important documents: Jacob Baral, who with continuous encouragement sent old Australian newspapers and the connected me with Anne Cooke, archivist, Children's Hospital at Westmead, Sydney, Australia, who provided access to Dr Reye's original handwritten notes; Graeme Morgan, who sent a copy of the original study data; and John Zwicky and Allison Seagram of the American Academy of Pediatrics and FDA staff, who graciously provided AAP and Freedom of Information documents, respectively. I am grateful to the librarians at the Lane Medical Library, Stanford University School of Medicine; the Louis

Acknowledgements

M. Darling Biomedical Library and the Hugh and Hazel Darling Law Library of the University of California, Los Angeles; the Duke University Medical Center Archives; and the Hathi Trust Digital Library.

My sincere gratitude goes to the professor and students of non-fiction at Stanford University who gave me the courage to include my personal experience and to those who provided guidance on publication and writing, Mildred Marmur, Amanda Mecke, Judy Kern, and Paula Roberts. A special thanks goes to Caren Rickhoff who, with grace, patience, and skill, volunteered to answer my many questions and assist with editing references. To my editor Julia Beaven, whose expertise, kindness, and a steady hand guided me to completion of the manuscript and to Michael Deves, who with patience and professionalism typeset the manuscript, I am deeply grateful.

My most heartfelt thanks goes to those who encouraged and supported me and without whom I would not have developed the skills and courage to pursue a career in medicine and write this book: my advisor at Gettysburg College Jack Shand, who during the 1960s, when few women entered medicine, suggested I consider a doctoral degree; my sisters at Gettysburg College for friendship and support in the early days and on; Temple University School of Medicine Dean Franklin Huber and advisor Bennett Lorber who supported a dream; Donald Francis who changed my path and introduced me to prevention; and physician-researcher Charles Bennett and author Mark Pendergrast, who supported my work over many years .

I am deeply grateful for the love and support of my dear friends Barbara Buchanan, John Buchanan, and Joseph Lynch, who have listened countless hours to my struggles and whose advice and friendship I cherish. And finally, no words can fully express my most deep gratitude for my family, especially my parents and children, whose love of learning and concern for others provide continuing inspiration, and to my grandson Alex, whose curiosity and humor lit my days during the writing of this book.

LIST OF MAIN INTERVIEWS

Baral, Jacob	March 2008
Baublis, Joan	22 September 2006
Berman, Wallace	11 August 2011
Brachman, Philip	11 September 2011
Campbell, Bob	21 October 2008
Cherry, James	11 April 2008
Conrad, J. Lyle	27 July 2011
Crawford, James	28 September 2011
Dowdle, Walter	28 July 2011
Eichenwald, Heinz	26 March 2007
Freudenburger, John	22 October 2008
Freudenburger, Terri	22 October 2008
Fitzgerald, Joseph	4 October 2011
Foege, William	22 July 2009
Forsythe, Brian	2 May 2012
Glick, Thomas	20 May 2009
Hall, Lois Hall	21 October 2008
Hilty, Milo	5 June 2009
Hime, Betty	2 March 2006
Hime, Raymond	2 March 1979 and 24 March 2006
Holtzhauer, Frank	21 October 2008
Jennison, M. Harry	19 & 30 August 2008
Kauffman, Ralph	12 February 2009
Linnemann, Calvin	12 December 2007
Lovejoy, Frederick	20 October 2010
Marks, James	14 September 2011
Marshall (Dieckman), Doris	8 August 2011
Monto, Arnold	14 August 2006
Morgan, Graeme	5 January 2009
Pettine, Louis	25 September 2006
Pollack, J. Dennis	5 June 2009

Acknowledgements

Quinan, Gerald	11 September 2011
Ray, C. George	24 March 2006
Riley, Harris	8 March 2007
Schubert, William	10 November 2011
Strain, James	27 September 2007
Strom, Brian	16 December 2006
Sullivan-Bolyai, John	11 September 2011
Waldman, Ronald	21 July 2011
Wilson, John	18 August 2009

Notes

Author's Note

1   Shannon, F.T. (1965). 'Aspirin medication in infancy and childhood'. *New Zealand Medical Journal*, 64, 571–573.

2   Goodman, L.S. & Gilman, A. (eds). (1970). *The pharmacological basis of therapeutics* (4th edition. p. 328). The MacMillan Company,

3   Lemasters, J.J. & Nieminen, A-L. (eds). (2001). *Mitochondria in pathogenesis*. Kluwer Academic/Plenum Publishers.

Preface

1   Vaughan, V.C., McKay, R.J., & Nelson, W.E. (eds). (1975). *Nelson textbook of pediatrics* (10th ed., pp. 1445–1446). W.B. Saunders Company.

2   Lichtenstein P.K., Heubi J.E., Daugherty C.C., Farrell M.K., Sokol R.J., Rothbaum R.J., Suchy F.J., Balistreri W.F. (1983). Grade I Reye's syndrome: a frequent cause of vomiting and liver dysfunction after varicella and upper-respiratory-tract infection. *New England Journal of Medicine*, 309, 133–139.

3   The American Academy of Pediatrics and the Children's Hospital Association. (30 December 2021). 'Children and COVID-19: State Data Report'. Retrieved 8 January 2022, from the American Academy of Pediatrics.

4   Monto A.S. (1999) The disappearance of Reye's syndrome—A public health triumph. *New England Journal of Medicine*, 340, 1423–1424.

5   Historical Archives Advisory Committee. (2001) Committee Report: American Pediatrics. Milestones at the Millennium. *Pediatrics*, 107, 1482–1491.

Chapter 1 – A Call

1   Shaw, B. (9 January 1979). Rodney's dad fights to turn loss into victory for others. *Arizona Daily Star.*

2   National Reye's Syndrome Foundation. (1977, 1979). A Medical Mystery. Reye's Syndrome. A Lethal Children's Disease. Cause and Cure Unknown [Brochures].

3   Shaw, B. (9 January 1979). Rodney's dad fights to turn loss into victory for others. *Arizona Daily Star.*

4   Vaughan, V.C., McKay, R.J., & Nelson, W.E. (eds). (1975). *Nelson textbook of pediatrics* (10th ed. pp. 1445–1446). W.B. Saunders Company.

5   Sartwell, P.E., & Last, J.M. (1980). Epidemiology. In Last, J.M. (ed.), *Public Health and Preventive Medicine* (pp. 13–14). Appleton-Century-Crofts.

Chapter 2 – The Arizona Study—A Suspect

1   Gibbons, P. (22 January 1979). 11-year-old with rare disease battling for her life. *Mesa Tribune.*

2   Vaughan, V.C., McKay, R.J., & Nelson, W.E. (eds). (1975). *Nelson Textbook of Pediatrics* (10th ed., pp. 1445–1446). W.B. Saunders Company.

Notes

3   Starko, K.M. (April 1979). *Salmonella gastroenteritis associated with milk.* Paper presented at the Epidemic Intelligence Service 28th Annual Conference of the Center for Disease Control, Atlanta, Georgia.

4   Ray, C.G. (1975). Viral infections of the central nervous system. In W.L. Drew (ed.), *Viral Infections—A Clinical Approach.* F.A. Davis Company.

5   US Food and Drug Administration. (1976). Reye's syndrome: Etiology uncertain but avoid antiemetics in children. *FDA Drug Bulletin, 6,* 40–41.

6   Starko, K.M., Ray, C.G., Dominguez, L.B., Stromberg, W.L., & Woodall, D.F. (1980). Reye's syndrome and salicylate use. *Pediatrics, 66* (6), 859–864.

7   Starko, K.M (Early 1979). Working list of medications taken by children with Reye's syndrome and ill control children, Arizona.

8   Nuzzo, R. (2014). Scientific method: Statistical errors. *Nature, 506,* 150–152.

9   Starko, K.M., Ray, C.G., Dominguez, L.B., Stromberg, W.L., & Woodall, D.F. (1980). Reye's syndrome and salicylate use. *Pediatrics, 66* (6), 859–864.

10   Vaughan, V.C., McKay, R.J., & Nelson, W.E. (eds). (1975). *Nelson textbook of pediatrics* (10th ed. p. 1719) W.B. Saunders Company.

11   Woodbury, D.M. (1970) Analgesic-antipyretics, anti-inflammatory agents, and inhibitors of uric acid synthesis. In L.S. Goodman & A. Gilman (eds) *The pharmacological basis of therapeutics* (4th ed., p. 328). The MacMillan Company.

12   Starko, K.M., Ray, C.G., Dominguez, L.B., Stromberg, W.L., & Woodall, D.F. (1980). 'Reye's syndrome and salicylate use'. *Pediatrics, 66* (6), 859–864.

13   Woodbury, D.M. (1970) Analgesic-antipyretics, anti-inflammatory agents, and inhibitors of uric acid synthesis. In L.S. Goodman & A. Gilman (eds) *The Pharmacological Basis of Therapeutics* (4th ed., p. 328). The MacMillan Company.

14   Langmead, F. (30 June 1906). Salicylate poisoning in children. *Lancet, 167* (4322), 1822–1825.

15   Starko, K. (5 February 1979). Memorandum to James Sarn. [Business memorandum EIS Officer, Field Services Division and Medical Epidemiologist, Arizona Department of Health Services to Assistant Director, Disease Control Services, Arizona Department of Health Services].

16   Suzanne Dandoy, Director, Arizona Department of Health Services) (27 February 1979). *News release.* [Press release].

17   Pesticide tie with disease is discounted. (2 March 1979). *Phoenix Gazette.*

18   Riley, H.D., & Worley, L. (October 1956). Salicylate intoxication. *Pediatrics, 18* (4):578–594.

19   ibid.

Chapter 3 – It Can't Be

1   Anderson, A.F. (1923). Report of five cases of acute encephalitis. *Boston Medical and Surgical Journal, 189,* 177–179.

2   Brain, W.R., Hunter, D., & Turnbull, H.M. (1929). Acute meningo-encephalitis of childhood: Report of six cases. *Lancet, 213* (5501), 221–227.

3   DeVivo, D.C., & Keating, J.P. (1976). Reye's syndrome. *Advances in Pediatrics, 22,* 175–229.

4   Low, A.A. (1930). Acute toxic (nonsuppurative) encephalitis in children. *Archives of Neurology & Psychiatry, 23,* 696–714.

5   Brown, C.L., & Symmers, D. (1925). Acute serous encephalitis: A newly recognized disease of children. *American Journal of Diseases of Children, 29,* 174–181.

6   Grinker, R.R., & Stone, T.T. (1928). Acute toxic encephalitis in childhood: A clinicopathologic study of thirteen cases. *Archives of Neurology & Psychiatry, 20,* 244–274.

7   Beverly, B.J. (1929). Encephalitis in children. *American Journal of Diseases of Children, 37,* 600–610.

8   Lyon, G., Dodge P.R., & Adams R.D. (1961). The acute encephalopathies of obscure origin in infants and children. *Brain, 8,* 680–708.

9   Brown, C.L., & Symmers, D. (1925). Acute serous encephalitis: A newly recognized disease of children. *American Journal of Diseases of Children, 29,* 174–181.

10   ibid.

11   Karsner, H.T. (1955). *Human pathology* (8th ed., pp. 42-51, 606–607). J.B. Lippincott & Co.

12   Beverly, B.J. (1929). Encephalitis in children. *American Journal of Diseases of Children, 37,* 600–610.

13   Brain, W.R., Hunter, D., & Turnbull, H.M. (1929). Acute meningo-encephalitis of childhood: Report of six cases. *Lancet, 213* (5501), 221–227.

14   Low, A.A. (1930). Acute toxic (nonsuppurative) encephalitis in children. *Archives of Neurology & Psychiatry, 23,* 696–714.

15   Lyon, G., Dodge, P.R., & Adams, R.D. (1961). The acute encephalopathies of obscure origin in infants and children. *Brain, 84,* 680–708.

16   Troll, M.M., & Menten, M.L. (1945). Salicylate poisoning. *American Journal of Diseases of Children, 69,* 37–43.

17   Jager, B.V., & Alway, R. (1946). The treatment of acute rheumatic fever with large doses of sodium salicylate; with special reference to dose management and toxic manifestations. *American Journal of Medical Sciences, 211,* 272–285.

18   Bove, K.E., McAdams, A.J., Partin, J.C., Partin, J.S., Hug, G., & Schubert, W.K. (September 1975). The hepatic lesion in Reye's syndrome. *Gastroenterology, 69* (3), 685–697.

19   Reye Papers –Children's Hospital Westmead Archives, Sydney, Australia.

20   Johnson, G.M. (1980). Reye's syndrome: Its American origins. *Journal of the National Reye's Syndrome Foundation, 1,* 56–62.

21   Johnson, G.M., Scurletis, T.D., & Carroll, N.B. (1963). A study of sixteen fatal cases of encephalitis-like disease in North Carolina children. *North Carolina Medical Journal, 24,* 464–473.

Chapter 4 – The Parents

1   Pollack, J.D. (ed.). (1975). *Reye's Syndrome. Proceedings of the Reye's Syndrome Conference Sponsored by the Children's Hospital Foundation, Columbus, Ohio.* Grune & Stratton.

2   Hilty M.D. (1974). Etiology of Reye's syndrome. In Pollack, J.D. (ed.). (1975). *Proceedings of the* [1974] *Reye's Syndrome Conference Sponsored by the Children's Hospital Foundation, Columbus, Ohio* (pp. 383–385). Grune & Stratton.

3   National Reye's Syndrome Foundation [Ohio]. (Fall 1979). NRSF Expansion. *National Reye's Syndrome Foundation in the News.* [Article in newsletter].

4   McCullough, B. (20 May 1979). The Syndrome of Death (Dedicated to the Memory of "A Husky" John S.E. Dieckman). *Detroit News.* (Reprinted in the *Congressional Record—Extension of Remarks.* 9 July 1979).

5   Chavez-Carballo, E., Gomez, M.R., & Sharbrough, F.W. (1975). Encephalopathy and fatty infiltration of the viscera (Reye-Johnson Syndrome). A 17-year experience. *Mayo Clinic Proceedings. 50,* 209–215.

6   McCullough, B. (20 May 1979). The Syndrome of Death (Dedicated to the Memory of "A Husky" John S.E. Dieckman). *Detroit News.* (Reprinted in the *Congressional Record—Extension of Remarks.* 9 July 1979).

7   ibid.

8   ibid.

9   ibid.

10   ibid.

11 National Reye's Syndrome Foundation [Michigan]. (June 1979). A concerned parent at work. *National Reye's Syndrome Foundation*, 2 (2), 9. [Article in newsletter].

12 US Food and Drug Administration. (1976). Reye's syndrome: Etiology uncertain but avoid antiemetics in children. *FDA Drug Bulletin*, 6, 40–41.

13 McCullough, B. (20 May 1979). The Syndrome of Death (Dedicated to the Memory of "A Husky" John S.E. Dieckman). *Detroit News*. (Reprinted in the *Congressional Record—Extension of Remarks*. 9 July 1979).

14 Children's Hospital (Columbus); Children's Hospital (Denver); Children Hospital of Philadelphia; Children's Hospital of Pittsburgh; Columbia Presbyterian Medical Center (New York City); C.S. Mott Children's Hospital (Ann Arbor); Detroit Children's Hospital; Emory University School of Medicine (Atlanta); Fitzsimmons Army Hospital (Pueblo); Jackson Memorial Hospital (Miami); Johns Hopkins Medical Center (Baltimore); National Medical Center (Washington, D.C.); New England Medical Center (Boston); Riley's Children's Hospital (Indianapolis); University of Chicago.

15 National Reye's Syndrome Foundation [Michigan]. (1979, June). Major research effort started. *National Reye's Syndrome Foundation*, 2 (2), 10. [Article in newsletter].

16 McCullough, B. (20 May 1979). The Syndrome of Death (Dedicated to the Memory of "A Husky" John S.E. Dieckman). *Detroit News*. (Reprinted in the *Congressional Record—Extension of Remarks*. 9 July 1979).

17 Jagt, G.V. (9 July 1979). A job that needs doing. *Congressional Record—Extension of Remarks* (p. 1767).

18 National Reye's Syndrome Foundation [Ohio]. (Fall 1981). Chronology of events 1979–80 (96th Congress). *National Reye's Syndrome Foundation in the News*. [Article in newsletter].

19 National Reye's Syndrome Foundation [Michigan]. (December 1979). The American Legion enters the battle. *National Reye's Syndrome Foundation*, 2 (3), 3. [Article in newsletter].

20 Including Michigan Reye's syndrome researchers Joe Baublis, Arnold Monto, Fay Luscombe, and William Hall; Ohio researchers Dennis Pollack, John Partin, Milo Hilty; and foundation founders Terri Freudenberger and John Dieckman.

21 LaMontagne, J.R. (1980). Summary of a Workshop on Influenza B Viruses and Reye's Syndrome [News from the National Institute of Allergy and Infectious Diseases]. *The Journal of Infectious Diseases 142* (3), 452–465.

Chapter 5 – Trusted: The Most Popular Medicine in the World and Early Alerts

1 Bayer's print attack on Tylenol campaign. (22 June 1977). *New York Times*.

2 Parascandola, J. (1992). *The development of American pharmacology: John J. Abel and the shaping of a discipline* (p. 26). The Johns Hopkins University Press.

3 McTavish J.R. (2004) The industrial history of analgesics: the evolution of analgesics and antipyretics. In Rainsford, K.D. (ed.) *Aspirin and related drugs* (pp. 25–43). Taylor & Francis.

4 IARC Working Group on the Evaluation of Carcinogenic Risks to Humans. Pharmaceuticals. Lyon (FR): International Agency for Research on Cancer; 2012. (IARC Monographs on the Evaluation of Carcinogenic Risks to Humans, No. 100A.) PHENACETIN. Accessed 14 March 2022, from the National Center for Biotechnology Information, National Library of Medicine, National Institutes of Health.

5 Antoni S., Soerjomataram I., Moore S., Ferlay J., Sitas F., Smith D.P., Forman D. (August 2014). The ban on phenacetin is associated with changes in the incidence trends of upper-urinary tract cancers in Australia. *Cancer, 38* (5), 455–458.

6 Sneader, W. (2000). The discovery of aspirin: A reappraisal. *British Medical Journal*, 321, 1591–1594.

7 Mann, C.C., & Plummer, M.L. (1991). *The aspirin wars: Money, medicine, and 100 years of rampant competition* (p. 26). Harvard Business School Press.

8   Dreser, H. (1899). Pharmakologisches über aspirin (Acetylsalicylsäure). *Pflugers Archiv, 76*, 306–318.

9   Jeffreys, D. (2005). *Aspirin: The remarkable story of a wonder drug aspirin* (p. 77). Bloomsbury.

10   Rainsford K.D. History and development of the salicylates. In Rainsford K.D., ed. (2004). *Aspirin and related drugs* (p. 17). Taylor and Francis.

11   Floeckinger (9 December 1899). Aspirin. *British Medical Journal, 2*, 96.

12   Mann, C.C., & Plummer, M.L. (1991). *The aspirin wars: Money, medicine, and 100 years of rampant competition* (p. 27). Harvard Business School Press.

13   ibid. p. 30.

14   ibid. p. 35.

15   Parascandola, J. (1992). *The development of American pharmacology: John J. Abel and the shaping of a discipline* (pp. 91–125). The Johns Hopkins University Press.

16   Wiley, W.H. (1906). Effect of salicylic acid as a food preservative on digestion and health. *The George Washington University Bulletin, 5*, 102–104.

17   Wiley, H.W. (1906). Influence of food and preservatives and artificial colors on digestion and health. Part II—Salicylic acid and salicylates. *US Department of Agriculture, Bureau of Chemistry—Bulletin No. 84, Part II* (pp. 754–756). Government Printing Office.

18   Hilts, P.J. (2004). *Protecting America's health: The FDA, business, and one hundred years of regulation* (pp. 35–55). University of North Carolina Press.

19   ibid.

20   Pure Food and Drug Act. An Act of 30 June 1906, Public Law Number 59-384, 34 STAT. 768.

21   Sigerist, H.E. (ed.). (1941). *Four treatises of Theophrastus von Hohenheim called Paracelsus. Translated from the original German with introductory essays by C. Lilian Temkin, George Rosen, Gregory Zilboorg, and Henry E. Sigerist* (p. 22). The Johns Hopkins University.

22   Wiley, H.W. (1911). *Foods and their adulteration; Origin, manufacture, and composition of food products; infants' and invalids' foods; detection of common adulterations, and food standards.* P. Blakiston's Son & Co.

23   US Food & Drug Administration. (2006). FDA's approach to the GRAS provision: A history of processes. Retrieved 3 June 2013, from the Food and Drug Administration.

24   ibid. p. 37.

25   Jeffreys, D. (2005). *The remarkable story of a wonder drug aspirin* (p. 151). Bloomsbury.

26   Mann, C.C., & Plummer, M.L. (1991). *The aspirin wars: Money, medicine, and 100 years of rampant competition* (p. 37). Harvard Business School Press.

27   ibid.

28   Hunt, T.C. *Frederick Samuel Langmead.* Accessed 22 June 2021, from Royal College of Physicians.

29   Langmead, F. (30 June 1906). Salicylate poisoning in children. *Lancet, 167 (4322)*, 1822–1825.

30   Lees, D.B. (1903). The Harveian Lectures on the treatment of some acute visceral inflammations. *British Medical Journal, 2 (2238)*, 1318–1322.

31   Lees, D.B. (16 January 1909). The effective treatment of acute and subacute rheumatism. *British Medical Journal, 1 (2507)*, 146–149.

32   Langmead, F. (30 June 1906). Salicylate poisoning in children. *Lancet, 167 (4322)*, 1822–1825.

33   Blanchier. (1879). Thése de Paris, No. 141. Quoted in Hanzlik, P.J. (1915). *The salicylates: A historical and critical review of the literature* (p. 41). American Medical Association. [Reprint from Annual Report (1914) of the Therapeutic Research

Notes

Committee of the Council on Pharmacy and Chemistry of the American Medical Association].

34   Connolly, C.A. (2018). *Children and drug safety* (p. 12). Rutgers University Press.

35   Hanzlik, P.J. (29 March 1913). A study of the toxicity of salicylates based on clinical statistics. *Journal of the American Medical Association, 60* (13), 957–962.

36   ibid.

37   Hanzlik, P.J., Scott, R.W., & Reycraft, J.I. (1917). The salicylates. VIII. Salicyl edema. *Archives of Internal Medicine, 22*, 329–340.

38   Special cable to the *New York Times*. (3 September 1923). Paris savant says aspirin revives withering flowers. *New York Times*, 1.

39   Hanzlik, P.J. (1927). *Actions and uses of the salicylates and cinchophen in medicine*. The Williams & Wilkins Company.

40   Bochefontaine and Chabbert. (1877). *Compt. Rend. Soc. Biol., 85*, 575. As described in Hanzlik, P.J. (1927). *Actions and uses of the salicylates and cinchophen in medicine* (p. 166). The Williams & Wilkins Company.

41   Laborde. (1877). *Bull. Gen. De Therap., 93*, 276. As described in Hanzlik, P.J. (1927). *Actions and uses of the salicylates and cinchophen in medicine* (p. 166). The Williams & Wilkins Company.

42   US Consumer Product Safety Commission. (2005). *Poison prevention packaging: A guide for healthcare professionals* [Brochure].

43   Mann, C.C., & Plummer, M.L. (1991). *The aspirin wars: Money, medicine, and 100 years of rampant competition* (p. 35). Harvard Business School Press.

44   ibid. p. 67.

45   ibid. p. 40.

46   Smith, R.G., & Barrie, A. (1976). *Aspro—How a family business grew up* (pp. 4–5). Nicholas International Limited.

47   ibid. p. 10.

48   ibid. pp. 12–13.

49   ibid. pp. 16–17.

50   ibid. p. 91.

51   Mann, C.C., & Plummer, M.L. (1991). *The aspirin wars: Money, medicine, and 100 years of rampant competition* (p. 37). Harvard Business School Press.

52   Jeffreys, D. (2005). *Aspirin: The remarkable story of a wonder drug aspirin* (p. 151). Bloomsbury.

53   Mann, C.C., & Plummer, M.L. (1991). *The aspirin wars: Money, medicine, and 100 years of rampant competition* (p. 37). Harvard Business School Press.

54   Bayer. (19 February 1917). One Real Aspirin. Bayer-Tablets of Aspirin [Advertisement]. *New York Times*.

55   *Bayer Co. v. United Drug Co.*, 272 F. 505 (S.D.N.Y. 1921)

56   Current Comment. Aspirin or acetylsalicylic acid—An important court decision. (14 May 1921). *Journal of the American Medical Association, 76*, 1356.

57   Takes steps to stop influenza spread. (14 September 1918). *New York Times*, 13.

58   US Navy. (WWI. No date). *Materia medica: The medicinal substances on the supply table of the Medical Department, United States Navy, and their principal properties, usage, and doses*. Retrieved 31 October 2021, from WWW Virtual Library, United States.

59   French, H. (1920). The clinical features of the influenza epidemic of 1918–19. In *Reports on public health and medical subjects, no. 4: Report on the pandemic of influenza, 1918–19* (pp. 66–109). Great Britain, Ministry of Health, His Majesty's Stationary Office.

60   Royal Society of Medicine. (30 November 1918). Resumed discussion of influenza: Morbid anatomy. *Lancet, 192* (4970), 742–744.

61 Monsanto Chemical (18 September 1918). We offer for prompt or future shipment. *Drug and Chemical Markets*, V (2), 1. [Advertisement]

62 Bayer Company, Inc. (18 September 1918). Completely under American Control [Advertisement]. Drug and Chemical Markets, V (2), 2.

63 Dewey, W.A. (1921). Homeopathy in influenza—A chorus of 50 in harmony. *Journal of the American Institute of Homeopathy.* 1038–1043.

64 Barry, J.M. (1999). *The great influenza.* Penguin Books.

65 Thisted, B., Krantz, T., Strom, J., & Sorensen, M.B. (May 1987). Acute salicylate self-poisoning in 177 consecutive patients treated in ICU. *Acta Anaesthesiologica Scandinavica, 31,* 312–316.

66 Starko, K.M. (1 November 2009). Salicylates and pandemic influenza mortality, 1918–1919 pharmacology, pathology, and historic evidence. *Clinical Infectious Diseases, 49* (9), 1405–1410.

67 Jeffreys, D. (2005). *Aspirin: The remarkable story of a wonder drug aspirin* (pp. 144–145). Bloomsbury.

68 Mann, C.C., & Plummer, M.L. (1991). *The aspirin wars: Money, medicine, and 100 years of rampant competition* (p. 51). Harvard Business School Press.

69 Jeffreys, D. (2005). *Aspirin: The remarkable story of a wonder drug aspirin* (p. 142). Bloomsbury.

70 Mann, C.C., & Plummer, M.L. (1991). *The aspirin wars: Money, medicine, and 100 years of rampant competition* (pp. 69–70). Harvard Business School Press.

71 Smith, R.G., & Barrie, A. (1976). *Aspro—How a family business grew up* (p. 17). Nicholas International Limited.

72 ibid. pp. 28–29.

73 ibid. pp. 34, 37–38.

Chapter 6 – Lost Warnings and Loopholes

1   Holt, L.E. & Howland, J. (1912). *The Diseases of infancy and childhood; For the use of students and practitioners of medicine* (6th ed., p. 300). D. Appleton and Company.

2   ibid. p. 518.

3   Holt, L.E., & Howland, J. (1918). *The diseases of infancy and childhood; For the use of students and practitioners of medicine* (7th ed., p. 524). D. Appleton and Company.

4   Libman, E. (November 1927). Obituary: Dr Henry Koplik. *Bulletin of the New York Academy of Medicine, 3* (11), 667–671.

5   Koplik, H. (1918). *The diseases of infancy and childhood: Designed for the use of students and practitioners of medicine* (4th ed.). Lea and Febiger.

6   Hilts, P.J. (2004). *Protecting America's health: The FDA, business, and one hundred years of regulation.* University of North Carolina Press.

7   US Food and Drug Administration (2018). A brief history of the Center for Drug Evaluation and Research. Retrieved 10 January 2022, from the Food and Drug Administration.

8   Meadows, M. (2006). Promoting safe and effective drugs for 100 years. *FDA Consumer Magazine* (The Centennial Edition/January –February 2006).

9   Mann, C.C., & Plummer, M.L. (1991). *The aspirin wars: Money, medicine, and 100 years of rampant competition* (pp. 138–148). Harvard Business School Press.

10 Government fines fifty misbranded medicines. (22 September 1915). *Weekly Drug Markets, II* (2), 18.

11 Mann, C.C., & Plummer, M.L. (1991). *The aspirin wars: Money, medicine, and 100 years of rampant competition* (p. 143). Harvard Business School Press.

12 ibid. p. 156.

13 ibid. p. 143.

14 ibid. p. 145.

Notes

15 Parascandola, J. (1992). *The development of American pharmacology: John J. Abel and the shaping of a discipline* (p. 100). The Johns Hopkins University Press.

16 US Food and Drug Administration. (2018). The American Chamber of Horrors. Retrieved 26 September 2021 from the Food and Drug Administration.

17 US Food and Drug Administration. (2018). 80 years of the Federal Food Drug and Cosmetic Act. Retrieved 26 September 2021 from the Food and Drug Administration.

18 Hill, L.F. (1928). The American Academy of Pediatrics—Its growth and development. *Pediatrics, 1,* 1–7.

19 Parascandola, J. (1992). *The development of American pharmacology: John J. Abel and the shaping of a discipline* (p. 93). The Johns Hopkins University Press.

20 Comments. (September 1934). *The Journal of Pediatrics, 5* (3), 432.

21 Carpenter, D. (2010). *Reputation and power: Organizational image and regulation at the FDA* (p. 80). Princeton University Press. As referenced in Connolly, C.A. (2018). *Children and drug safety* (p. 19). Rutgers University Press.

22 Mann, C.C., & Plummer, M.L. (1991). *The aspirin wars: Money, medicine, and 100 years of rampant competition* (p. 149). Harvard Business School Press.

23 ibid. p. 150.

24 ibid. p. 152.

25 ibid. pp. 159–161.

26 ibid. p. 161.

27 ibid. p. 162.

28 Bart, P. (26 March 1961). Aspirin consumption increases with the nation's headaches; Huge gain shown in use of aspirin. *New York Times.*

29 Mann, C.C., & Plummer, M.L. (1991). *The aspirin wars: Money, medicine, and 100 years of rampant competition* (p. 334). Harvard Business School Press.

30 Brodie, B.B., Udenfriend, S., & Coburn, A.F. (January 1944). The determination of salicylic acid in plasma. *Journal of Pharmacology and Experimental Therapeutics, 80,* 114–117.

31 Coburn, A.F. (1943). Salicylate therapy in acute rheumatic fever. *Bulletin of the Johns Hopkins Hospital, 73,* 435–464.

32 ibid. p. 445.

33 Woodbury, D. (1970). Analgesic-antipyretic, anti-inflammatory agents, and inhibitors of uric acid synthesis. In L.S. Goodman and A. Gilman (eds), *The pharmacological basis of therapeutics* (4th ed., p. 328). The MacMillan Company.

34 Fashena, G.J., & Walker, J.N. (December 1944). Salicylate intoxication: Studies on the effect of sodium salicylate on prothrombin time and alkali reserve. *American Journal of Diseases of Children, 68,* 369–375.

35 Link K.P., Overman R.S., Sullivan W.R., Huebner CF, Scheel L.D. (1943). Studies on the hemorrhagic sweet clover disease. XI. Hypoprothrombinemia in the rat induced by salicylic acid. *Journal of Biological Chemistry, 147,* 463–474.

36 Rapoport, S., & Guest, G.M. (September 1945). The effect of salicylates on the electrolyte structure of the blood plasma. I. Respiratory alkalosis in monkeys and dogs after sodium and methyl salicylate: The influence of hypotonic drugs and of sodium bicarbonate on salicylate poisoning. *The Journal of Clinical Investigations, 24* (5), 759–769.

37 Guest, G.M., Rapoport, S., & Roscoe, C. (September 1945). The effect of salicylates on the electrolyte structure of the blood plasma. II. The action of therapeutic doses of sodium salicylate and of acetysalicylic acid in man. *Journal of Clinical Investigations, 24* (5), 770–774.

38 Smull, K., Wegria, R., & Leland, J. (26 August 1944). The effect of sodium bicarbonate on the serum salicylate level during salicylate therapy of patients with acute rheumatic fever. *Journal of the American Medical Association,125* (17), 1173–1175.

39 Stevens, D.L, & Kaplan, D.B. (November 1945). Salicylate intoxication in children. Report of four cases. *American Journal of Diseases of Children, 68*, 331–335.

40 ibid.

41 Dubow, E., & Solomon, N.H. (April 1948). Salicylate tolerance and toxicity in children. *Pediatrics,* 1: 495–504.

42 Lester, D., Lolli, G., & Greenberg, L.A. (August 1946). The fate of acetylsalicylic acid. *Journal of Pharmacology and Experimental Therapeutics, 87* (4), 329–342.

43 ibid.

44 Smith, P.K., Gleason, H.L., Stoll, C.G., & Ogorzalek, S. (July 1946). Studies on the pharmacology of salicylates. *Journal of Pharmacology and Experimental Therapeutics, 87* (3), 237–255.

45 Dubow, E., & Solomon, N.H. (April 1948). Salicylate tolerance and toxicity in children. *Pediatrics,* 1: 495–504.

46 Acetylsalicylic acid deaths. (1940). [Editorial]. *Journal of the American Medical Association, 115* (14):1199–1200.

47 Gross, M., & Greenburg, L.A. (1948). *The salicylates. A critical bibliographic review* (p. 167). Hillhouse Press.

48 Dubow, E., & Solomon, N.H. (April 1948). Salicylate tolerance and toxicity in children. *Pediatrics,* 1: 495–504.

49 Erganian, J.A., Gorbes, G.B., & Case, D.M. (February 1947). Salicylate intoxication in the infant and young child; A report of thirteen cases. *The Journal of Pediatrics, 30* (2), 129– 145.

50 ibid. p. 141.

51 Wyckoff, A.S. (24 August 2016). Did you know? The green and the gray: *Pediatrics* and *The Journal of Pediatrics. AAP News* [Official Newsmagazine of the American Academy of Pediatrics].

52 Lester, D., Lolli, G., & Greenberg, L.A. (August 1946). The fate of acetylsalicylic acid. *Journal of Pharmacology and Experimental Therapeutics, 87* (4), 329–342.

53 Gross M. & Greenburg L.A. (1948). *The salicylates. A critical bibliographic review.* Hillhouse Press.

54 Mann, C.C., & Plummer, M.L. (1991). *The aspirin wars: Money, medicine, and 100 years of rampant competition* (p. 186). Harvard Business School Press.

55 Miles Laboratories, Inc. (1952) When you need relief with speed ... [Advertisement].

56 Ballabriga, A. (1991). One century of pediatrics in Europe. In B.L. Nichols, A. Ballabriga, & N. Kretchmer (eds) *History of pediatrics 1850–1950* (pp. 6–10). Raven Press.

57 Wood, H.C. (1947). The origin of Young's rule. *Journal of the American Pharmaceutical Association, 8*, 35–36.

58 Deseille, J. (1879). *De la médication salicylée dans le rhumatisme chez les enfants. Thése de Paris* No. 494. A. Parent.

59 Archambault (1878). Cited by Deseille, J. (1879) in *Thése de Paris* No. 494. As referenced in Hanzlik, P.J. (1927). *Actions and uses of the salicylates and cinchophen in medicine* (p. 166). The Williams and Wilkins Company.

60 Archambault (1878), as quoted in Sollmann, T.H. (1936). *A manual of pharmacology and its application to therapeutics and toxicology* (p. 594). W.B. Saunders Company.

61 Altman, L.K. (28 November 2000). Dr Louis S. Goodman, 94, chemotherapy pioneer, dies. *New York Times.*

62 L.S. Goodman & A. Gilman (eds). (1941). *The pharmacological basis of therapeutics* (1st ed., p. 231). The MacMillan Company.

63 L.S. Goodman & A. Gilman (eds). (1955). *The pharmacological basis of therapeutics* (2nd ed.). The MacMillan Company.

64 Chapin, H.D., & Royse, L.T. (1925). *Diseases of infants and children*. Hamilton Printing Co.

65 Fischer, L. (1928). *Diseases of infancy and childhood: Their dietetic, hygienic, and medical treatment; A text-book designed for practitioners and students in medicine* (11th ed., Vol. 1.). F.A. Davis Company.

66 Holt, L.E., & Howland, J. (1920). *The diseases of infancy and childhood; For the use of students and practitioners of medicine* (7th ed., p. 1139). D. Appleton and Company.

67 Lucas, W.P. (1923). *Children's diseases for nurses* (p. 541). The MacMillan Company.

68 ibid.

69 G.W.G. (1945). Charles Gilmore Kerley, M.D. 1863–1945. *Am J Dis Child, 70*(5), 359.

70 Kerley, C.G., & Graves, G.W. (1924). *The practice of pediatrics* (3rd ed., p. 87). W.B. Saunders Company.

71 Shaw, H.L.K. (1928). *Infectious diseases of infancy and childhood*. D. Appleton and Company.

72 Holt, L.E. & Howland, J., revised by L. Emmett Holt, Jr & Rustin McIntosh. (1933). *Holt's Diseases of infancy and childhood; A textbook for the use of students and practitioners of medicine* (10th ed., p. 372). D. Appleton and Company.

73 Jeans, P.C., & Rand, W. (1936). *Essentials of pediatrics for nurses* (2nd ed., p. 97). J.B. Lippincott.

74 Nelson, W.E., (ed.) (1950). *Mitchell-Nelson textbook of pediatrics* (5th ed., pp. 222–224). W.B. Saunders Company.

75 Astin, A.V., & Karo, H.A. (1959). US National Bureaus of Standards. Refinement of values for the yard and pound. Retrieved 7 August 2021, from the National Geodetic Survey (NGS), National Oceanic and Atmospheric Association.

76 Vaughan, V.C., McKay, R.J., & Nelson, W.E. (eds). (1975). *Nelson textbook of pediatrics* (10th edition, p. 1719). W.B. Saunders Company.

77 Done, A.K., Yaffe, S.J., & Clayton, J.M. (1979). Aspirin dosage for infants and children. *The Journal of Pediatrics, 95*(4), 617–625.

78 Hill, L.F., Hubbard, J.P., Harris, T.N., Jackson, R.L., & Wheatley, G.M. (May 1949). Rheumatic fever: Summary of present concepts [Panel discussion]. *Pediatrics, 3*(5), 680–710.

79 Woodbury D. (1970). Analgesic-antipyretic, anti-inflammatory agents, and inhibitors of uric acid synthesis. In L.S. Goodman & A. Gilman (eds). *The pharmcological basis of therapeutics*. 4th ed., p. 328). The MacMillan Company.

80 Greenburg L.A. (1950). An evaluation of reported poisonings by acetylsalicylic acid. *New England Journal of Medicine*, 243,124–129.

81 Aspirin consumption quadrupled since '29. (20 February 1948). *New York Times*.

82 United States Census Bureau. Decennial Census by Decade. Retrieved 23 June 2021, from the United States Census Bureau.

83 Olsen, P.C. (11 August 1952). Three year report on 222 drug store product lines. Drug Topics, 96. As described in Bain, K. (June 1954). Death due to accidental poisoning in young children. *The Journal of Pediatrics, 44*(6), 616–623.

84 Bain, K. (June 1954). Death due to accidental poisoning in young children. *Journal of Pediatrics, 44*(6), 616–623.

Chapter 7 – Accidents: Unsupervised Children?

1 Lewis, S. (1 March 2018). Abe Plough (1892–1984). *Tennessee encyclopedia*. Retrieved 3 March 2022, from the Tennessee Historical Society.

2 Chapin, H.D., & Royster, L.T. (1925). *Diseases of infants and children*. Hamilton Printing Co.

3   Fischer, L. (1928). *Diseases of infancy and childhood: Their dietetic, hygienic, and medical treatment; A text-book designed for practitioners and students in medicine* (11th ed., Vol. 1.). F.A. Davis Company.

4   Committee on Toxicology. (7 May 1955). Candy medication and accidental poisoning. [Report to the Council on Pharmacology and Chemistry]. *Journal of the American Medical Association, 158*(1), 44–45.

5   *Child safety act and personnel training. (1966). Hearings, Eighty-ninth Congress, second session, June 24, August 15, 29, September 12, 19, 1966* (p. 133). US Government Printing Office.

6   Plough, Inc. (October 1947). Preferred by millions [Advertisement]. *Lansing State Journal,* 5.

7   Duke University Medical Center Archives. Gifford, J. (28 February 1984). *Jay Arena, Professor of Pediatrics and Community Health and Director of Duke Poison Control Center, an oral history interview* [Transcript]. Published 17 June 2004.

8   ibid.

9   ibid.

10 Tots treated for eating aspirin. (8 February 1950). *Long Beach Press.*

11 Sunland child dies from eating aspirin. (31 March 1958). *Long Beach Press.*

12 Sterling Drug (9 July1950). New ... Bayer Aspirin in Children's Size [Advertisement]. *Long Beach Press,* 74.

13 Sterling Drug (November 1951). Now Bayer Aspirin in Children's Size [Advertisement]. *Women's Day,* 185.

14 Sterling Drug, Inc. History (1988). In *International directory of company histories* (Vol. 1). St James Press. Retrieved 23 June 2021, from Funding Universe.

15 ibid.

16 Bayer aspirin plant opened. (18 September 1947). *New York Times.*

17 Sterling Drug (September 1951). Mothers Are Talking and Buying [Advertisement]. *Chain Store Age,* 26.

18 Sterling Drug. (15 June 1952). New, Flavored Children's Size BAYER ASPIRIN [Advertisement]. *The Reading Eagle.*

19 Sterling Drug. (14 March 1953). Gentle as a Mother's Kiss [Advertisement]. *Saturday Evening Post,* 70.

20 Nagle, J.J. News of the advertising and marketing fields. (21 June 1953). *New York Times.*

21 ibid.

22 Jeffreys, D. (2005). *Aspirin: The remarkable story of a wonder drug aspirin* (pp. 209–210). Bloomsbury.

23 ibid. p. 211.

24 Jeffreys, D. (2005). *Aspirin: The remarkable story of a wonder drug aspirin* (pp. 205–206). Bloomsbury.

25 Reckitt and Colman. (December 1955). Disprin for children [Advertisement]. *Journal of Tropical Medicine.*

26 Bart, P. (26 March 1961). Aspirin consumption increases with the nation's headaches; Huge gain shown in use of aspirin. *New York Times.*

27 Palmer, B. & Clegg, D.J. (25 June 2020). Salicylate toxicity. *New England Journal of Medicine 382*(26), 2544–2555.

28 Goodman, L.S., & Gilman, A. (eds). (1975). *The pharmacological basis of therapeutics* (5th ed., p. 238). The MacMillan Company.

29 Federal Caustic Poison Act. (4 March 1927). Title 15, Chapter 489, Section 1, 44 Stat. 1406, Section 402.

30 Stevenson, C.S. (1937). Oil of wintergreen (methyl salicylate) poisoning. Report of three cases, one with autopsy, and a review of the literature. *American Journal of Medical Sciences, 193,* 772–788.

Notes

31 Federal Register. (10 April 1954). Labeling of drug preparations containing significant portions of wintergreen oil. Title 21, Chapter 1, Part 3, Section 3.35, 2085.

32 Dietrich, H.F., Wheatley, G.M., Brooks, G.L., Kotte, R.H., & Wyvell, D. (1951). Round table discussion: Childhood accidents and their prevention. *Pediatrics,8*, 426–430.

33 ibid.

34 Marshall, J.T. (July 1949). The sixth revision of the international lists of diseases and causes of death. *The Milbank Memorial Fund Quarterly, 27*(3), 289–298.

35 Bain, K. (June 1954). Death due to accidental poisoning in young children. *Journal of Pediatrics, 44*(6), 616–623.

36 ibid.

37 Burda, A.M. & Burda, N.M. (April 1997). The nation's first poison control center: Taking a stand against accidental childhood poisoning in Chicago. *Veterinary and Human Toxicology, 39*, 115–119.

38 Cann, H.M., Neyman, D.S., & Verhulst, H.L. (11 October 1958). Control of accidental poisonings—A progress report. *Journal of the American Medical Association, 168*, 717–724.

39 ibid.

40 Orenstein, W.A., Papania, M.J., & Wharton, M.E. (2004). Measles elimination in the United States. *The Journal of Infectious Diseases, 189*(Supple 1), S1–3.

41 City reports 10% hit by Asian flu. (2 January 1958). *New York Times.*

42 Committee on Toxicology. (7 May 1955). Candy medication and accidental poisoning. [Report to the Council on Pharmacology and Chemistry]. *Journal of the American Medical Association, 158*(1), 44–45.

43 Singer, H. (1901). Ueber aspirin. *Pflugers Archiv, 84*, 527–546. As described in Denis, W., & Means, J.H. (1916). The influence of salicylate on metabolism in man, *Journal of Pharmacology and Experimental Therapeutics, 8*, 273–283.

44 Denis, W. & Means, J.H. (1916). The influence of salicylate on metabolism in man. *Journal of Pharmacology and Experimental Therapeutics, 8*, 273–283.

45 Cutting, W.C., Mehrtens, H.G., & Tainter, M.L. (15 July 1933). Actions and uses of dinitrophenol: Promising metabolic applications. *Journal of the American Medical Association, 101*(3),193–195.

46 Astwood, E.B. (1970). Thyroid and antithyroid drugs. In L.S. Goodman and A. Gilman (eds), *The pharmacological basis of therapeutics* (4th ed., p. 1482). The MacMillan Company.

47 ibid.

48 Tainter, M.L., Stockton, A.B., & Cutting, C.C. (3 August 1935). Dinitrophenol in the treatment of obesity: Final report. *Journal of the American Medical Association, 105*, 332–337.

49 Tainter, M.L., Cutting, W.C., & Stockton, A.B. (October 1934). Use of dinitrophenol in nutritional disorders: A critical survey of clinical results. *American Journal of Public Health, 24*(10),1045–1053.

50 Boardman, W.W. (13 July 1935). Rapidly developing cataract after dinitrophenol. *Journal of the American Medical Association, 105*(2),108.

51 Horner, W.D., Jones, R.B., & Boardman, W.W. (13 July 1935). Cataracts following the use of dinitrophenol. *Journal of the American Medical Association, 105*(2), 108–110.

52 Parascandola, J. (15 November 1974). Dinitrophenol and bioenergetics: An historical perspective. *Molecular and Cellular Biochemistry, 5*, 69–77.

53 Andersson, B. (10 December 1997). The Nobel Prize in Chemistry 1997 Award Ceremony Speech. Retrieved 6 May 2022, from The Nobel Prize.

54 ibid.

55 The Nobel Foundation. (15 October 1997). Nobel Prize in Chemistry 1997. [Press release]

56 The Nobel Prize in Chemistry 1997. Retrieved 6 May 2022, from The Nobel Prize.

57   Brody, T.M. (1955). The uncoupling action of the salicylates in brain and liver mitochondrial preparations. *Journal of Pharmacology and Experimental Therapeutics, 113*, 335–363.

58   Brody, T.M. (1956). Action of sodium salicylate and related compounds on tissue metabolism *in vitro. Journal of Pharmacology and Experimental Therapeutics, 117* (1), 39–51.

59   Lutwak-Mann, C. (1942). The effect of salicylate and cinchophen on enzyme and metabolic processes. *Biochemical Journal, 36*(10–12): 706–728.

60   *Child safety act and personnel training. Hearings before the Subcommittee on Public Health and Welfare of the Committee on Interstate and Foreign Commerce House of Representatives*, Eighty-ninth Congress, second session, June 24, August 15, 29, September 12, 19, 1966. US Government Printing Office (p. 174).

61   Clarke, A., & Walton, W.W. (1979). Effect of safety packaging on aspirin ingestion by children. *Pediatrics, 63* (5), 687–693.

62   Kerlan, I. (6 April 1957). Health problems occurring from household chemicals, including drugs. *Journal of the American Medical Association, 163* (14): 1254–1257.

63   *Child safety act and personnel training. Hearings before the Subcommittee on Public Health and Welfare of the Committee on Interstate and Foreign Commerce House of Representatives*, Eighty-ninth Congress, second session, June 24, August 15, 29, September 12, 19, 1966. US Government Printing Office (p. 15).

64   Federal Register. (15 October 1955). Labeling of drug preparations containing salicylates. Title 21, Chapter 1, Part 3, Section 3.43, 7792.

65   *Child safety act and personnel training. Hearings before the Subcommittee on Public Health and Welfare of the Committee on Interstate and Foreign Commerce House of Representatives*, Eighty-ninth Congress, second session, June 24, August 15, 29, September 12, 19, 1966. US Government Printing Office (p. 15).

66   Federal Register. (15 October 1955). As stated in Kerlan, I. (6 April 1957). Health problems occurring from household chemicals, including drugs. *Journal of the American Medical Association, 163* (14), 1254–1257.

67   Code of Federal Regulations (13 April 1979). Administrative Practices and Procedures. CFR, Title 21, Volume 1, Part 10.

68   Kerlan, I. (6 April 1957). Health problems occurring from household chemicals, including drugs. *Journal of the American Medical Association, 163* (14), 1254–1257.

69   Physicians call aspirin major childhood peril. (5 April 1957). *New York Times.*

70   Plough, Inc. (1958). More and more children are victims of colds and the Asian flu [Advertisement]. *New York News.* Retrieved 15 March 2022, Duke University Digital Collection, Medicine, and Madison Avenue.

71   Plough, Inc. (2 December 1957). When Asian Flu and cold miseries strike … [Advertisement], *LIFE*, 22.

72   Cann, H.M, Neyman, D.S., & Verhulst, H.L. (11 October 1958). Control of accidental poisonings—A progress report. *Journal of the American Medical Association, 168*, 717–724.

73   ibid.

74   Arena, J.M. (14 March 1959). Safety closure caps: Safety measure for prevention of accidental drug poisoning in children. *Journal of the American Medical Association, 169* (11),1187–1188.

75   Duke University Medical Center Archives. Gifford, J. (28 February 1984). *Jay Arena, Professor of Pediatrics and Community Health and Director of Duke Poison Control Center, an oral history interview* [Transcript, p. 17]. Published 17 June 2004.

76   Connolly, C.A. (2018). *Children and drug safety* (p. 109). Rutgers University Press.

77   *Child safety act and personnel training. Hearings before the Subcommittee on Public Health and Welfare of the Committee on Interstate and Foreign Commerce House of*

Representatives, Eighty-ninth Congress, second session, June 24, August 15, 29, September 12, 19, 1966. US Government Printing Office (p. 16).

78　ibid. pp. 307–308.

79　"Child Protection" in *CQ Almanac 1966* (22nd ed., pp. 325–327). Congressional Quarterly, 1967.

80　ibid.

81　*Child safety act and personnel training. Hearings before the Subcommittee on Public Health and Welfare of the Committee on Interstate and Foreign Commerce House of Representatives*, Eighty-ninth Congress, second session, June 24, August 15, 29, September 12, 19, 1966. US Government Printing Office (pp. 87–89).

82　Martin D. (2 January 2010). James L. Goddard, crusading FDA leader, dies at 86. *New York Times.*

83　US Consumer Product Safety Commission. (2005). *Poison prevention packaging: A guide for healthcare professionals* [Brochure].

84　US Consumer Product Safety Commission. (1999). *Poison prevention packaging: A text for pharmacists and physicians* [Brochure].

85　Clarke, A., & Walton, W.W. (1979). Effect of safety packaging on aspirin ingestion by children. *Pediatrics, 63* (5), 687–693.

86　ibid.

87　Rodgers, G.B. (September 2002). The effectiveness of child-resistant packaging for aspirin. *Archives of Pediatrics and Adolescent Medicine, 156* (9), 929–933.

88　Riley, H.D., & Worley, L. (October 1956). Salicylate intoxication. *Pediatrics, 18* (4):578–594.

Chapter 8 – Poisoning During Therapy at Home: Overdose or Wrong Dose?

1　Dodd, K., Minot, A.S., & Arena, J.M. (June 1937). Salicylate poisoning: An explanation of the more serious manifestations. *American Journal of Diseases of Children, 53* (6),1435–1446.

2　ibid.

3　Jeffreys, D. (2005). *Aspirin: The remarkable story of a wonder drug aspirin* (p. 219). Bloomsbury.

4　Lucas, W.P. (1923). *Children's diseases for nurses* (p. 541). The MacMillan Company.

5　Kerley, C.G., & Graves, G.W. (1924). *The practice of pediatrics* (3rd ed., p. 87). W.B. Saunders Company.

6　Marriott, W.M. (1930). *Infant nutrition.* C.V. Mosby Company.

7　Marriott, W.M. (1935). *Infant nutrition* (2nd ed.). C.V. Mosby Company.

8　Marriott, W.M. (1941). *Infant nutrition* (3rd ed.). P.C. Jeans (rev.). C.V. Mosby Company.

9　Jeans, P.C., & Marriott, W.M. (1947). *Infant nutrition* (4th ed.). C.V. Mosby Company.

10　Barnett, H.L, Powers, J.R, Benward, J.H, & Hartmann, A.F. (1 August 1942). Salicylate intoxication in infants and children. *Journal of Pediatrics, 21* (2), 214–223.

11　Erganian, J.A., Forbes, G.B., & Case, D.M. (February 1947). Salicylate intoxication in the infant and young child: A report of thirteen cases. *Journal of Pediatrics, 30,* 129–145.

12　Aspirin held infant peril: 3 Baby deaths in St Louis tied to dosages, doctors warn. (22 November 1952). *New York Times.*

13　Nelson, W.E. (ed.). (1950). *Mitchell-Nelson textbook of pediatrics* (5th ed.). W.B. Saunders Company.

14　The Bayer Company, Inc. (27 June 1919). "Bayer Cross" on Aspirin [Advertisement]. *The Richmond* [Richmond, Madison County, Kentucky] *Daily Register.*

15   Infant deaths from aspirin. (February 1953). [Editorial]. *Journal of Pediatrics, 42*(2), 276.

16   Hoffman W.S. (1953). Pitfalls of acetylsalicylic acid medication. *American Journal of Diseases of Children*, 85, 58.

17   Hoffman, W.S. (1954). *The biochemistry of clinical medicine* (p. 208). The Yearbook Publishers, Inc.

18   ibid. p. 210.

19   Wallace, W. (1954). The use of salicylates in pediatrics. *Quarterly Review of Pediatrics, 9*, 135–141.

20   Riley, H.D., & Worley, L. (October 1956). Salicylate intoxication. *Pediatrics, 18*(4):578–594.

21   Plough, Inc. (2 December 1957). When Asian flu and cold's miseries strike ... [Advertisement]. *LIFE*, 22.

22   Done, A.K. (April 1959). Uses and abuses of antipyretic therapy. *Pediatrics, 23*(4), 774–780.

23   ibid.

24   Done, A.K. (31 May 1965). Salicylate poisoning. *Journal of the American Medical Association, 192*(9),770–772.

25   Done, A.K., & Temple, A.R. (August 1971). Treatment of salicylate poisoning. *Modern Treatment, 8*(3), 528–551.

26   Segar, W.E., & Holliday, M.A. (18 December 1958). Physiologic abnormalities of salicylate intoxication. *New England Journal of Medicine, 259*(25), 1191–1198.

27   Wood H.C. & Reichert E.T. (1882). *Journal of Physiology, 3*, 321-326.

28   Barbour H.G. & Devenis M.M. (1919). Antipyretics II. Acetylsalicylic acid and heat regulation in normal individuals. *Archives of Internal Medicine, 24, 617-623.*

29   Winters, R.W., White, J.S., Hughes, M.C., & Ordway, N.K. (February 1959). Disturbances of acid-base equilibrium in salicylate intoxication. *Pediatrics, 23*(2), 260–285.

30   Crichton, J.U., & Elliott, G.B. (26 November 1960). Salicylate—A dangerous drug in infancy and childhood: A survey of 58 cases of salicylate poisoning. *Canadian Medical Association Journal, 83*(22), 1144–1147.

31   Bayer aspirin with instant flaking action. (1960s). [Television advertisement]. Retrieved 4 August 2020, from YouTube at https://youtu.be/K07fW589Czw

32   Sterling Drug (9 December 1960). You can give flavored BAYER Aspirin for Children with your doctor's blessing [Advertisement]. *Catholic Advance.*

33   US Food and Drug Administration. (February 1977). Safety and effectiveness of over-the-counter drugs: The FDA's OTC drug review. *Pediatrics, 59*(2), 309–311.

34   Gill, P.F. (1 June 1950). Agranulocytopenia following "chloromycetin:" Report on two cases. *Medical Journal of Australia, 1*(23), 768–769.

35   Hilts, P.J. (2004). *Protecting America's health: The FDA, business, and one hundred years of regulation* (pp. 115–116). University of North Carolina Press.

36   Including William P. Barba, Temple University School of Medicine (Philadelphia); Alan Done, University of Utah (Salt Lake City); Horace Hodes, Sydenham Hospital (Baltimore); Philip Charles Jeans, University of Iowa School of Medicine (Iowa City); Harry C. Shirkey, Children's Hospital Medical Center (Cincinnati); Helen Taussig, Johns Hopkins University (Baltimore); Sumner Yaffe, State University of New York (Buffalo).

37   Connolly, C.A. (2018). *Children and drug safety*. Rutgers University Press.

38   Miller, L. (1953). Lloyd Miller's handwritten notes of a meeting with USP president Windsor Cutting, 14 October 1953, box 149, folder, USP archives. As referenced in Connolly, C.A. (2018). *Children and drug safety* (p. 46). Rutgers University Press.

39   Connolly, C.A. (2018). *Children and drug safety* (p. 77). Rutgers University Press.

40 Charles C. Edwards. American Academy of Pediatrics Keynote, 16 October 1972, 11, MSS O 447m Box, folder 1, Charles C. Edwards Papers Mandeville Special Collections Library, Geisel Library, University of California, San Diego, La Jolla, California. As referenced in Connolly, C.A. (2018). *Children and drug safety* (p. 85). Rutgers University Press.

41 Dodd, K., Minot, A.S., & Arena, J.M. (June 1937). Salicylate poisoning: An explanation of the more serious manifestations. *American Journal of Diseases of Children, 53* (6), 1435–1446.

42 Graham, J.D.P., & Parker, W.A. (April 1948). The toxic manifestations of sodium salicylate therapy. *Quarterly Journal of Medicine, 17* (66), 153–163.

43 Wallace, W. (1954). The use of salicylates in pediatrics. *Quarterly Review of Pediatrics, 9*, 135–141.

44 Riley, H.D., & Worley, L. (October 1956). Salicylate intoxication. *Pediatrics, 18* (4), 578– 594.

45 Done, A.K. (November 1960). Salicylate intoxication: Significance of measurements of salicylate in blood in cases of acute ingestion. *Pediatrics, 26* (5), 800–807.

46 Limbeck, G.A., Ruvalcaba, R.H.A., Samols, E., & Kelley, V.C. (February 1965). Salicylates and hypoglycemia. *American Journal of Diseases of Children, 109* (2), 165–167.

47 Levy, G., & Tsuchiya, T. (31 August 1972). Salicylate accumulation kinetics in man. *New England Journal of Medicine, 287*, 430–432.

48 Harvey, E.N. (26 June 1914). Cell permeability for acids. *Science, 39* (1017), 947–949.

49 Binns, T.B. (ed.). (1964). *Absorption and distribution of drugs.* Williams and Wilkins Company.

50 Hill, J.B. (24 May 1973). Current concepts: Salicylate intoxication. *New England Journal of Medicine, 288*, 1110–1113.

51 Levy, G., & Yaffe, S.J. (December 1974). Relationship between dose and apparent volume of distribution in salicylate of children. *Pediatrics, 54* (6), 713–717.

52 Done, A.K. (1974). Salicylate, pharmacokinetics, and the pediatrician. *Pediatrics, 54*, pp. 670–672.

53 Ibid.

Chapter 9 – An Unfolding Disaster and an Unsuspected Culprit, 1950s

1 Breen, G.E., & Emond, R.T.D. (15 September 1954). Chickenpox associated with fulminating hepatitis. *The Medical Press, 251.*

2 Wright, E.M., Lipson, M.J., & Mortimer, E.A. (1 November 1956). Varicella and severe hypoglycemia. [Abstract in Society Transactions of the American Pediatric Society]. *American Medical Association Journal of Diseases of Children, 92* (5), 512.

3 Karsner, H.T. (1955). *Human pathology* (8th ed., pp. 42–51, 606–607). J.B. Lippincott Company.

4 Dodd, K., Minot, A.S., & Arena, J.M. (June 1937). Salicylate poisoning: An explanation of the more serious manifestations. *American Journal of Diseases of Children, 53* (6), 1435–1446.

5 Barnett, H.L., Powers, J.R., Benward, J.H., & Hartmann, A.F. (1 August 1942). Salicylate intoxication in infants and children. *Journal of Pediatrics, 21* (2), 214–223.

6 Lutwak-Mann, C. (December 1942). The effect of salicylate and cinchophen on enzymes and metabolic processes. *Biochemical Journal, 36* (10–12), 706–728.

7 Mortimer, E.A., & Lepow, M.L. (1 April 1962). Varicella with hypoglycemia possibly due to salicylates. *American Journal of Diseases of Children,103* (4), 91–98.

8 ibid.

9 Bourne, W.A. (November 1962). Liver disease in infancy. Clinico-pathological Conference held at the Royal Alexandra Hospital for Sick Children, Brighton. *Postgraduate Medical Journal, 38* (445), 642–652.

10   Anderson, R. McD. (20 April 1963). Encephalitis in childhood: Pathological aspects. *Medical Journal of Australia,* 573–575.

11   How accidents cost children's lives. (27 December 1955). *Sydney Morning Herald.*

12   Warning on aspirin. (9 July 1960). *Age.* [Australian newspaper].

13   Aspirin is not safe for the young. (8 July 1960). *Herald.* [Australian newspaper].

14   Warning on use of aspirin. (9 July 1960). *Age* [Australian newspaper].

15   McIlraith, S. (16 December 1964). Danger in self-medication. Aspirin may cause internal bleeding. *People.*

16   They took 400 tons of aspirin a year. (18 September 1962). *Courier-Mail.* [Australian newspaper].

17   Nicholas Product. (26 August 1950). Get straight to work with 'Aspro.' [Advertisement for Aspro]. *Courier-Mail* [Australian newspaper].

18   Nicholas Product (19 August 1950). The best way to buy. [Advertisement for Aspro]. *Courier Mail.* [Australian newspaper]

19   Coroner warns on aspirin for babies. (1 May 1960). *Sun.* [Australian newspaper].

20   Those who suffer. (1 May 1962). *Herald.* [Australian newspaper].

21   Doctors say children could suffer. (1 May 1962). *Herald.* [Australian newspaper].

22   Coroner warns on aspirin for babies. (1 May 1960). *Sun.* [Australian newspaper].

23   ibid.

24   ibid.

25   Aspirin baby is in danger. (3 May 1962). *Herald.* [Australian newspaper].

26   Nurses to debate use of aspirin. (2 May 1962). *Herald.* [Australian newspaper].

27   Parents warned on pills. (11 September 1962). *Sydney Morning Herald.* [Australian newspaper].

28   Doctors say children could suffer. (1 May 1962). *Herald.* [Australian newspaper].

29   No need to give children aspirin. (2 May 1962). *Age.* [Australian newspaper].

30   'Give them aspirin.' (4 May 1962). *Herald* [Letter to editor, name withheld]. [Australian newspaper].

31   Child danger, doctors say. (1 May 1962). *Herald.* [Australian newspaper].

32   ibid.

33   ibid.

34   Warning on aspirin use. (2 May 1962). *Canberra Times.*

35   Doctors set maximum child doses. (21 June 1962). *Sun.* [Australian newspaper].

36   ibid.

37   Statewide move on aspirin labels. (19 September 1962). *Herald.* [Australian newspaper].

38   Headache powders. (22 August 1962). *Australian Women's Weekly.*

39   McIlraith, S. (16 December 1964). Danger in self-medication. Aspirin may cause internal bleeding. *People,* 4–6.

40   Shannon, F.T. (October 1965). Aspirin medication in infancy and childhood. *New Zealand Medical Journal, 64,* 571–573.

41   Cilento, P. (10 June 1966). Lady Cilento, medical mother's opinion: Aspirin can be danger to baby. *Courier-Mail* [Australian newspaper].

42   Craig, J.O., Ferguson, I.C., & Syme, J. (26 March 1966). Infants, toddlers, and aspirin. *British Medical Journal, 1* (5490), 757–761.

43   Aspirin, a child killer. (26 March 1966). *Canberra Times.*

44   Danks, D.M. (10 October 1987). Reye's syndrome and aspirin [Letter to editor]. *Lancet, 330* (8563), 864.

45   Shannon, F.T. (1965). Aspirin medication in infancy and childhood. *New Zealand Medical Journal, 64,* 571–573.

46 Newgreen D.B. (February 1998) Review of non-prescription analgesics, prepared for the Therapeutic Goods Administration.

47 Orlowski, J.P, Gillis, J., & Kilham, H.A. (5 November 1987). A catch in the Reye. *Pediatrics, 80*(5), 638–642.

48 Jeffreys, D. (2005). *Aspirin: The remarkable story of a wonder drug aspirin* (p. 209). Bloomsbury.

49 Mann, C.C., & Plummer, M.L. (1991). *The aspirin wars: Money, medicine, and 100 years of rampant competition* (pp. 190–191). Harvard Business School Press.

50 Jeffreys, D. (2005). *Aspirin: The remarkable story of a wonder drug aspirin* (pp. 207–209). Bloomsbury.

Chapter 10 – Reye's Syndrome and Its Calling Card, 1963

1   Reye, R.D.K., Morgan, G., & Baral, J. (12 October 1963). Encephalopathy and fatty degeneration of the viscera. A disease entity in childhood. *Lancet, 2*(7311), 749–752.

2   Altman, L.K. (11 May 1999). Tale of triumph on every aspirin bottle. *New York Times.*

3   Reye Papers –Children's Hospital Westmead Archives, Sydney, Australia.

4   Schubert, W.K., Bobo, R.C., Partin, J.C., & Partin, J.S. (December 1975). Reye's syndrome. In D.F. Dowling (ed.), *Disease-a-month* (p. 15) [Monthly clinical monographs on current medical problems]. Year Book Medical Publishers, Inc.

5   Baral, J. (6 June 2009). Oral presentation by Dr Jacob Baral, guest of honor and key speaker, National Reye's Syndrome Foundation's 35th Annual Meeting Columbus, Ohio. [Oral presentation]. Retrieved 29 September 2021 from YouTube: https://www.youtube.com/watch?v=Repw3pJyj0M

6   Reye, R.D.K., Morgan, G., & Baral, J. (12 October 1963). Encephalopathy and fatty degeneration of the viscera. A disease entity in childhood. *Lancet, 282*(7311), 749–752.

7   Ibid.

8   Gonzales, T.A., Vance, M., Helpern, M., & Umberger, C.J. (1954). Legal medicine, pathology, and toxicology (2nd ed., p. 824). Appleton-Century-Crofts, Inc.

9   Editorial. (12 October 1963). Acute fatty liver and coma in children. *Lancet, 282*(7311), 772–773.

10 Brain & Hunter, D. (26 October 1963). Encephalopathy and fatty degeneration of the viscera [Letter to the editor]. *Lancet, 282* (7313), 881-882

Chapter 11 – Mother, The Perfect Scapegoat, 1960s

1   Knightly, P., Evans, E., Potter, E., & Wallace, M. [*Sunday Times of London* Insight Team] (1979). *Suffer the children: The story of thalidomide* (pp. 5–9). Viking Press.

2   Hilts, P.J. (2004). *Protecting America's health: The FDA, business, and one hundred years of regulation* (p. 158). University of North Carolina Press.

3   The drug that left a trail of heartbreak: The full story of thalidomide. (10 August 1962). *LIFE, 53*(6), 24–36.

4   US Food and Drug Administration. (February 1977). Safety and effectiveness of over-the-counter drugs: The FDA's OTC drug review. *Pediatrics, 59*(2), 309–311.

5   Dixon, A.St.J., Martin, B.K., Smith, M.J.H., & Wood, P.H.N. (eds) (1963). *Salicylates. An International Symposium.* Sponsored by the Empire Rheumatism Council, with the support of the Nicholas Research Institute. Held at the Postgraduate Medical School of London, 13–15 September 1962. Little, Brown and Company.

6   Including those from Beecham Research Laboratories of Betchworth, Surrey, England; Boots Pure Drug Company of Nottingham, England; J.R. Geigy SA of Basel, Switzerland; Miles Laboratories Inc. of Elkhart, Indiana; Nicholas Research Institute Ltd of Slough, England; Parke Davis and Company of Hounslow, Middlesex, England, and Ann Arbor, Michigan; and Wellcome Research Laboratories ofBeckenham, Kent, England.

7   Done, A.K. (1962). Maturational influences in salicylate intoxication. In C.D. May (ed.), *Report of 41st Ross Conference on Pediatric Research* (p. 83).

8   Done, A.K. (1963). Ontogenetic studies of salicylate intoxication. In A.St.J. Dixon, B.K. Martin, M.J.H. Smith, & P.H.N. Wood (eds). *Salicylates. An International Symposium.* Sponsored by the Empire Rheumatism Council, with the support of the Nicholas Research Institute. Held at the Postgraduate Medical School of London, 13–15 September 1962. Little, Brown and Company.

9   Davis, L.E., Westfall, B.A., & Short, C.R. (1968). Comparative study of biotransformation and pharmacokinetics of salicylate during the neonatal period. *Pharmacologist, 10*, 167.

10 Levy, G. (July 1965). Pharmacokinetics of elimination of salicylate in man. *Journal of Pharmaceutical Sciences, 54*(7), 959–967.

11 Binns, T.B. (ed.). (1964). *Absorption and distribution of drugs.* Williams and Wilkins Company.

12 ibid. p. 169.

13 Levy, G. (July 1965). Pharmacokinetics of elimination of salicylate in man. *Journal of Pharmaceutical Sciences, 54*(7), 959–967.

14 Sprowls, J.B. (ed.) (1963). Prescription pharmacy. dosage formulation and pharmaceutical adjuncts. J.B. Lippincott Company.

15 Levy, G. (July 1965). Pharmacokinetics of elimination of salicylate in man. *Journal of Pharmaceutical Sciences, 54*(7), 959–967.

16 Bedford, C., Cummings, A.J., & Martin, B.K. (April 1965). A kinetic study of the elimination of salicylate in man. *British Journal of Pharmacology, 24*(2), 418–431.

17 Levy, G., Tsuchiya, T., & Amsel, L.P. (March 1972). Limited capacity for salicyl phenolic glucuronide formation and its effect on the kinetics of salicylate elimination in man. *Clinical Pharmacology & Therapeutics, 13*(2), 258–268.

18 Levy, G., & Tsuchiya, T. (31 August 1972). Salicylate accumulation kinetics in man. *New England Journal of Medicine, 287*, 430–432.

19 Levy, G., & Yaffe, S.J. (December 1968). The study of salicylate pharmacokinetics in intoxicated infants and children. *Clinical Toxicology, 1*(4), 409–424.

20 Furst, D.E., Gupta, N., & Paulus, H.E. (July 1977). Salicylate metabolism in twins. *Journal of Clinical Investigation, 60*(1), 32–42.

21 Levy, G., & Yaffe, S.J. (December 1968). The study of salicylate pharmacokinetics in intoxicated infants and children. *Clinical Toxicology, 1*(4), 409–424.

22 Furst, D.E., Gupta, N., & Paulus, H.E. (July 1977). Salicylate metabolism in twins. Evidence suggesting a genetic influence and induction of salicylurate formation. *Journal of Clinical Investigation, 60*, 32–42.

23 Sterling Drug. (November 1962). When anyone in your family has a cold or flu … [Advertisement]. *Ladies Home Journal*, 127.

24 Levy, G., & Hollister, L.E. (August 1964). Variation in rate of salicylate elimination by humans. *British Medical Journal, 2*, 286–288.

25 Levy, G. (November 1978). Clinical pharmacokinetics of aspirin. *Pediatrics, 62*(5s), 867– 872.

26 Gupta, N., Sarkissian, E., & Paulus, H.E. (1975). Correlation of plateau serum salicylate level with rate of salicylate metabolism. *Clinical Pharmacology & Therapeutics, 18*(3), 350–355.

27 Shirkey, H.C. (ed.) (1964). *Pediatric therapy.* The C.V. Mosby Company.

28 Gellis, S.S., & Kagan, B.M. (eds) (1964). *Current pediatric therapy.* W.B. Saunders Company.

29 Shirkey, H.C. (ed.) (1964). *Pediatric therapy.* The C.V. Mosby Company.

30 Shirkey, H.C. (1965). Drug dosage for infants and children. *Journal of the American Medical Association, 193*(6), 105–108.

31   Tainter, M.L., & Ferris, A.J. (1969). *Aspirin in modern therapy. A review* (pp. 85–104). Bayer Company Division of Sterling Drug Inc.

32   *Child safety act and personnel training. (1966). Hearings*, Eighty-ninth Congress, second session, June 24, August 15, 29, September 12, 19, 1966. US Government Printing Office (pp. 176–177).

33   Lamont-Havers, R.W., & Wagner, B.M. (eds). (1968). *Proceedings of the conference on effects of chronic salicylate administration*. Held in New York, New York, 1966. US Department of Health, Education and Welfare, National Institutes of Health, National Institute of Arthritis and Metabolic Diseases. US Government Printing Office.

34   For example, Case Western Reserve University, Children's Hospital of Philadelphia, Children's Seashore House, Columbia University, Hahnemann Medical College, McGill University, New Jersey College of Medicine, New York Medical College, New York University, Ohio State University, Philadelphia College of Science and Pharmacy, Robert B. Brigham Hospital, Rockefeller University, Texas Children's Hospital, University of British Columbia, University of Cincinnati, University of London, University of Manchester, University of Pennsylvania, University of Utah, University of Washington, and Yale University.

35   Lamont-Havers, R.W., & Wagner, B.M. (eds). (1968). *Proceedings of the conference on effects of chronic salicylate administration*. Held in New York, New York, 1966. US Department of Health, Education and Welfare, National Institutes of Health, National Institute of Arthritis and Metabolic Diseases. US Government Printing Office. p. 151.

36   ibid. p. 152.

37   *Child safety act and personnel training. (1966). Hearings,* Eighty-ninth Congress, second session, June 24, August 15, 29, September 12, 19, 1966. US Government Printing Office (p. 189).

38   Sterling Drug. (1960s). My mother gives me orange flavored Bayer® Aspirin for Children ... [Advertisement].

39   Breslin, M.M. (12 December 1998). Joan Beck, 75, pioneering journalist. *Chicago Tribune.*

40   Beck, J. (9 May 1967). Notes on aspirin for children. *Chicago Tribune.*

Chapter 12 – Algorithm Think: If It's One, It Can't Be the Other, 1960s

1   Utian, H.L., Wagner, J.M., & Sichel, R.J.S. (14 November 1964). "White liver" disease. *Lancet, 284* (7368), 1043–1045.

2   Elliot, R.I.K., Mann, T.P., & Nash, F.W. (26 October 1963). Encephalopathy and fatty degeneration of the viscera [Letter to the editor]. *Lancet, 282* (7313), 882.

3   Corlett, K. (2 November 1963). Encephalopathy and fatty degeneration of the viscera [Letter to the editor]. *Lancet, 282* (7314), 938.

4   Maloney, A.F.J. (23 November 1963). Encephalopathy and fatty degeneration of the viscera [Letter to the editor]. *Lancet, 282* (7317), 1122.

5   Stejskal, J., & Kluska, V. (14 March 1964). Encephalopathy and fatty degeneration of the viscera [Letter to the editor]. *Lancet, 283* (7333), 615.

6   Utian, H.L., Wagner, J.M., & Sichel, R.J.S. (14 November 1964). "White liver" disease. *Lancet, 284* (7368), 1043–1045.

7   Giles, H.Mc.C. (15 May 1965). Encephalopathy and fatty degeneration of the viscera [Letter to the editor]. *Lancet, 285* (7394), 1075.

8   Mann, T.P. (September 1965). Less common syndromes associated with hypoglycemia. *Proceedings of the Royal Society of Medicine, 59*, 805–810.

9   Golden, G.S., & Duffell, D. (July 1965). Encephalopathy and fatty change in the liver and kidney. *Pediatrics, 36* (1), 67–74.

10 Randolph, M., Kranwinkel, R., Johnson, R., & Gelfman, N.A. (July 1965). Encephalopathy, hepatitis and fat accumulation in viscera. *American Journal of Diseases of Children, 110*(1), 95–99.

11 Jabbour, J.T., Howard, P.H., & Jaques, W.E. (13 December 1965). Encephalopathy and fatty degeneration of the liver and kidneys. *Journal of the American Medical Association, 194*(11), 1245–1247.

12 Winograd, H.L. (13 December 1965). Encephalopathy with hypoglycemia and degeneration of the liver. *Journal of the American Medical Association, 194*(11), 1247–1249.

13 Becroft, D.M.O. (16 July 1966). Syndrome of encephalopathy and fatty degeneration of viscera in New Zealand children. *British Medical Journal, 2*, 135–140.

14 ibid.

15 Simpson, H. (10 December 1966). Encephalopathy and fatty degeneration of viscera. Acid-base observations. *Lancet, 288*(7476), 1274–1277.

16 ibid.

17 Shakespeare, W.D. (10 September 1966). Encephalopathy and fatty degeneration of viscera [Correspondence]. *British Medical Journal, 2*(5514), 642.

18 Simpson, H. (10 December 1966). Encephalopathy and fatty degeneration of viscera. Acid-base observations. *Lancet, 288*(7476), 1274–1277.

19 Dvorackova, I., Vortel, V., Hroch, M., & Kralove, H. (March 1966). Encephalitic syndrome with fatty degeneration of viscera. *Archives of Pathology, 81*, 240–246.

20 ibid.

21 Becroft, D.M.O. (16 July 1966). Syndrome of encephalopathy and fatty degeneration of viscera in New Zealand children. *British Medical Journal, 2*(5506), 135–140.

22 Jenkins, R., Dvorak, A., & Patrick, J. (May 1967). Encephalopathy and fatty degeneration of the viscera associated with chickenpox. *Pediatrics, 39*(5), 769–771.

23 Bradford, W.D., & Latham, W.C. (August 1967). Acute encephalopathy and fatty hepatomegaly. *American Journal of the Diseases of Children, 114*(2), 152–156.

24 Norman, M.G., Lowden, J.A., Hill, D.E., & Bannatyne, R.M. (21 September 1968). Encephalopathy and fatty degeneration of the viscera in childhood: II. Report of a case with isolation of influenza B virus. *Canadian Medical Association Journal, 99*(11), 549–554.

25 Norman, M.G. (21 September 1968). Encephalopathy and fatty degeneration of the viscera in childhood: I. Review of cases at the Hospital for Sick Children, Toronto (1954–1966). *Canadian Medical Association Journal, 99*(11), 522–526.

26 Randolph, M., & Gelfman, N.A. (September 1968). Acute encephalopathy in children associated with acute hepatocellular dysfunction: Reye's syndrome revisited. *American Journal of Diseases of Children, 116*(3), 303–307.

27 Glasgow, J.F.T., & Ferris, J.A.J. (2 March 1968). Encephalopathy and visceral fatty infiltration of probable toxic aetiology. *Lancet, 291*(7540), 451–453.

28 Fronstin, M.H., Moore, L.W., Ruffolo, E.H., & Hooper, G.S. (1968). Encephalopathy and fatty degeneration of the viscera. *American Journal of Clinical Pathology, 49*(5), 704–709.

29 Barr, R., Glass, I.H.J, & Chawla, G.S. (1 June 1968). Reye's syndrome: Massive fatty metamorphosis of the liver with acute encephalopathy. *Canadian Medical Association Journal, 98*(22), 1038–1044.

30 Laxdal, O.E., Sinha, R.P., Merida, J., Wong, L.C., & Stephen, J.D. (June 1969). Reye's syndrome. Encephalopathy in children associated with fatty change in the viscera. *American Journal of Diseases of Children, 117*(6), 717–721.

31 Bornhofen, J.H., Hankins, E., & Araoz, C. (1970). Acute encephalopathy with fatty change of viscera. *Journal of the Arkansas Medical Society, 67*(2), 60–65.

32 Vorse, H., LaFont, D., Rubio, T., Reynolds, D., & Riley, H.D. (1970). Reye's syndrome, an encephalopathy with fatty infiltration of viscera: A report of 6 cases. *Clinical Research, 18*, 85.

Notes

33 Guillette, R., Berlin, C.M., & Finkelstein, J.D. (1971). Reye's syndrome. Clinical aspects. *Clinical Proceedings of Children's Hospital (Washington, D.C.), 27,* 224–238.

34 Zavala Romero, J.E., Cilliani, G., & Cilliani, I. (1970). *Síndrome de Reye: Encefalopatía y degeneración grasa de las vísceras. Prensa Médica Argentina, 57,* 1767–1771.

35 Cullity, G.J., & Kakulas, B.A. (1970). Encephalopathy and fatty degeneration of the viscera. *Brain, 93* (1), 77–88.

36 Burns, R.R., & Silverberg, S.G. (February 1970). Encephalopathy and fatty degeneration of the viscera. (Reye's syndrome). A clinicopathologic entity? *Southern Medical Journal, 63* (2), 183–188.

37 Severy, P.R. (1969). Reye's disease: A syndrome of unexplained death in childhood. *Journal of Forensic Sciences, 14* (1), 111–119.

38 Bergman, A.B. (1 March 2003). Obituary: Sydney S. Gellis, MD (1914–2002). *Archives of Pediatrics & Adolescent Medicine, 157* (3), 218.

39 Gellis, S.S., & Jones, W.A. (5 January 1967). Case 1-1967—Varicella in a six-year-old boy, with coma and gastrointestinal bleeding. (Case records of the Massachusetts General Hospital). *New England Journal of Medicine, 276* (1), 47–55.

40 Gellis, S.S. (ed.). (1968). *Year book of pediatrics, 1968* (pp. 223–225). Year Book Medical Publishers.

41 ibid.

42 Gellis, S.S. (ed.). (1970). *Year book of pediatrics, 1970* (p. 252). Year Book Medical Publishers.

43 Dodge, P.R., Kissane, J.M., Prensky, A.L., & Kahn, L.I. (1969). Acute encephalopathy with severe liver dysfunction. How common is this syndrome? *Clinical Pediatrics, 8* (3), 154–160.

44 Pross, D.C, Bradford, W.D., & Krueger, R.P. (May 1970). Reye's syndrome treated by peritoneal dialysis. *Pediatrics, 45* (5), 845–847.

45 Shaw, E.B. (December 1979). Reye's syndrome and salicylate intoxication [Letter to the editor]. *Pediatrics, 46* (6), 976–977.

46 Mortimer, E.A. (1970). Reye's syndrome and salicylate intoxication [Letter to the editor]. *Pediatrics, 46* (6), 977.

47 Gellis, S.S. (ed.). (1971). *Year book of pediatrics, 1971* (p. 280). Year Book Medical Publishers.

48 Gellis, S.S. (ed.). (1971). *Year book of pediatrics, 1971* (p. 204). Year Book Medical Publishers.

49 Gellis, S.S. (ed.). (1977). *Year book of pediatrics, 1977* (p. 198). Year Book Medical Publishers.

50 Gellis, S.S. (ed.). (1978). *Year book of pediatrics, 1978* (p. 189). Year Book Medical Publishers.

51 Huttenlocher, P.R., Schwartz, A.D., & Klatskin, G. (March 1969). Reye's syndrome: Ammonia intoxication as a possible factor in the encephalopathy. *Pediatrics, 43* (3), 443–454.

52 Olsen, L.C., Bourgeois, C.H., Cotton, R.B., Harikul, S., Grossman, R.A., & Smith, T.J. (April 1971). Encephalopathy and fatty degeneration of the viscera in northeastern Thailand. Clinical syndrome and epidemiology. *Pediatrics, 47* (4), 707–716.

53 Bourgeois, C.H., Keschamras, N., Comer, D.S., Harikul, S., Evans, H., Olson, L., Smith, T., & Beck, M.R. (1969). Udorn encephalopathy. Fatal cerebral edema and fatty degeneration of the viscera in Thai children. *Journal of the Medical Association of Thailand, 52* (7), 553–563.

54 Bourgeois, C.H., Keschamras, N., Comer, D.S., Harikul, S., Evans, H., Olson, L., Smith, T., & Beck, M.R. (1969). Udorn encephalopathy. Fatal cerebral edema and fatty degeneration of the viscera in Thai children. *Journal of the Medical Association of Thailand, 52* (7), 553–563.

55 Evans, H., Bourgeois, C.H., Comer, D.S., & Keschamras, N. (1970, December). Brain lesions in Reye's syndrome. *Archives of Pathology, 90,* 543–546.

56   Bourgeois, C.H., Keschamras, N., Comer, D.S., Harikul, S., Evans, H., Olson, L., Smith, T., & Beck, M.R. (1969). Udorn encephalopathy. Fatal cerebral edema and fatty degeneration of the viscera in Thai children. *Journal of the Medical Association of Thailand, 52* (7), 553–563.

57   Tainter, M.L., & Ferris, A.J. (1969). *Aspirin in modern therapy. A review* (p. 26). Bayer Company Division of Sterling Drug Inc.

58   Silverman, A., Roy, C.C., & Cozzetto, F.J. (1971). Reye's syndrome. *Pediatric clinical gastroenterology* (pp. 345–350). The C.V. Mosby Company.

59   ibid.

60   Schubert, W.K., Partin, J.C., & Partin, J.S. (1972). Encephalopathy and fatty liver (Reye's syndrome). In H. Popper & F. Schaffner (eds), *Progress in liver diseases, Volume IV* (pp. 489–510). Grune and Stratton.

Chapter 13 – A Gordian Knot, 1970s

1   Luscombe, F., Monto, A.S., & Baublis, J.V. (September 1980). Mortality due to Reye's syndrome in Michigan: Distribution and longitudinal trends. *Journal of Infectious Diseases, 142* (3), 363–371.

2   Pierce, A.W. (September 1974). Salicylate poisoning. *Pediatrics, 54* (3), 342–347.

3   Glick, T.H., Likosky, W.H., Levitt, L.P., Mellin, H., & Reynolds, D.W. (1970). Reye's syndrome: An epidemiologic approach. *Pediatrics, 46* (3), 371–377.

4   Leonnig C., & Rucker P. (2021). *I Alone Can Fix It* (p. 15). Penguin Press.

5   Partin, J.C., Schubert, W.K., & Partin, J.S. (9 December 1971). Mitochondrial ultrastructure in Reye's syndrome (encephalopathy and fatty degeneration of the viscera). *New England Journal of Medicine, 285* (24), 1339–1343.

6   Partin, J.C., Partin, J.S., & Schubert, W.K. (September 1973). Fatty liver in Reye's syndrome: Is it a distinct morphologic entity? *Gastroenterology,* A-39/563.

7   Dr Harris Riley, Jr [Obituary]. (29 March 2010). *The Atlanta Journal Constitution.*

8   Riley, H.D., & Worley, L. (October 1956). Salicylate intoxication. *Pediatrics, 18* (4), 578–594.

9   Reynolds, D.W., Riley, H.D., LaFont, D.S., Vorse, H., Stout, L.C., & Carpenter, R.L. (March 1972). An outbreak of Reye's syndrome associated with influenza B. *Journal of Pediatrics, 80* (3), 429–432.

10   Riley, H.D. (1972). Reye's syndrome [Editorial]. *Journal of Infectious Diseases, 125* (1), 77–81.

11   Segar, W.E., & Holliday, M.A. (18 December 1958). Physiologic abnormalities of salicylate poisoning. *New England Journal of Medicine, 259* (25), 1191–1198.

12   Riley, H.D. (1972). Reye's syndrome [Editorial]. *Journal of Infectious Diseases, 125* (1), 77–81.

13   Hart, J.C., Fiumara, N.J., Smith, V., Hinman, A.R., Cannon, J.E., & Aiken, R.B., & the Neurotropic Disease Unit of the CDC. (27 March 1971). Reye's syndrome—New England and New York State. *Morbidity and Mortality, 20* (12), 101–102.

14   Hochberg, F.H., Nelson, K., & Jenzen, W. (24 February 1975). Influenza type B-related encephalopathy. The 1971 outbreak of Reye syndrome in Chicago. *Journal of the American Medical Association, 231* (8), 817–821.

15   Altman, L.K. (24 February 1974). Child's disease spurs research. Rare aliment affects brain and liver—cases increase. *New York Times.*

16   Corey, L., Ruben, R.J., Hattwick, M.A.W., Noble, G.R., & Cassidy, E. (November 1976). A nationwide outbreak of Reye's syndrome. Its epidemiological relationship to influenza B. *American Journal of Medicine, 61* (5), 615–625.

17   Hall, B.D., Hughes, W.T., & Kmetz, D. (April 1969). Reye's syndrome: An association with influenza A infection. *Journal of the Kentucky Medical Association, 67* (4), 269–271.

Notes

18 Horner, F.A. (15 May 1958). Neurologic disorders after Asian influenza. *New England Journal of Medicine, 258* (20), 983–985.

19 Kapila, C.C., Kaul, S., Kapur, S.C., Kalayanam, T.S. & Banerjee, D. (29 November 1958). Neurological and hepatic disorders associated with influenza. *British Medical Journal, 2* (5108), 1311–1314.

20 McConkey, B. and Daws, R.A. (5 July 1958). Neurologic Disorders associated with Asian influenza. *Lancet, 270* (6984), 15–17.

21 Nelson, D.B, Hurwitz, E.S., Sullivan-Bolyai, J.Z., Morens, D.M., & Schonberger, L.B. (September 1979). Reye's syndrome in the United States in 1977–1978, a non-influenza B virus year. *Journal of Infectious Diseases, 140* (3), 436–439.

22 DeVivo, D.C., & Keating, J.P. (1976). Reye's syndrome. In I. Schulman (ed.), *Advances in Pediatrics* (Vol. 22, pp. 175–229). Year Book Medical Publishers. The list is modified after Corey, L. (1975). Reye's syndrome—an epidemiological approach. In J.D. Pollack (ed.), *Reye's Syndrome. Proceedings of the* [1974] *Reye's Syndrome Conference Sponsored by the Children's Hospital Foundation, Columbus, Ohio* (p. 180). Grune and Stratton.

23 Morens, D.M., & Noble, G.R. (9 April 1977). Reye's syndrome and influenza [Letter to editor]. *Lancet, 309* (8015), 807–808.

24 DeVivo, D.C., & Keating, J.P. (1976). Reye's syndrome. In I. Schulman (ed.), *Advances in pediatrics* (Vol. 22, pp. 175–229). Year Book Medical Publishers.

25 ibid..

26 Hilty, M.D., McClung H.J., Haynes R.E., Romshe, C.A., & Sherard, E.S. (April 1979). Reye syndrome in siblings. *The Journal of Pediatrics, 94* (4), 576–579.

27 Chin, J., Hausler, W., Herron, C.A., Bahn, A., & the Viral Diseases Division, Bureau of Epidemiology, and the International Influenza Center for the Americas, CDC. (16 February 1976). Influenza surveillance: Reye's syndrome and viral infections—United States. *Morbidity and Mortality Weekly Report, 23* (7), 58.

28 Chavez-Carballo, E., Gomez, M.R., & Sharbrough, F.W. (April 1975). Encephalopathy and fatty infiltration of the viscera (Reye-Johnson syndrome). A 17-year experience. *Mayo Clinic Proceedings, 50*, 209–215.

29 Westchester youth, 16, dies of Reye's syndrome. (25 February 1977). *New York Times*.

30 Huttenlocher, P.R., & Trauner, D.A. (1 July 1978). Reye's syndrome in infancy. *Pediatrics, 62* (1), 84–90.

31 Sullivan-Bolyai, J.Z., Nelson, D.B., Morens, D.M., Schonberger, L.B., Marks, J.S., Johnson, D., Holtzhauer, F., Bright, F., Kramer, T., & Halpin, T.J. (1 March 1980). Reye syndrome in children less than 1 year old: Some epidemiologic observations. *Pediatrics, 65* (3), 627–629.

32 Corey, L., Rubin, R.J., Hattwick, M.A.W., Noble, G.R., & Cassidy, E. (November 1976). A nationwide outbreak of Reye's syndrome. Its epidemiologic relationship to influenza B. *American Journal of Medicine,61* (5), 615–625.

33 Brown, R.E., & Madge, G.E. (November 1972). Fatty acids and metabolic disturbances in Reye's syndrome [Letter to the editor]. *Archives of Pathology, 94*, 475–476.

34 Johnson, P.G.B. (22 September 1973). Aetiology of Reye's syndrome [Correspondence]. *British Medical Journal, 3*, 640.

35 Lombardi, B. (January 1966). Considerations on the pathogenesis of fatty liver. *Laboratory Investigation, 15* (1, Pt 1), 1–20.

36 Crocker, J.F.S., Rozee, K.R., Ozere, R.L., Digout, S.C., & Hutzinger, O. (6 July 1974). Insecticide and viral interaction as a cause of fatty visceral changes and encephalopathy in the mouse [Preliminary communications]. *Lancet, 304* (7871), 22–24.

37 Rare children's disease tied to solvents used in pesticides. (10 April 1976). *New York Times* (p. 28).

38 DeVivo, D.C., & Keating, J.P. (1976). Reye's syndrome. In I. Schulman (ed.), *Advances in pediatrics* (Vol. 22, pp. 175–229). Year Book Medical Publishers.

39 ibid.

40 Strauss, R.G., & McAdams, A.J. (July 1970). Arthritis, aspirin, and coma [Clinical-Pathological Conference]. *Journal of Pediatrics, 77* (1), 156–163.

41 Linnemann, C.C., Shea, L., Kauffman, C.A., Schiff, G.M., Partin, J.C., & Schubert, W.K. (27 July 1974). Association of Reye's syndrome with viral infection. *Lancet, 304* (7874), 179–182.

42 Hilty M. (1974). Etiology of Reye's syndrome. In Pollack, J.D. (ed). (1975). Reye's Syndrome. *Proceedings of the [1974] Reye's Syndrome Conference Sponsored by the Children's Hospital Foundation*, Columbus, Ohio (p. 384). Grune & Stratton.

43 Linnemann, C.C., Shea, L., Partin, J.C., Schubert, W.K., & Schiff, G.M. (1975). Reye's syndrome: Epidemiologic and viral studies, 1963–1974. *American Journal of Epidemiology, 101* (6), 517–526.

44 Cotton, E.K., & Fahlberg, V.J. (1 August 1964). Hypoglycemia with salicylate poisoning: A report of two cases. *American Journal of Diseases of Children, 108* (2), 171–173.

45 Rich, R.R., & Johnson, J.S. (January–February 1973). Salicylate hepatotoxicity in patients with juvenile rheumatoid arthritis. *Arthritis Rheumatology, 16* (1), 1–9.

46 Loveday, C., & Eisen, V. (22 September 1973). Suppression of lymphocyte transformation by salicylates [Letter to the editor]. *Lancet, 302* (7830), 276.

47 Waldman, J.D., Given, G.Z., & Schwartz, A.D. (February 1973). "Therapeutic success" in Reye's syndrome [Letter to the editor]. *Journal of Pediatrics, 82* (2), 343–344.

48 Decision-making (Adults). (7 September 2021). In *Wikipedia*.

49 Combes, B. (8 May 1975). Reye's syndrome. *Medical Grand Rounds Parkland Memorial Hospital*.

50 Lyon, L.J., & Nevins, M.A. (1974). Viral hepatitis and salicylism simulating Reye's syndrome. *Journal of the Medical Society of New Jersey, 71* (9), 657–660.

51 Rosenfeld, R.G., & Leibhaber, M. (March 1976). Acute encephalopathy in siblings: Reye syndrome vs salicylate intoxication. *American Journal of Diseases of Children, 130* (3), 295–297.

52 Sillanpää, M., Mäkelä, A., & Koivikko, A. (1975). Acute liver failure and encephalopathy (Reye's syndrome?) during salicylate therapy. *Acta Paediatrica Scandinavica, 64*, 877–880.

53 ibid.

54 Linnemann, C.C. (1 November 1981). Salicylates and Reye's syndrome [Letter to the editor]. *Pediatrics, 68* (5), 747–748.

55 Linnemann, C.C., Ueda, K., Hug, G., Schaeffer, A., Clark, A., & Schiff, G.M. (1979). Salicylate intoxication and influenza in ferrets. *Pediatric Research, 13*, 44–47.

56 Hilty, M.D., & Romshe, C.A. (1974). Reye's syndrome and hyperaminoacidemia. *Journal of Pediatrics, 84* (3), 362–365.

57 Brown, T., Hug, G., Lansky, L., Bove, K., Scheve, A., Ryan, M., Brown, H., Schubert, W.K., Partin, J.C., & Lloyd-Still, J. (15 April 1976). Transiently reduced activity of carbamyl phosphate synthetase and ornithine transcarbamylase in liver of children with Reye's syndrome. *New England Journal of Medicine, 294* (16), 861–867.

58 Corey, L., Rubin, R.J., Bregman, D., Gregg, M.B. (1 November 1981). Diagnostic criteria for influenza B-associated Reye's syndrome: Clinical vs. pathologic criteria. *Pediatrics, 60* (5), 702–708.

59 American Academy of Pediatrics, Committee on Infectious Diseases. (October 1974). *News and Comment*.

60 American Academy of Pediatrics, Committee on Infectious Diseases, Katz, S.L., Chairman. (January 1975). Statement on Reye's syndrome. *Pediatrics, 55* (1), 139.

61 Barker E. US Food and Drug Administration, Bureau of Drugs. (10 January 1976). Minutes of the Panel on Reye Syndrome of the Neurologic Drugs Advisory Committee meeting.

62 Gellis S. & Barker E.F. US Food and Drug Administration, Bureau of Drugs (10 January 1977). Minutes of the Panel on Reye Syndrome and Appropriate Use of Antiemetics in Children meeting.

63 Gellis S.S. (19 January 1976) Recommendations of the Ad Hoc Panel on Reye Syndrome to the Neurologic Drugs Advisory Committee.

64 Reye's Syndrome—Avoid Antiemetics in Children. (November–December 1976). *FDA Drug Bulletin, 6,* 40–41.

Chapter 14 – The Telltale Tiny Fat Drops, September 1979

1 Starko, K.M. (12 September 1979). Letter to George Ray. [Business letter from EIS Officer, Field Services Division, Center for Disease Control and Acting State Epidemiologist, Arizona to Professor, Pathology and Pediatrics, University of Arizona Health Sciences Center].

2 Starko, K.M. (3 September 1979). Letter to Tim Dondero. [Business letter from EIS Officer, Field Services Division, Center for Disease Control and Acting State Epidemiologist, Arizona to Assistant Director, Field Services Division, Center for Disease Control].

3 Center for Disease Control, Viral Disease Division and Chronic Diseases Division, Bureau of Epidemiology. (17 September 1979). Investigation of aflatoxin in children with Reye Syndrome in 7 southeastern states. Memo to Director, CDC.

4 Fashena, G.J., & Walker, J.N. (1944). Salicylate intoxication. Studies on the effects of sodium salicylate on prothrombin time and alkali reserve. *American Journal of Diseases of Children, 68* (6), 369–375.

5 Manso, C., Nydick, I., & Taranta, A. (October 1956). Effect of aspirin administration on serum glutamic oxaloacetic and glutamic pyruvic transaminases in children. *Proceedings of the Society for Experimental Biology and Medicine, 93* (1), 84–88.

6 Gross, M., & Greenberg, L.A. (1948). *The salicylates. A critical bibliographic review.* Hillhouse Press.

7 Karsner, H.T. (1955). *Human pathology* (8th ed., pp. 44, 606–607). J.B. Lippincott Company.

8 Huttenlocher, P.R., Schwartz, A.D., & Klatskin, G. (March 1969). Reye's syndrome: Ammonia intoxication as a possible factor in the encephalopathy. *Pediatrics, 43* (3), 443– 454.

9 Russell, A.S., Sturge, R.A., & Smith, M.A. (May 1971). Serum transaminases during salicylate therapy. *British Medical Journal, 2* (5759), 428–429.

10 Arthreya, B.H., Moser, G., Cecil, H.S., & Myers, A.R. (July–August 1975). Aspirin-induced hepatotoxicity in juvenile rheumatoid arthritis. A prospective study. *Arthritis and Rheumatology, 18* (4), 347–352.

11 Russell, A.S., Sturge, R.A., & Smith, M.A. (22 May 1971). Serum transaminases during salicylate therapy. *British Medical Journal, 2* (5759): 428–429.

12 Zimmerman, H.J. (1 January 1974 1). Aspirin-induced hepatic injury [Editorial]. *Annals of Internal Medicine, 80* (1), 103–105.

13 Does aspirin harm the liver? (13 April 1974). [Editorial]. *Lancet,303* (7859), 667.

14 Rich R.R. and Johnson J.S. (1973). Salicylate hepatotoxicity in juvenile rheumatoid arthritis. *Arthritis & Rheumatology. 16* (1), 1–9.

15 Arthreya, B.H., Moser, G., Cecil, H.S., & Myers, A.R. (July–August 1975). Aspirin induced hepatotoxicity in juvenile rheumatoid arthritis. A prospective study. *Arthritis and Rheumatology, 18* (4), 347–352.

16 Seaman, W.E., Ishak, K.G., Plotz, P.H. (1974). Aspirin-induced hepatotoxicity in patients with systemic lupus erythematosus. *Annals of Internal Medicine. 80,* 1–8.

17   Zucker, P., Daum F., Cohen, M.I. (1975). Aspirin hepatitis. *American Journal of Diseases of Childhood.129* (12), 1433–1434.

18   Saltzman, D.A., Gall, E.P., Robinson S.F. (1976). Aspirin-induced hepatic dysfunction in a patient with adult rheumatoid arthritis. Digestive Diseases. *21* (9), 815–820.

19   O'Gorman T. and Koff, R.S. (1977). Salicylate hepatitis. *Gastroenterology. 72* (4), 726–728.

20   Sbarbaro, J.A. and Bennett, R.M. (1977). Aspirin hepatotoxicity and disseminated intravascular coagulation. *Annals of Internal Medicine. 86* (2), 183–185.

21   Bernstein, B.H., Singsen, B.H., King, K.K., Hansen, V. (1977). Aspirin-induced hepatotoxicity and its effect on juvenile rheumatoid arthritis. *American Journal of Diseases of Childhood.* 131, 659–663.

22   Ulshen, M.H., Grand, R.J., Crain, J.D., Gelfand, E.W. (1978). Hepatotoxicity with encephalopathy associated with aspirin therapy. *Journal of Pediatrics, 93* (6) 1034–1037.

23   Arthreya, B.H., Moser, G., Cecil, H.S., & Myers, A.R. (July–August 1975). Aspirin-induced hepatotoxicity in juvenile rheumatoid arthritis. A prospective study. *Arthritis and Rheumatology, 18* (4), 347–352.

24   Furst, D.E, Gupta, N., & Paulus, H.E. (July 1977). Salicylate metabolism in twins. Evidence suggesting a genetic influence and induction of salicylurate formation. *Journal of Clinical Investigation, 60,* 32–42.

25   Day, R.O., Furst, D.E., Dromgoole, S.H., & Paulus, H.E. (May/June 1988). Changes in salicylate serum concentration and metabolism during chronic dosing in normal volunteers. *Biopharmaceutics & Drug Disposition, 9* (3), 273–283.

26   US Food and Drug Administration, Department of Health, Education, and Welfare. (8 July 1977). Over-the-counter drugs. Establishment of a monograph for OTC internal analgesic, antipyretic, and antirheumatic products. *Federal Register, 42* (131), 2 of 2 books, p. 35408.

27   Bove, K.E., McAdams, A.J., Partin, J.C., Partin, J.S., Hug, G., & Schubert, W.K. (September 1975). The hepatic lesion in Reye's syndrome. *Gastroenterology, 69* (3), 685–697.

28   Paisseau, G., Friedmann, E., & Vaille, C. (1934). *Bulletins et mémoires de la Société Médicale des Hôpitaux de Paris, 50,*1201. As discussed in Williams, S.W. & Panting, R.M. (13 March 1937). Treatment of aspirin poisoning with intravenous sodium lactate solution. *British Medical Journal, 1* (3975), 550–552.

29   Paisseau, G., Freedman, E., & Vaille, C. (16 July 1934). Fatal intoxication by sodium salicylate. *Bulletins et mémoires de la Société Médicale des Hôpitaux de Paris,* 1201. Provided as Abstract 294 (27 October 1937) in Epitome of current medical literature. *British Medical Journal, 2* (3851), E61.

30   Gross, M., & Greenberg, L.A. (1948). *The salicylates. A critical bibliographic review.* Hillhouse Press.

31   Wetzel, N.C., & Nourse, J.D. (1926). Wintergreen poisoning. *Archives of Pathology & Laboratory Medicine, 1,* 182–188.

32   Olmstead, J.G.M., & Aldrich, C.A. (1928). Acidosis in methyl salicylate poisoning: Report of two cases and a review of the literature. *Journal of the American Medical Association, 90* (18), 1438–1440.

33   Eimas, A. (October 1938). Methyl salicylate poisoning in an infant. *Journal of Pediatrics, 13* (4), 550–554.

34   Meyerhoff, I.S. (31 May 1930). Methyl salicylate poisoning in infancy. Necropsy observations. *Journal of the American Medical Association, 94* (22), 1751–1753.

35   Stevenson, C.S. (1937). Oil of wintergreen (methyl salicylate) poisoning. Report of three cases, one with autopsy, and a review of the literature. *American Journal of Medical Sciences, 193,* 772–788.

Notes

36 McCready, R.A. (4 February 1943). Methyl salicylate poisoning. *New England Journal of Medicine, 228* (5), 155–156.

37 Troll, M.M, & Menten, M.L. (January 1945). Salicylate poisoning. Report of four cases. *American Journal of Diseases of Children, 69* (1), 37–43.

38 Krasnoff, S.O., & Bernstein, M. (15 November 1947). Acetylsalicylic acid poisoning: With a report of a fatal case. *Journal of the American Medical Association, 135* (11), 712–714.

39 Lipman, B.L, Krasnoff, S.O., & Schless, R.A. (1949). Acute acetylsalicylic acid intoxication. *American Journal of Diseases of Children, 78* (4), 477–483.

40 Winters, R.W., White, J.S., Hughes, M.C., & Ordway, N.K. (1 February 1959). Disturbances of acid-base equilibrium in salicylate intoxication. *Pediatrics, 23* (2), 260–285.

41 Moeschlin, S. (1965). *Poisoning, diagnosis and treatment.* (J. Bickel, Trans; 1st American ed., p. 419). Grune & Stratton. (Translated from the 4th German Edition).

42 Schiff, L. (ed.). (1969). *Diseases of the liver* (3rd ed.). J.B. Lippincott.

43 Tainter, M.L., & Ferris, A.J. (1969). *Aspirin in modern therapy. A review.* Bayer Company Division of Sterling Drug, Inc.

44 Woodbury, D. (1970). Analgesic-antipyretic, anti-inflammatory agents, and inhibitors of uric acid synthesis. In L.S. Goodman & A. Gilman (eds), *The pharmacological basis of therapeutics* (4th ed.). The Macmillan Company.

45 Starko, K.M., & Mullick, F.G. (12 February 1983). Hepatic and cerebral pathology findings in children with fatal salicylate intoxication: Further evidence for a causal relation between salicylate and Reye's syndrome. *Lancet, 321* (8320), 326–329.

46 Saltzman, D.A., Gall, E.P., & Robinson, S.F. (September 1976). Aspirin-induced hepatic dysfunction in a patient with adult rheumatoid arthritis. *American Journal of Digestive Diseases, 21* (9), 815–820.

47 Bernstein, B.H., Singsen, B.H., King, K.K., & Hanson, V. (June 1977). Aspirin-induced hepatotoxicity and its effect on juvenile rheumatoid arthritis. *American Journal of Diseases of Children, 131* (6), 659–653

48 Cincinnati Children's. History of the Medical Center. Retrieved 16 August 2021, from Cincinnati Children's.

49 Bove, K.E., McAdams, A.J., Partin, J.C., Partin, J.S., Hug, G., & Schubert, W.K. (September 1975). The hepatic lesion in Reye's syndrome. *Gastroenterology, 69* (3), 685–697.

50 Mitchell R.A., Ram M.L., Arcinue E.L., Chang C.H. (1980). Comparison of cytosolic and mitochondrial hepatic enzyme alteration in Reye's syndrome. *Pediatric Research, 14*, pp. 1216–1221.

51 Pessayre, D., Fromenty, B., & Mansouri, A. (2001). Drug-induced microvesicular steatosis and steatohepatitis. In J.J. Lemasters & A.L. Nieminen (eds) *Mitochondria in pathogenesis* (pp. 489–571). Kluwer Academic/Plenum Publishers, 2001.

52 Morales, A.R., Bourgeois, C.H., Trapukdi, S., & Chulacharit, E. (1969). Encephalopathy and fatty degeneration of the viscera. An electron microscopic study. *American Journal of Clinical Pathology, 52* (6), 755 [Abstract from Scientific Sessions of the Annual Meeting of the American Society of Clinical Pathologists, 14–21 September 1969].

53 Partin, J.C., Schubert, W.K., & Partin, J.S. (1971, December 9). Mitochondrial ultrastructure in Reye's syndrome (encephalopathy and fatty degeneration of the viscera). *New England Journal of Medicine, 285* (24), 1339–1343.

54 Brown, R.E., & Madge, G.E. (December 1972). Hepatic ultrastructure in Reye's syndrome. *Virginia Medical Monthly, 99*, 1295–1300.

55 Chang, L.W., Gilbert, E.F., Tanner, W., & Moffat, H.L. (August 1973). Reye syndrome. Light and electron microscopic studies. *Archives of Pathology, 96*, 127–132.

56   Tang, T.T., Siegesmund, K.A., Sedmak, G.V., Casper, J.T., Varma, R.R., & McCreadie, S.R. (30 June 1975). Reye syndrome. A correlated electron-microscopic, viral, and biochemical observation. *Journal of the American Medical Association, 232* (13), 1339–1346.

57   Iancu, T.C., Mason, W.H., & Neustein, H.B. (July 1977). Ultrastructural abnormalities of liver cells in Reye's syndrome. *Human Pathology, 8* (4), 421–431.

58   Partin, J.C., Schubert, W.K., & Partin, J.S. (9 December 1971). Mitochondrial ultrastructure in Reye's syndrome (encephalopathy and fatty degeneration of the viscera). *New England Journal of Medicine, 285* (24), 1339–1343.

59   Tolman, K.G., Peterson, P., Gray, P., & Hammar, S.P. (February 1978). Hepatotoxicity of salicylates in monolayer cell cultures. *Gastroenterology, 74* (2), 205–208.

60   Iancu, T., & Elian, E. (September 1976). Ultrastructural changes in aspirin hepatotoxicity. *American Journal of Clinical Pathology, 66* (3), 570–575.

61   Schubert, W.K., Partin, J.C., & Partin, J.S. (1972). Encephalopathy and fatty liver (Reye's syndrome). In H. Popper and F. Schaffner (eds), *Progress in liver disease* (Volume IV, pp. 489–510). Grune & Stratton.

62   Evans, H., Bourgeois, C.H., Comer, D.S., & Keshamras, N. (December 1970). Brain lesions in Reye's syndrome. *Archives of Pathology, 90,* 543–546.

63   Partin, J.C., Partin, J.S., Schubert, W.K., & McLaurin, R.L. (1975). Brain ultrastructure in Reye's syndrome: (Encephalopathy and fatty alteration of the viscera). *Journal of Neuropathology & Experimental Neurology, 34* (5), 425–444.

64   ibid.

65   Schubert, W.K., Partin, J.C., & Partin, J.S. (1972). Encephalopathy and fatty liver (Reye's syndrome). In H. Popper and F. Schaffner (eds), *Progress in liver disease* (Volume IV, pp. 489–510). Grune & Stratton.

66   Partin, J.C., Partin, J.S., & Schubert, W.K. (1 September 1973). Fatty liver in Reye's syndrome: Is it a distinct morphologic entity? *Gastroenterology, 65* (3), A-39/563 [Abstracts of papers submitted to the American Association for the Study of Liver Diseases].

67   Schubert, W.K. (December 1975). Commentary: The diagnosis of Reye syndrome. *Journal of Pediatrics, 87* (6), 867.

68   *Bove, K.E.* Education and Training. Retrieved 15 March 2022, from Cincinnati Children's.

69   Bove, K.E. The character and specificity of the hepatic lesion in Reye's syndrome. In J.D. Pollack (ed.). (1975) *Reye's Syndrome. Proceedings of the [1974] Reye's Syndrome Conference Sponsored by the Children's Hospital Foundation, Columbus, Ohio* (pp. 93–116). Grune & Stratton.

70   ibid.

71   Schubert, W.K. (December 1975). Commentary: The diagnosis of Reye syndrome. *Journal of Pediatrics, 87* (6), 867.

72   Schubert, W.K., Bobo, R.C., Partin, J.C., & Partin, J.S. (December 1975). Reye's syndrome. In D.F. Dowling (ed.), *Disease-a-month* (p. 15) [Monthly clinical monographs on current medical problems]. Year Book Medical Publishers, Inc.

73   ibid.

74   Partin, J.C., Partin, J.S., & Schubert, W.K. (1 September 1973 1). Fatty liver in Reye's syndrome: Is it a distinct morphologic entity? *Gastroenterology, 65* (3), A-39/563 [Abstracts of papers submitted to the American Association for the Study of Liver Diseases].

75   DeVivo, D.C., & Keating, J.P. (1976). Reye's syndrome. In I. Schulman (ed.), *Advances in pediatrics* (Vol. 22, pp. 175–229). Year Book Medical Publishers.

76   Schubert, W.K., Partin, J.C., & Partin, J.S. (1972). Encephalopathy and fatty liver (Reye's syndrome). Chapter 28 in H. Popper and F. Schaffner (eds), *Progress in liver disease* (Vol. IV, p. 506).

77   Wilson, M.L., & Reller, L.B. (1 October 2005). The proposed closing of the Armed Forces Institute of Pathology. *Clinical Infectious Diseases, 41* (7), 1003–1004.

78   Starko, K.M. (28 September 1979). Letter to Michael B. Gregg. [Business letter EIS Officer, Field Services Division, Center for Disease Control and Acting State Epidemiologist, Arizona to Deputy Director, Bureau of Epidemiology, Center for Disease Control].

79   Aprille, J.R. (26 August 1977). Reye's syndrome: Patient serum alters mitochondrial function and morphology in vitro. *Science, 197* (43060), 908-910.

80   Glick, T.H., Likosky, W.H., Levitt, L.P., Mellin, H., & Reynolds, D.W. (September 1970). Reye's syndrome: an epidemiologic approach. *Pediatrics, 46* (3), 371–377.

81   Corey, L., Rubin, R.J., Hattwick, M.A.W., Noble, G.R., & Cassidy, E. (November 1976). A nationwide outbreak of Reye's syndrome. Its epidemiologic relationship to influenza B. *American Journal of Medicine, 61* (5), 615–625.

82   Corey, L., Rubin, R.J., Bregman, D., Gregg, M.B. (November 1977). Diagnostic criteria for influenza B-associated Reye's syndrome: Clinical vs. pathologic criteria. *Pediatrics, 60* (5), 702–708.

83   Gregg, M.B. (9 October 1979). Letter to the author. [Business letter Deputy Director, Bureau of Epidemiology, Center for Disease Control to EIS Officer, Field Services Division, Center for Disease Control and Acting State Epidemiologist, Arizona.].

84   S.1794. Reye's syndrome Act of 1979. (21 September 1979). *Congressional Record—Senate* (pp. 25738–25741).

85   Berman, W.F. (19 October 1979). Letter to Guy Vander Jagt. [Business letter from Chief, Pediatric Gastroenterologist, Medical College of Virginia to Member of Congress, House of Representatives].

86   National Reye's Syndrome Foundation [Michigan]. (December 1979). Multi Center Study Group. *National Reye's Syndrome Foundation, 2* (3), 6. [Article in newsletter].

87   National Reye's Syndrome Foundation [Ohio]. (1979, all). *National Reye's Syndrome Foundation in the News*, p. 1–8. [Newsletter].

88   Subak-Sharpe, G.J. (1 November 1979). Reye's syndrome: Baffling killer of children. *Family Circle*, T 2.

89   Sterling Drug. (February 1980). When mother has to be the "doctor" … [Advertisement]. *Good Housekeeping.*

90   ibid.

Chapter 15 – Now What?

1   Heath, C. (28 December 2019). Letter to the author. [Business letter from Director, Chronic Disease Division to EIS Officer, Field Services Division, Center for Disease Control and Acting State Epidemiologist, Arizona].

2   Dalen J.E. (2006). Aspirin to prevent heart attack and stroke: what's the right dose? *American Journal of Medicine, 119* (3), 198-202.

3   Schonberger, L.B., Bregman, D.J., Sullivan-Bolyai, J.Z., Keenlyside, R.A., Ziegler, D.W., Retailliau, H.F., Eddins, D.L., & Bryan, J.A. (August 1979). Guillain-Barre syndrome following vaccination with National Influenza Immunization Program, United States, 1976–1977. *American Journal of Epidemiology, 110* (2), 105–123.

4   Johnson, G.M. (1980). Reye's syndrome: Its American origins. *Journal of the National Reye's Syndrome Foundation, 1* (2), 56–62.

5   Starko, K.M. (10 December 1979). Monthly report for October and November 1979 to J. Lyle Conrad, Director, and Stanley I. Music, Deputy Director, Field Services Division, Bureau of Epidemiology, Center for Disease Control.

6   Mortimer, E.A. (7 February 1980). Letter to the author. [Business communication Professor of Community Health and Pediatrics, Case Western Reserve University to EIS Officer, Field Services Division, Center for Disease Control and Acting State Epidemiologist, Arizona.].

7   Foege, W.H. (28 November 1979). Letter to Guy Vander Jagt. [Business letter Director, Center for Disease Control to Member of Congress, House of Representatives.].

8   Obituary of Brenda Dee Moore Newman. (1 January 1980). *Arizona Republic*.

9   Starko, K.M. (3 January 1980). Letter to Mel Cohen, Alan Kaplan, and C. George Ray. [Business letter EIS Officer, Field Services Division, Center for Disease Control and Acting State Epidemiologist, Arizona to Deputy Director, Bureau of Epidemiology, Center for Disease Control to Chief, Department of Pediatrics, St Joseph's Hospital, Phoenix, Pediatric Neurology, Good Samaritan Hospital, Phoenix, and Professor, Pathology and Pediatrics, University of Arizona Health Sciences Center].

10   Hospitals slow in giving Reye's syndrome data. (25 February 1980). *Tuscan Citizen*.

11   ibid.

12   Schonberger, L.B, (19 February 1980). Letter to the author. [Business communication from Chief, Enteric and Neurotropic Viral Disease Branch, Viral Diseases Division, Bureau of Epidemiology, Center for Disease Control to EIS Officer, Field Services Division, Center for Disease Control and Acting State Epidemiologist, Arizona.].

13   Munro, I. (25 February 1980). Letter to the author [Business letter from Editor, *Lancet* to EIS Officer, Field Services Division, Center for Disease Control and Acting State Epidemiologist, Arizona].

14   Malone, T.E. (January 1980). *NIH research activities on Reye's syndrome*. Report prepared by Deputy Director, National Institutes of Health, Department of Health Education and Welfare, Public Health Service in response to request from the US Senate Appropriations Committee.

15   Watson, W.C. (13 April 1979). Letter to John Melcher. Entered into the Congressional Record for S. 1794. Reye's syndrome act of 1979. *Congressional Record—Senate* (pp. 25738–25741), 21 September 1979.

16   Associated Press. Schools for 12,000 shut in Michigan due to flu. (25 February 1980).

17   Reye's syndrome stalking children again, but death rate is lower. (28 February 1980). *Arizona Daily Star.*

18   15 in state struck by Reye's syndrome since January 1. (2 March 1980). *New York Times*.

19   Sullivan-Bolyai, J.Z., Nelson, D.B., Morens, D.M., Schonberger, L.B., Marks, J.S., Johnson, D., Holtzhauer, F., Bright, F., Kramer, T., & Halpin, T.J. (March 1980). Reye syndrome in children less than 1 year old: Some epidemiologic observations. *Pediatrics, 65*(3), 627–629.

20   Varma, R.R., Riedel, D.R., Komorowski, R.A., Harrington, G.J., & Nowak T.V. (28 September 1979). Reye's syndrome in nonpediatric age groups. *Journal of the American Medical Association, 242*(13), 1373–1375.

21   Davis, L.E., & Kornfield, M. (June 1980). Influenza A virus and Reye's syndrome in adults. *Journal of Neurology, Neurosurgery, and Psychiatry, 43*(6), 516–521.

22   ibid.

23   Christoffersen, P., Faarup, P., Geertinger, P., & Krogh, P. (March–April 1980). Reye's syndrome in a child on long-term salicylate medication. *Forensic Science International, 15*(2), 129–133.

24   Kolata, G. (28 March 1980). Reye's syndrome: A medical mystery. *Science, 207*(4438), 1453–1454.

Chapter 16 – The FDA's 1977 Draft Monograph—*Shh*

1   US Food and Drug Administration, Department of Health, Education, and Welfare. (8 July 1977). Over-the-counter drugs. Establishment of a monograph for OTC internal analgesic, antipyretic, and antirheumatic products. *Federal Register, 42*(131), 2 of 2 books.

2   Panel members included Henry W. Elliot, MD (Chairman, died 1976); J. Weldon Bellville, MD (Chairman from August 1976); William H. Barr, PhD; Julius M. Coon,

MD, PhD; Ninfa I. Redmond, PhD (resigned January 1977); Naomi F. Rothfield, MD; and George Sharpe, MD.

3   US Food and Drug Administration. (1977). Safety and efficacy of over-the-counter drugs: The FDA's OTC drug review. *Pediatrics, 59* (2), 309–311.

4   ibid.

5   US Food and Drug Administration, Department of Health, Education, and Welfare. (8 July 1977). Over-the-counter drugs. Establishment of a monograph for OTC internal analgesic, antipyretic, and antirheumatic products. *Federal Register, 42* (131), 2 of 2 books.

6   ibid. p. 35355.

7   ibid. p. 35356.

8   ibid. pp. 35407–35408.

9   ibid. p. 35356.

10   ibid. p. 35356.

11   ibid. p. 35360.

12   ibid. p. 35360.

13   ibid. p. 35366.

14   Done, A.K., Yaffe, S.J., & Clayton, J.M. (1979). Aspirin dosage for infants and children. *The Journal of Pediatrics, 95* (4), 617–625.

15   US Food and Drug Administration, Department of Health, Education, and Welfare. (8 July 1977). Over-the-counter drugs. Establishment of a monograph for OTC internal analgesic, antipyretic, and antirheumatic products. *Federal Register, 42* (131), 2 of 2 books, p. 35367.

16   ibid. pp. 35366–35368.

17   ibid. p. 35358.

18   Mann, C.C., & Plummer, M.L. (1991). *The aspirin wars: Money, medicine, and 100 years of rampant competition* (p. 206). Harvard Business School Press.

19   Swann J., & Ottes R.T. (12 November 1997) Oral history interview of J. Richard Crout. [FDA Historian interview of former, Director, Bureau of Drugs, FDA]. Retrieved 29 November 2021, from the Food and Drug Administration.

20   US Food and Drug Administration. (January 2018). A Brief History of the Center for Drug Evaluation and Research. Retrieved 19 March 2022, from the FDA.

21   Done, A.K., Yaffe, S.J., & Clayton, J.M. (1979). Aspirin dosage for infants and children. *The Journal of Pediatrics, 95* (4), 617–625.

Chapter 17 – Replication—The Ohio and Michigan Studies

1   Rubin, F.L., Streiff, E.J., Neal, M., & Michaels, R.H. (1976). Epidemiologic studies of Reye's syndrome: Cases seen in Pittsburgh, October 1973–April 1975. *American Journal of Public Health, 66* (11), 1096–1098.

2   Corey, L, Rubin, R.J., Thompson, T.R., Noble, G.R., Cassidy, E., Hattwick, M.A.W., Gregg, M.B., & Eddins, D. (March 1977). Influenza B-associated Reye's syndrome. *Journal of Infectious Diseases, 135* (3), 398–407.

3   Center for Disease Control, Viral Diseases Division, Bureau of Epidemiology. (17 March 1979). Outbreak of Reye's syndrome in Ohio. Memorandum to Director, Center for Disease Control.

4   Sullivan-Bolyai, J.Z., Marks, J.S., Johnson, D., Nelson, D.B., Holtzhauer, F., Bright, F., Kramer, T., Halpin, T.J. (November 1980). Reye's syndrome in Ohio, 1973–1980. *American Journal of Epidemiology, 112* (5), 629–638.

5   Center for Disease Control, Viral Diseases Division, Bureau of Epidemiology. (4 June 1979). Outbreak of Reye Syndrome in Ohio. Memorandum to Director, Center for Disease Control.

6   Nationwide Realty Investors, Ltd. (2006) *The Arena District, A neighborhood 170 years in the making.*

7   Hughes, B. (6 April 1982). Tragedy leads to activism. Parents with a cause. *The Argus Press* [Owosso, Michigan].

8   Experts confirm all exposed to PBB carry chemical in blood, fat. (11 July 1979). *Ironwood Daily Globe*

9   Fear, frustration draws parents to Reye's syndrome meeting. (21 February 1980). *Ironwood Daily Globe.*

10   ibid.

11   Palmida Discount Center coupon for St Joseph's Children's Aspirin. (1 March 1980). *Ironwood Daily Globe.*

12   Galton, L.A. (11 May 1980). Mysterious disease that attacks children. *Parade.*

13   Goldman, A.I. (11 February 1980). New York flu outbreak is put at 'epidemic' level. *New York Times.*

14   Starko, K.M. (3 April 1980). Letter to Floribel Mullick. [Business letter from EIS Officer, Field Services Division, Center for Disease Control and Acting State Epidemiologist, Arizona to Physician, Department of Environmental and Drug-induces Pathology, Armed Forces Institute of Pathology].

15   Correa-Villasenor A. (18 April 1980). *Epidemiologic aspects of Reye syndrome in Ohio, December 1978–November 1979.* Presentation at the 29th Annual EIS Conference, 14–18 April 1980. Center for Disease Control, Atlanta, Georgia.

16   Starko, K.M. (18 April 1980). *Reye syndrome associated with salicylate consumption.* Presentation at the 29th Annual EIS Conference, 14–18 April 1980. Center for Disease Control, Atlanta, Georgia.

17   Hurwitz, E.S. (28 January 1982). *Studies concerning Reye's syndrome and salicylates.* Memorandum for the record from Eugene S. Hurwitz, Medical Epidemiologist, Viral Diseases Division, Centers for Disease Control.

Chapter 18 – Enough, Summer 1980

1   United Press International. (28 April 1980). Flu epidemic spurs feared child illness. *Arizona Republic.*

2   United Press International. (23 May 1980). Aspirin-Reye's syndrome link found. *Mesa Tribune.*

3   Vesell, E.S. (1 May 1980). Sounding board. Why are toxic reactions to drugs so often undetected initially? *New England Journal of Medicine, 302* (18), 1027–1029.

4   Nelson, D.B., Sullivan-Bolyai, J.Z., Morens, D.M., Hurwitz, E.S., Schonberger, L.B. (January–June 1980). The epidemiology of Reye's syndrome: A review—with emphasis on recent observations. *University of Michigan Medical Center Journal, XLVI* (1–2), 4–8.

5   Starko, K.M. (23 June 1980). Letter to J. Lyle Conrad. [Business letter from EIS Officer, Field Services Division, Center for Disease Control and Acting State Epidemiologist, Arizona to Director, Field Services Division, Bureau of Epidemiology, Center for Disease Control].

6   Conrad, J.L. (27 June 1980). Memorandum from Director of the Field Service Division to Phillip Brachman, Director of the Bureau of Epidemiology, Center for Disease Control.

7   Starko, K.M. (24 June 1980). Letter to Gerhardt Levy. [Business letter from EIS Officer, Field Services Division, Center for Disease Control and Acting State Epidemiologist, Arizona to Distinguished Professor, Department of Pharmaceutics, State University of New York at Buffalo].

8   National Reye's Syndrome Foundation [Ohio]. (Winter 1981). *National Reye's Syndrome Foundation in the News.*

9   Correa A. (1980). Epidemiologic aspects of Reye's syndrome in Ohio: November 1978-December 1979. *Journal of the National Reye's Syndrome Foundation, 1* (2), 126.

10 State and Territorial Epidemiologists, K. Starko & Enteric and Neurotropic Viral Disease Branch, Viral Diseases Division, Bureau of Epidemiology, Center for Disease Control. (11 July 1980). Follow-up on Reye Syndrome—United States. *Morbidity and Mortality Weekly Report, 29* (27), 321–332.

11 Todd, J., Fishaut, M., Kapral, F., & Welch, T. (25 November 1978). Toxic-shock syndrome associated with the phage-group-I Staphylococci. *Lancet, 312* (8100), 1116–1168.

12 Donawa, M.E., Schmid, G.R., & Osterholm, M.T. (July–August 1984). Toxic shock syndrome: Chronology of state and federal epidemiologic studies and regulatory decision-making. *Public Health Reports, 99* (4), 42–50.

13 Center for Disease Control. (23 May 1980). Toxic-shock syndrome—United States. *Morbidity and Mortality Weekly Report, 29* (20), 229–230.

14 Center for Disease Control. (27 June 1980). Follow-up on toxic-shock syndrome— United States. *Morbidity and Mortality Weekly Report, 29* (25), 297–299.

15 Centers for Disease Control. (29 June 1990). Historical perspectives reduced incidence of menstrual toxic-shock syndrome—United States, 1980–1990. *Morbidity and Mortality Weekly Report, 39* (25), 421–423.

16 Davis, D.L., & Buffler, P. (24 October 1992). Reduction of deaths after drug labelling for risk of Reye's syndrome [Letter to the editor]. *Lancet, 340* (8826), 1042.

17 Gibson, P. (19 June 1948). Salicylic acid for coronary thrombosis? *Lancet, 251* (6512), 965.

18 Craven, L.L. (February 1950). Acetylsalicylic acid, possible preventive of coronary thrombosis. *Annals of Western Medicine and Surgery, 4* (2), 95–99.

19 Poole, J.C.F., & French, J.E. (8 July 1961 8). Thrombosis. *Journal of Atherosclerosis Research, 1* (4) 251–282.

20 Vane, J.R. (23 June 1971). Inhibition of prostaglandin synthesis as a mechanism of action for aspirin-like drugs. *Nature: New Biology, 231* (25), 232–235.

21 Elwood, P.C., Cochrane, A.L., Burr, P.M., Sweetnam, P.M., Williams, G., Welsby, E., Hughes, S.J., & Renton, R. (9 March 1974). A randomized controlled trial of acetyl salicylic acid in the secondary prevention of mortality from myocardial infarction. *British Medical Journal, 1* (5905), 436–440.

22 Mann, C.C., & Plummer, M.L. (1991). *The aspirin wars: Money, medicine, and 100 years of rampant competition* (pp. 291–293). Harvard Business School Press.

23 Ravven, W. (7 November 2003). New leader for center for consumer self care at UCSF. Retrieved 19 March 2022, at University of California, San Francisco News.

Chapter 19 – Warnings—with Caveats, Late 1980

1   Jones, J.K. (29 October 1980). Memorandum from Director, Division of Drug Experience, FDA, to the record.

2   Vaughan, V.C., McKay, R.J., & Nelson, W.E. (eds). (1975). *Nelson textbook of pediatrics* (10th edition, pp. 1445–1446). W.B. Saunders Company.

3   Luscombe, F.A., Monto, A.S., & Baublis, J.V. (September 1980). Mortality due to Reye's syndrome in Michigan: Distribution and longitudinal trends. *Journal of Infectious Diseases, 142* (3), 363–371.

4   Engelhardt, S.J., Halsey, N.A., Eddins, D.L., & Hinman, A.R. (November 1980). Measles mortality in the United States 1971–1975. *American Journal of Public Health, 70* (11), 1166 –1169.

5   Sullivan-Bolyai, J.Z., Marks, J.S., Johnson, D., Nelson, D.B., Holtzhauer, F., Bright, F., Kramer, T., & Halpin, T.J. (November 1980). Reye's syndrome in Ohio, 1973–1977. *American Journal of Epidemiology, 112* (5), 629–638.

6   Jones, J.K. (29 October 1980). Memorandum from Director of Drug Experience, FDA, for the Record.

7   Centers for Disease Control, Division of Viral Diseases and Field Services Division. (9 November 1982). Use of antipyretics in children with chickenpox. Wayne County, Tennessee. Memorandum to Director, CDC.

8   Jones, J.K. (29 October 1980). Memorandum of telephone conversation of Director, Division of Drug Experience, FDA, with Eileen Barker, Division of Neurological Drug Products, FDA.

9   Jones, J.K. (29 October 1980). Memorandum of telephone conversation of Director, Division of Drug Experience, FDA, with Sam Drage, Developmental Neurology, National Institutes of Health.

10 Jones, J.K. (30–31 October 1980). Memoranda of telephone conversations of Director, Division of Drug Experience, FDA, with Gene Hurwitz, CDC.

11 ibid.

12 Jones, J.K. (5 November 1980 5). Memorandum of telephone conversation of Director, Division of Drug Experience, FDA, with Gene Hurwitz, CDC.

13 Freudenberger, J. (Winter 1981). Presidential notes. *National Reye's Syndrome Foundation in the News* (p. 2). National Reye's Syndrome Foundation.

14 Freudenberger, T. (28 March 2008). List of accomplishments of the National Reye's Syndrome Foundation of Bryan, Ohio, of 28 March 2008. [List provided to the author].

15 "Reye" is sometimes used rather than "Reye's."

16 Halpin, T.J., Holtzhauer, F., & Hayner, N. (7 November 1980). Reye Syndrome— Ohio, Michigan. *Morbidity and Mortality Weekly Report, 29* (44), 532, 537–539.

17 Aspirin link to Reye's syndrome revealed. (8 November 1980). *Chicago Tribune.*

18 Studies warn parents about link of aspirin to childhood disease. (9 November 1980). *New York Times.*

19 Sterling Drug, Inc. (17 February 1982). *Detailed comments on epidemiologic studies of Reye's syndrome* (p. 37). Report submitted to the Food and Drug Administration.

20 ibid.

21 ibid.

22 ibid.

23 Kauffman, R.E. (18 March 1981). Letter to June Lockhart. [Business letter from Associate Professor, Pediatrics and Pharmacology, Wayne State University School of Medicine, to June Lockhart, Director of Health Care and Pediatric Practice, AAP].

24 Jones, J.K. (21 November 1980). Memorandum from Director, Division of Drug Experience, FDA, to Associate Director for New Drug Evaluation, FDA.

25 Jones, J.K. (3 December 1980). Memorandum of telephone conversation of Director, Division of Drug Experience, FDA, and Dr Releigh [*sic*], CDC.

26 Mann, C.C., & Plummer, M.L. (1991). *The aspirin wars: Money, medicine, and 100 years of rampant competition* (pp. 292–293). Harvard Business School Press.

27 Starko, K.M., Ray, C.G., Dominguez, L.B., Stromberg, W.L., & Woodall, D.F. (December 1980). Reye's syndrome and salicylate use. *Pediatrics, 66* (6), 859–864.

28 Snodgrass, W., Rumack, B.H., Peterson, R.G., & Holbrook, M.L. (March 1981). Salicylate toxicity following therapeutic doses in young children. *Clinical Toxicology, 18* (3), 247–259.

Chapter 20 – Smackdown, Early 1981

1   Kotulak, R. (4 January 1981). Reye's disease linked to aspirin. *Chicago Tribune.*

2   Remedies for influenza stress rest and aspirin. (7 January 1981). *New York Times.*

3   Brody, J.E. (9 January 1981). Health officials report widespread outbreaks of flu. *New York Times.*

Notes

4   Takes steps to stop influenza spread. Surgeon General Blue says it can be controlled only by intelligent action of the public. Gives advice to doctors. (14 September 1918). *New York Times.*

5   Asian flu in city called epidemic; 150,000 pupils ill. (3 October 1957). *New York Times.*

6   Profit rises 9.8% at Sterling drug; quarter's net up to a new high of 64 cents a share, against 58 in 1957. (2 May 1958). *New York Times.*

7   Plough, Inc., lifts half-year profit. (14 July 1958). *New York Times.*

8   Dougherty, P.H. (6 January 1969). Advertising: Flu pushes home-remedy sales to fever heights. *New York Times.*

9   Sullivan, R. (19 February 1978). Flu expected to hit state public schools. *New York Times.*

10   Goldman, A.L. (11 February 1980). New York flu outbreak is put at "epidemic" level. *New York Times.*

11   Clayton, J.M. (12 February 1982). Letter to Thomas J. Halpin. [Business letter from Vice President, Quality Control and Clinical and Regulatory Services, Plough, Inc., to Chief, Division of Preventive Medicine and State Epidemiologist, Ohio Department of Health].

12   Hall, W.M. (23 February 1981). Letter to John Clayton. [Business letter from Chief, Division of Disease Surveillance, Michigan Department of Public Health, to the Vice President, Quality Control and Clinical and Regulatory Services, Plough, Inc].

13   Sterling Drug, Inc. (17 February 1982). *Detailed comments on epidemiologic studies of Reye's syndrome.* Report submitted to the Food and Drug Administration.

14   Young W.M. (7 January 1981). Unpublished letter to Jerold F. Lucey, Editor, *Pediatrics,* forwarded to K.M. Starko for response to comment regarding the article Starko, K.M., Ray, C.G., Dominguez, L.B., Stromberg, W.L., & Woodall, D.F. (December 1980). Reye's syndrome and salicylate use. *Pediatrics, 66* (6), 859–864.

15   Young, W.M. (September 1981). Doubts relationship of salicylate and Reye's syndrome. [Letter to the editor]. *Pediatrics, 68* (3), 466–467.

16   Clark, J.H., & Fitzgerald, J.F. (September 1981). Doubts relationship of salicylate and Reye's syndrome. [Letter to the editor]. *Pediatrics, 68* (3), 467.

17   Gall, D.G., Barker, G., & Cutz, E. (September 1981). Doubts relationship of salicylate and Reye's syndrome. [Letter to the editor]. *Pediatrics, 68* (3), 467–468.

18   Pascoe, J.M. (October 1981). Salicylate and Reye's syndrome. [Letter to the editor]. *Pediatrics, 68* (4), 661–662.

19   Symposium on Analgesics. (February 1981). Georgetown University Symposium on Analgesics. Aspirin and acetaminophen. *Archives of Internal Medicine, 141* (3 Spec. No.), 273–406.

20   Winchester, J.F. (February 1981). Georgetown University Symposium on analgesics. *Archives of Internal Medicine, 141* (3 Spec. No.), 273–274.

21   Temple, A.R. (February 1981). Acute and chronic effects of aspirin toxicity and their treatment. *Archives of Internal Medicine, 141* (3 Spec. No.), 364–369.

22   American Academy of Pediatrics. (9 January 1981). Interim decisions of the Executive Committee in minutes of the Executive Board Meeting, Evanston, Illinois, 23–25 January 1981.

23   American Academy of Pediatrics. (March 1981). Policy Statement. Reye's syndrome and Aspirin. *News and Comment* [Newsletter], *32* (3), 15.

24   Lockhart, J.D. (31 March 1981). Memorandum from the Director, Department of Health Care and Pediatric Practice to the Committee on Drugs, American Academy of Pediatrics, regarding aspirin and Reye's syndrome.

25   Snodgrass, W., Rumack, B.H., Peterson, R.G., & Holbrook, M.L. (March 1981). Salicylate toxicity following therapeutic doses in young children. *Clinical Toxicology, 18* (3), 247–259.

26   Done, A.K. (September 1981). [Letter to the editor]. *Clinical Toxicology, 18*(9), 1125–1126.

27   In Memoriam. (September 1998). Alan Kimball Done, MD, 1926–1998. *Journal of Toxicology: Clinical Toxicology, 36*(4), vii–viii.

28   Done, A.K., Cohen, S.N., & Strebel, L. (1977). Pediatric clinical pharmacology and the "therapeutic orphan." *Annual Review of Pharmacology Toxicology, 17*, 561–573.

29   Reagan, R. (20 January 1981). Inaugural address.

30   Hilts, P.J. (2004). *Protecting America's health: The FDA, business, and one hundred years of regulation* (p. 214). University of North Carolina Press.

31   ibid. p. 215.

32   ibid. p. 216.

33   Chayet, N.L. (1967). Power of the package insert. *New England Journal of Medicine, 277*, 1253–1254.

34   Stolley, P.D. (November–December 1982). The use of vital and morbidity statistics for the detection of adverse drug reactions and for monitoring of drug safety. *Journal of Clinical Pharmacology, 22*(11), 499–504.

35   Goyan, J. (May 1981). Fourteen fallacies about patient package inserts. *The Western Journal of Medicine, 134*, 463–468.

36   ibid.

37   Hevesi, D. (1 March 2010 1). Arthur Hayes Jr, who led F.D.A. in Tylenol case, is dead at 76. *New York Times*.

38   Hilts, P.J. (2004). *Protecting America's health: The FDA, business, and one hundred years of regulation* (p. 216). University of North Carolina Press.

39   ibid. pp. 216–217.

40   Consensus Conference. (27 November 1981). Diagnosis and treatment of Reye's syndrome. *Journal of the American Medical Association, 246*(21), 2441–2444.

41   Sterling Drug, Inc. (17 February 1982). *Detailed comments on epidemiologic studies of Reye's syndrome*. Report submitted to the Food and Drug Administration.

42   ibid.

43   Rossiter, A. (5 March 1981). Study urges caution with aspirin. Warning sounded on flu, chickenpox. United Press International.

44   ibid.

45   Salicylates, fever, and Reye's syndrome—An etiologic triad? (April 1981). *Forefronts of Neurology/Canada, 2*(2), 6.

46   Abramowicz, M. (4 June 1981). Letter to Karen M. Starko. [Business letter from the editor of *The Medical Letter*].

47   Starko, K.M. (29 June 1981). Letter to Mark Abramowicz. [Business letter to the editor of *The Medical Letter*].

48   Partin, J.S., Partin, J.C., Schubert, W.K., & Hammond, J. (April 1981). 619 Salicylates and Reye's syndrome [abstract]. *Pediatric Research, 15*(4, part 2), 543.

49   Aspirin products. (24 July 1981). *The Medical Letter, 23*(15), 65–67.

50   Haley, C.E., & Starko, K.M. (4 September 1981). Letter to the editor. [Unpublished business letter to the editor of the *New England Journal of Medicine* from Fellow, Division of Epidemiology/Virology, School of Medicine, University of Virginia and former EIS officer, Field Services Division, CDC].

51   Centers for Disease Control. (5 June 1981). *Pneumocystis* pneumonia—Los Angeles. *Morbidity and Mortality Weekly Report, 30*(21), 250–252.

52   Centers for Disease Control. (1 June 2001). First report of AIDS. *Morbidity and Mortality Weekly Report, 50*(21), 429.

53   Shilts, R. (1987). *And the bank played on* (pp. 73–74). St Martin's Press.

Notes

54 ibid.

55 Good, L., & Conrad, J.L. (28 May 1982). CDC Information Clearance sheet indicating Good and Conrad's approval of abstract entitled *Hepatic and cerebral lesions of children with fatal salicylate intoxication* by Karen M. Starko and Floribel G. Mullick submitted for presentation at Reye's Syndrome Conference, to be held at Vail, Colorado, 19 June 1981.

56 Starko, K.M. (19 June 1982). *Hepatic and cerebral lesions of children with fatal salicylate intoxication*. Oral presentation at the Reye's Syndrome Conference, a Joint Annual Meeting of the National Reye's Syndrome Foundation and the American Reye's Syndrome Foundation, 19–20 June 1981, Vail, Colorado.

57 Program. (19 June 1981). Reye's Syndrome Conference, a Joint Annual Meeting of the National Reye's Syndrome Foundation and the American Reye's Syndrome Foundation. 19–20 June 1981, Vail, Colorado.

58 Pollack, J.D. (ed.). (1981). Proceedings of the Seventh Annual Meeting of the National Reye's Syndrome Foundation, Bryan, Ohio, Co-sponsored by the American Reye's Syndrome Foundation, Denver, Colorado. 19–20 June 1981, Vail, Colorado. *Journal of the National Reye's Syndrome Foundation, 2*, 1–70.

59 Miller, T. (31 March 1984). The O.M.B. writes a prescription. *The Nation*, 383–385.

60 Aspirin or paracetamol? (8 August 1981). [Editorial]. *Lancet, 318*(8241), 281–288.

61 Associated Press. (24 August 1981). New center in Ohio will seek a cure for Reye's syndrome. *New York Times*.

62 Sydenham, T., as cited in Kluger, M.J. (1979). *Fever: Its biology, evolution, and function* (p. 130). Princeton University Press.

63 Sterling Drug, Inc. (17 February 1982). *Detailed comments on epidemiologic studies of Reye's syndrome* (p. 7). Report submitted to the Food and Drug Administration. (FOI. Ref.23)

64 Meeting on Reye's syndrome. (13 April 1982). Summary of meeting among FDA, Sterling Drug Inc., Bristol-Myers Co., the Dow Chemical Company, and Monsanto (p. 4).

65 ibid.

66 National Reye's Syndrome Foundation [Ohio]. (1980). Medical mystery: Reye's syndrome. Because You Need to Know [Brochure].

67 Wilson, J.T. (3 September 1981). Letter to Karen M. Starko. [Business letter from Professor, Departments of Pharmacology and Pediatrics, Louisiana State University Medical Center, to former EIS Officer, Field Services Division, CDC].

68 Starko, K.M. (16 September 1981). Letter to John T. Wilson. [Business letter from Medical Epidemiologist, Bureau of Disease Control, Maricopa County Health Department].

69 Wilson, J.T., & Brown, R.D. (June 1982). Reye's syndrome and aspirin use: The role of prodromal illness severity in the assessment of relative risk. *Pediatrics, 69*(6), 822–825.

70 Arrowsmith, J.B., Kennedy, D.L., Kuritsky, J.N., & Faich, G.A. (June 1987). National patterns of aspirin use and Reye syndrome reporting, United States, 1980–1985. *Pediatrics, 79*(6), 858–863.

71 Millenson, M.L. (21 November 1982). J&J gains admiration, strength. *Chicago Tribune.*

72 Arrowsmith, J.B., Kennedy, D.L., Kuritsky, J.N., & Faich, G.A. (June 1987). National patterns of aspirin use and Reye syndrome reporting, United States, 1980–1985. *Pediatrics, 79*(6), 858–863.

73 Millenson, M.L. (21 November 1982). J&J gains admiration, strength. *Chicago Tribune.*

Chapter 21 – Would You Give This? Late 1981

1   Dowdle, W. (16 September 1981). Letter to Karen M. Starko. [Business letter from Director, Center for Infectious Diseases, Centers for Disease Control, to Medical Epidemiologist, Bureau of Disease Control, Maricopa County Health Department].

2   ibid.

3   Alexander, E.R. (12 November 1981). Letter from Chief, Section of Pediatric Infectious Diseases, the University of Arizona Health Sciences Center to Walter Dowdle, Director, Center for Infectious Diseases, CDC, with attachment titled *Review of case-control studies of Reye syndrome and salicylates. Summary of Reye syndrome consultants* (dated 13–14 October 1981).

4   Linnemann, C.C. (November 1981). Salicylates and Reye's syndrome [Letter to the editor]. *Pediatrics, 68* (5), 748.

5   Tonsgard, J.H., & Huttenlocher, P.R. (November 1981). Salicylates and Reye's syndrome. *Pediatrics, 68* (5), 747–748.

6   Foege, W.H. (4 December 1981). Letter from Director, CDC to Arthur H. Hayes, Jr, Commissioner, FDA.

7   Conner, P. (25 August 1985). Stalling for time. *San Francisco Chronicle.*

8   Conner, P. (25 August 1985). Stalling for time. *San Francisco Chronicle.*

9   Sterling Drug, Inc. (17 February 1982). *Detailed comments on epidemiologic studies of Reye's syndrome.* Report submitted to the Food and Drug Administration.

10 Handwritten note on file at the FDA. (11 February 1982). Reye's syndrome.

11 Director, Bureau of Drugs, FDA. (1 February 1982). Memorandum to Executive Communication Committee, FDA.

Chapter 22 – Misbranded, Early 1982

1   Partin, J.S., Partin, J.C., Schubert, W.K., & Hammond, J.G. (23 January 1982). Serum salicylate concentrations in Reye's disease. A study of 130 biopsy-proven cases. *Lancet, 319* (8265), 191–194.

2   Rodgers, G.C., Weiner, L.B., & McMillan, J.A. (13 March 1982). Salicylate and Reye's syndrome [Letter to the editor]. *Lancet, 319* (8272), 616.

3   Andresen, B.D., Alexander, M.S., Ng, K.J., & Bianchine J.R. (17 April 1982). Aspirin and Reye's disease: A reinterpretation [Letter to the editor]. *Lancet, 319* (8277), 903.

4   Bianchine, J.R., Alexander, M.S., Andresen, B.D., & Ng, K.D. (11 December 1982). The aspirin/Reye's syndrome link [Letter to the editor]. *Lancet, 320* (8311), 1333.

5   Editorial. (24 April 1982). Reye's syndrome—epidemiologic considerations. *Lancet, 319* (8278), 941–943.

6   American Academy of Pediatrics, Committee on Infectious Diseases. Draft minutes of meeting, Washington, DC, 10 May 1982.

7   American Academy of Pediatrics, Committee on Drugs. (9 February 1982). Draft minutes of meeting, Willamsburg, Virginia, 4–5 February 1982.

8   American Academy of Pediatrics, Committee on Infectious Diseases. Draft minutes of meeting, Washington, DC, 10 May 1982.

9   Doyle, L. (31 May 1987). Aspirin-Reye's chronology: Threat of suits delayed warning process. *Los Angeles Times.* 383–385.

10 Jennison, M.H. (3 February 1982). Memo to Committee on Infectious Diseases, American Academy of Pediatrics. As referenced in Mortimer, E.A. (10 April 1987). Reye's syndrome, salicylates, epidemiology, and public health policy. *Journal of the America Medical Association, 257* (14), 1941.

11 Conner, K.P. (25 August 1985). Stalling for time. *SF Chronicle.*

12 ibid.

13 American Academy of Pediatrics, Committee on Infectious Diseases. Draft minutes of meeting, Washington, DC, 10 May 1982.

Notes

14 American Academy of Pediatrics, Executive Board (February 1982). Memo to the American Academy of Pediatrics membership. *News and Comment.*

15 Finkle, M.J. (9 February 1982 9). Memo of telecon between Dr Solar [*sic*], Vice President for Scientific Affairs of Glenbrook Laboratories Division of Sterling Drug, and Marion J. Finkle, Associate Director of NDE/BD [New Drug Evaluation/ Bureau of Drugs] of the Food and Drug Administration.

16 Brady, R.P. (11 February 1982). Memorandum of meeting: Reye's syndrome/prior ingestion of aspirin.

17 Centers for Disease Control. (February 1982). National surveillance for Reye syndrome, 1981: Update, Reye syndrome and salicylate usage. *Morbidity and Mortality Weekly Report, 31* (5), 53–56, 61.

18 US Food and Drug Administration. (12 February 1982). Aspirin and Reye syndrome. *Talk Paper,* T82–10.

19 Harris, G. (15 February 2005). Drug industry's longtime critic says "I told you so". *New York Times.*

20 Public Citizen (11 February 1982). *Statement by Sidney M. Wolfe, M.D. Director, Public Citizen's Health Research Group.* [Press release].

21 Seabrook, C. (12 February 1982). CDC accused of not warning on child illness. *The Atlanta Journal.*

22 Rosa, F. (27 February 1982). Memorandum of a telephone conversation with Sidney Wolfe, Director, Health Research Group.

23 Public Citizen (11 February 1982). *Statement by Sidney M. Wolfe, M.D. Director, Public Citizen's Health Research Group.* [Press release].

24 Bishop, J. (28 September 1982). Aspirin makers fight national test of link with a children's disease. *Wall Street Journal.*

25 Attorneys for Plough, Inc., & Sterling Drug, Inc. (22 June 1982). Reye syndrome and salicylates. Memorandum to Department of Health and Human Services.

26 Congressional Research Service. (29 January 2008). *The Food and Drug Administration: Budget and statutory history, FY1980–FY2007* (pp. 1–56). [CRS report for congress].

27 CDC spared from major cuts. (11 February 1982). *The Atlanta Constitution.*

28 Sterling Drug, Inc. (17 February 1982). *Detailed comments on epidemiologic studies of Reye's syndrome.* Report submitted to the Food and Drug Administration.

29 Aprille, J. (1981). Salicylate has several effects on mitochondrial function. *Journal of the National Reye's Syndrome Foundation, 2* (1), 56–60.

30 Lee, S.H., Laltoo, M., Crocker, J.F., & Rozee, K.R. (October 1980). Emulsifiers that enhance susceptibility to virus infections: Increased virus penetration and reduced interferon response. *Applied and Environmental Microbiology, 40* (4), 787–793.

31 Romshe, C.A., Hilty, M.D., McClung, H.J., Kerzner, B., & Reiner, C.B. (May 1981). Amino acid patterns in Reye syndrome: Comparison with clinically similar entities. *Journal of Pediatrics, 98* (5), 788–790.

32 McClung, H.J., Nahata, M., Andresen, B., Hilty, M., & Kerzner, B. The use of hepatic drugs in Reye's syndrome. (1981). *Journal of the National Reye's Syndrome Foundation,* 47–53.

33 Sterling Drug, Inc. (17 February 1982). *Detailed comments on epidemiologic studies of Reye's syndrome.* Report submitted to the Food and Drug Administration.

34 Food and Drug Administration. (24 May 1982). *Scientific workshop on Reye's syndrome and its possible association with salicylate use* (p. 176) [Transcript]. Wilson Hall, Building 1, National Institutes of Health, Bethesda, Maryland.

35 Wayne State University School of Medicine. (2021). Historic timeline. Retrieved 28 December 2021, from the School of Medicine, Wayne State University.

36 U.S Food and Drug Administration. (24 May 1982). *Scientific workshop on Reye's syndrome and its possible association with salicylate use* [Transcript]. Held at the National Institutes of Health, Bethesda, Maryland.

37 Drug companies accused of "misleading advertising." (6 May 1969 6). *Bennington Banner.*

38 Chayet, N.L. (May 1982). Great danger, great opportunity. *The Internist, 23,* 6–8.

39 Conner, K.P. (25 August 1985). Stalling for time. *San Francisco Chronicle.*

40 Hilts, P.J. (2004). *Protecting American's health: The FDA, business, and one hundred years of regulation* (p. 221). The University of North Carolina Press

41 Wilson, J.T. (August 2009). Curriculum vitae dated 11 August 2009, provided by Andrea Driver, Department of Pediatrics/Clinical Pharmacology, Louisiana State University Health Sciences Center.

42 Edlavitch, S.A. (12 February 1982). Memorandum of telephone conversation with John M. Clayton, Vice President, Schering Plough.

43 Angell, M. (8 March 1982). Letter to Karen M. Starko. [Business letter from Deputy Editor, *New England Journal of Medicine,* to Medical Epidemiologist, Bureau of Disease Control, Maricopa County Health Department.].

44 Garfunkel, J.M. (13 May 1982). Letter to Karen M. Starko. [Business letter from Editor, *Journal of Pediatrics,* to Medical Epidemiologist, Bureau of Disease Control, Maricopa County Health Department].

45 Lucey, J.F. (17 July 1982). Letter to Karen M. Starko. [Business letter from Editor of *Pediatrics to* Medical Epidemiologist, Bureau of Disease Control, Maricopa County Health Department].

46 Halperin, J.A. (5 March 1982). Reye's syndrome working group targeted dates. Memorandum from Deputy Director, Bureau of Drugs, FDA, to Mark Novitch, Deputy Commissioner, FDA.

47 Wolfe, S.M. (9 March, 8 April 1982). Petitions from Director, Public Citizens' Health Research Group, to the FDA as quoted in *Public Citizen Health Research Group v. Commissioner, Food & Drug Administration,* 740 F.2d 21 (D.C. Cir. 1984).

48 Federal Food, Drug, and Cosmetic Act, 21 USC (United States Code), §352 (1938).

49 *Public Citizen Health Research Group v. Commissioner, Food & Drug Administration,* 740 F.2d 21 (D.C. Cir. 1984).

50 Clayton, J.M. (12 March 1982). A blank "Dear Doctor" form letter from Vice President, Clinical Research, Plough, Inc., to physicians.

51 American Academy of Pediatrics. Committee on Drugs. (8 March 1982). Minutes of meeting in Alexandria, Virginia, 5–6 March 1982.

52 Strain, J.E. Report to the Executive Board on Academy Affairs by Vice President of the American Academy of Pediatrics James E. Strain, included as Appendix 1 in minutes of Executive Board Meeting, Maui, Hawaii, 15–18 March 1982.

53 ibid.

54 Sterling Drug, Inc., Bristol-Myers Co., The Dow Chemical Co., & Monsanto. (13 April 1982). Comments to the FDA on "Meeting on Reye's Syndrome". [Meeting attended by Sterling, Bristol Meyers, Dow, Monsanto, and the FDA].

55 *Public Citizen Health Research Group v. Commissioner, Food & Drug Administration,* 740 F.2d 21 (D.C. Cir. 1984).

56 deCourcy Hinds, M. (28 April 1982). Aspirin linked to children's disease. *New York Times* (p. 67).

57 American Academy of Pediatrics, Committee on Infectious Diseases. Draft minutes of meeting, Washington, DC, 10 May 1982.

58 US Food and Drug Administration. (24 May 1982). *Scientific workshop on Reye's syndrome and its possible association with salicylate use* [Transcript]. Held at the National Institutes of Health, Bethesda, Maryland.

59 Waldman, R.J., Hall, W.N., McGee, H., & Van Amburg, G. (11 June 1982). Aspirin as a risk factor in Reye's syndrome. *Journal of the American Medical Association, 247* (22), 3089–3094.

60 Halpin, T.J., Holtzhauer, F.J., Campbell, R.J., Hall, L.J., Correa-Villaseñor A., Lanese, R., Rice, J., & Hurwitz, E.S. (13 August 1982). Reye's syndrome and medication use. *Journal of the American Medical Association, 248* (8), 687–691.

61 U.S Food and Drug Administration. (24 May 1982). *Scientific workshop on Reye's syndrome and its possible association with salicylate use* (p. 41) [Transcript]. Held at the National Institutes of Health, Bethesda, Maryland.

62 Starko, K.M. (3 June 1982). Letter to Harry M. Meyer. [Business letter from Medical Epidemiologist, Bureau of Disease Control, Maricopa County Health Department to Director, Bureau of Biologics, FDA].

Chapter 23 – Stand Don't Walk, Late 1982

1   Minutes of Executive Board meeting, Itasca, Illinois, 18–20 June 1982.

2   Committee on Infectious Diseases, Fulginiti, V.A., Brunell, P.S., Cherry, J.D., Ector, W.L., Gershon, A.A., Gotoff, S.P., Hughes, W.T., Mortimer, E.A., & Peter, G. (1 June 1982). Special report. Aspirin and Reye's syndrome. *Pediatrics, 69* (6), 810–812.

3   Strain, J.E. (June 1982). Interim Report of the Executive Committee by President-Elect of the American Academy of Pediatrics James E. Strain, included as Appendix 15 in the minutes of Executive Board Meeting, Itasca, Illinois, 18–20 June 1982.

4   Wilson, J.T., & Brown, R.D. (June 1982). Reye syndrome and aspirin use: The role of prodromal illness severity in the assessment of relative risk. *Pediatrics, 69* (6), 822–825.

5   Wilson, J.T., Brown, R.D., Bocchini, J.A., & Kearns, G.L. (June 1982). Efficacy, disposition and pharmacodynamics of aspirin, acetaminophen and choline salicylate in young febrile children. *Therapeutic Drug Monitoring, 4* (2), 147–180.

6   ibid.

7   US Food and Drug Administration. (4 June 1982 4). *HHS News.* [Press release].

8   Millenson, M.L. (7 November 1982). Consumers turn to aspirin after Tylenol poisonings. *Chicago Tribune* (p. N3).

9   Mann, C.C., & Plummer, M.L. (1991). *The aspirin wars: Money, medicine, and 100 years of rampant competition* (p. 291). Harvard Business School Press.

10 Trueman, C.N. (15 May 2015). *Blitzkrieg.* The History Learning Site. Retrieved 3 April 2022.

11 deCourcy Hinds, M. (5 June 1982). Warning issued on giving aspirin to children. *New York Times.*

12 OSU Research, Ohio State University. (5 June 1982). Link between aspirin and Reye's syndrome discounted. [Press release].

13 Bianchine, J.R., Alexander, M.S., Andresen, B.D., & Ng, K.J. (December 1982). The aspirin/Reye's syndrome link [Letter to the editor]. *Lancet, 320* (8311), 1333.

14 Reye's Foundation talks about care, treatment. (19 July 1982). *Bryan Times* (p. 3).

15 United Press International. (6 June 1982). Aspirin tie to rare children's diseases disputed; warning called premature. *Arizona Republic.*

16 Ringuette, A.L. (September 1988). Joseph M. White. [Vignette.]. *Regulatory Toxicology and Pharmacology, 8* (3), 376–378.

17 United Press International. (12 January 1985). Makers of aspirin endorse warning: Manufacturers agrees to label telling of risks of Reye's syndrome in children. *New York Times* (p. 26).

18 United Press International. (6 June 1982). Aspirin tie to rare children's diseases disputed; warning called premature. *Arizona Republic.*

19 Attorneys for Plough, Inc., & Sterling Drug, Inc. (22 June 1982). Reye syndrome and salicylates. Memorandum to Department of Health and Human Services.

20   Patterson, F.T. (8 July 1982). Minutes of meeting. [Minutes by the Office of General Counsel, FDA, of meeting attended by FDA staff and industry representatives].

21   Reye's Foundation talks about care, treatment. (19 July 1982). *Bryan Times.*

22   Freudenberger, J. (spring 1982). Presidential notes. *National Reye's Syndrome Foundation in the News, 6*, 2.

23   Boyd, L. (fall 1982). National Reye's Syndrome Foundation opens Washington office. *National Reye's Syndrome Foundation in the News, 6*, 3.

24   Mathias, B.J. (1982). Public awareness: The first step toward early diagnosis. *Journal of the National Reye's Syndrome Foundation, 3* (1), 2–10.

25   ibid.

26   ibid.

27   RS Working Group. (1 July 1982). Reye syndrome and salicylates: A spurious association. *Pediatrics, 70* (1), 158–160.

28   Reye's foundation talks about care treatment. (19 July 1982). *Bryan Times.*

29   Horwitz, N. (14 July 1982). House panel probes aspirin-Reye's warning. *Medical Tribune.*

30   Krushat, W.M. (22 July 1982). Further analysis of the data pertaining to the reported association between salicylate use and Reye's syndrome. Memorandum from mathematical statistician, Division of Biometrics, Food and Drug Administration, to Stanley A. Edlavitch, FDA.

31   deCourcy Hinds, M. (25 July 1982). Food and Drug Administration says some risk must be accepted. [Interview with Arthur Hull Hayes, Jr, FDA commissioner.] *New York Times.*

32   US Food and Drug Administration. (August 1982). Salicylate labeling may change because of Reye's syndrome. *FDA Drug Bulletin, 12* (2), 1, 9.

33   Biometrics Research Institute. (20 August 1982). *Review of the Ohio Department of Health case-control study of Reye's syndrome. Phase I review.* [Report prepared for Glenbrook Laboratories, Inc., and Schering-Plough].

34   Temko, S.L. (31 August 1982). Letter to Juan del Real, General Counsel, Department of Health and Human Services, enclosing a draft protocol for a cooperative Case/Control Study on Reye's Syndrome.

35   Starko, K.M. (25 August 1982). Letter to Mary Magsitza. [Business letter from Medical Epidemiologist, Bureau of Disease Control, Maricopa County Health Department to Sterling Drug, indicating enclosure of copy of draft manuscript].

36   Gelb, B.S. (7 September 1982). Letter to Richard S. Schweiker. [Business letter from President, Consumer Products Group, Bristol-Myers Company, to Secretary of Health and Human Services].

37   Orlowski, J.P. (2, 3 September 1982). Business letters to Monroe Trout. [Business Letters from Assistant Director, Pediatric and Surgical ICU, The Cleveland Clinic Foundation, to Senior Vice President, Sterling Drug, Inc.].

38   Quinnan, G.V. (15 September 1982). Memorandum from Director, Division of Virology, FDA, to Harry M. Meyer, Director of the National Center for Drugs and Biologics, FDA.

39   Lucey J. (17 September 1982). Letter to Karen M. Starko. [Business letter from Editor, *Pediatrics*, to Medical Epidemiologist, Bureau of Disease Control, Maricopa County Health Department].

40   Mortimer, E.A. (7 October 1982 7). Letter to Jerald Lucey. [Business letter from Elisabeth Severance Prentiss Professor of Community Health and Pediatrics, School of Medicine, Case Western Reserve University to Editor, *Pediatrics*].

41   Lucey, J. (11 October 1982). Letter to Ted Mortimer. [Business letter from Editor, *Pediatrics,* to Elisabeth Severance Prentiss Professor of Community Health and Pediatrics, School of Medicine, Case Western Reserve University, to Editor, *Pediatrics*].

Notes

42 Jonah Shacknai. (14 November 2021). In *Wikipedia.*

43 *Reye's syndrome: Hearing before the Subcommittee on Natural Resources, Agriculture Research, and Environment of the Committee on Science and Technology,* US House of Representatives, Ninety-seventh Congress, second session. (17, 29 September 1982). US Government Printing Office [published in 1983].

44 Pear, R. (September 1982). Schweiker assails curb on Medicare. Opposes tying aid to need—Seeks warning on Reye's syndrome and aspirin. *New York Times.*

45 Pippert, W.G. (20 September 1982). United Press International article describing plans of Health Secretary Schweiker to warn parents that giving aspirin to children with flu or chickenpox could lead to Reye's syndrome.

46 ibid.

47 ibid.

48 ibid.

49 ibid.

50 ibid.

51 ibid.

52 Fulginiti, F.A. (28 September 1982). Letter to the author. [Business letter from the Head of the Department of Pediatrics, University of Arizona Health Sciences Center to the Medical Epidemiologist, Bureau of Disease Control, Maricopa County Health Department].

53 Starko, K.M. (February 1983). Aspirin consumption and severity of Reye's syndrome [Letter to the editor]. *Pediatrics, 71* (2), 293–295.

54 La Montagne, J.R. (November 1983). From the National Institute of Allergy and Infectious Diseases: Summary of a workshop on disease mechanisms and prospects for prevention of Reye's syndrome. *Journal of Infectious Diseases, 148* (5), 943–950.

55 Bishop, J.E. (28 September 1982). Aspirin makers fight national test of link with a children's disease. *Wall Street Journal.*

56 *Reye's syndrome: Hearing before the Subcommittee on Natural Resources, Agriculture Research, and Environment of the Committee on Science and Technology, US House of Representatives,* Ninety-seventh Congress, second session. (17, 29 September 1982). US Government Printing Office (published in 1983), p. 94.

57 Beck, M., Monroe, S., Prout, L.R., Hagar, M., & LaBreque R. (11 October 1982). The Tylenol Scare. *Newsweek* (p. 32).

58 Mullen, W. (23 October 1983). The Hunt. *Chicago Tribune.*

59 Mullen, W. (2 October 1983). The Hunt. *Chicago Tribune.*

60 Beck, M., Monroe, S., Prout, L.R., Hagar, M., & LaBreque, R. (11 October 1982). The Tylenol Scare. *Newsweek* (p. 32).

61 Mullen, W. (2 October 1983). The Hunt. *Chicago Tribune.*

62 Beck, M., Monroe, S., Prout, L.R., Hagar, M., & LaBreque, R. (11 October 1982). The Tylenol Scare. *Newsweek* (p. 32).

63 ibid. p. 36.

64 Changes in packages for drugs possible to deter tampering. (4 October 1982). *Wall Street Journal.*

65 Beck, M., Monroe, S., Prout, L.R., Hagar, M., & LaBreque, R. (11 October 1982). The Tylenol Scare. *Newsweek* (p. 36).

66 Millenson, M.L. (21 November 1982). J&J gains admiration, strength. *Chicago Tribune.*

67 ibid.

68 Millenson, M.L. (7 November 1982 7). Consumers turn to aspirin after Tylenol poisonings. *Chicago Tribune.*

Chapter 24 – Keep Parents in the Dark, Late 1982

1   *Public Citizen Health Research Group v. Commissioner, Food & Drug Administration*, 740 F.2d 21 (D.C. Cir. 1984). Refers to letter from James C. Morrison to Sidney M. Wolfe, M.D. (4 October 1982) [at 2, JA 20], that FDA labeled a "second interim response" and that indicated that publication had been delayed pending review by the Office of Management and Budget pursuant to Executive Order 12291.

2   Miller, T. (31 March 1984). The O.M.B. writes a prescription. *The Nation*, 383–385.

3   deCourcy Hinds, M. (5 June 1982). Warning issued on giving aspirin to children. *New York Times*.

4   US Food and Drug Administration, Department of Health and Human Services. (28 December 1982). 21 CFR Part 201 (Docket No. 82N-0158): Labeling for salicylate-containing drug product. II. Educational activities. *Federal Register, 47* (249), 57897.

5   US Food and Drug Administration, Department of Health and Human Services. (1982). Reye's syndrome. [Brochure, HHS Publication No. (FDA) 82-3126].

6   School Awareness Bulletin. (October 1982). Reye's syndrome information.

7   Abramowicz, M. (6 October 1982). Letter to Karen M. Starko requesting review of preliminary draft of article on aspirin and Reye syndrome for *The Medical Editor*. [Business letter from Editor, *The Medical Letter*, to Medical Epidemiologist, Bureau of Disease Control, Maricopa County Health Department].

8   Starko, K.M. (26 October 1982). Letter to Mark Abramowicz with comments on preliminary draft of article on aspirin and Reye syndrome for *The Medical Editor*. [Business letter from Medical Epidemiologist, Bureau of Disease Control, Maricopa County Health Department, to Editor, *The Medical Letter*].

9   Shacknai, J. (15 October 1982). Aspirin and the danger of childhood disease. *Wall Street Journal*.

10 Starko, K.M. (21 October 1982). Letter to Jerold Lucey. [Business letter from Medical Epidemiologist, Bureau of Disease Control, Maricopa County Health Department, to Editor, *Pediatrics*].

11 Brown, R.D. & Wilson, J.T. (February 1983) Aspirin consumption and severity of Reye's syndrome [Letter to the editor]. *Pediatrics, 71* (2), 293–294.

12 Starko, K.M. (February 1983). Aspirin consumption and severity of Reye's syndrome [Letter to the editor]. *Pediatrics, 71* (2), 294–295.

13 Aspirin-Reye's syndrome linkage termed tenuous. (October 1982). *Hospital Practice* (p. 50M).

14 ibid.

15 American Academy of Pediatrics (11 November 1982). Minutes of Executive Board meeting in New York City, NY, 27 October 1982.

16 ibid.

17 James Strain of Denver, Colorado; Paul F. Wehrle of Los Angeles, California; Richard M. Narkewicz of South Burlington, Vermont; James G. Lione of Little Neck, New York; Arthur Maron of West Orange, New Jersey; Martin H. Smith of Gainesville, Georgia; William C. Montgomery of Detroit, Michigan; Edmond C. Burke of Rochester, Minnesota; William A. Daniel of Birmingham, Alabama, Donald W. Schiff of Littleton, Colorado; and Birt Harvey of Palo Alto, California.

18 Starko, K.M. (10 November 1982). Letter to the editor of *Lancet*. [Business letter from Medical Epidemiologist, Bureau of Disease Control, Maricopa County Health Department to Editor, *Lancet*].

19 Munro, I. (29 November 1982). Letter to Karen M. Starko. [Business letter from Editor, *Lancet* to Medical Epidemiologist, Bureau of Disease Control, Maricopa County Health Department].

20 DeMuth, C.C. (June 2020). Curriculum vitae. Retrieved 12 January 2022, from https://ccdemuth.com/wp-content/uploads/2020/10/DeMuth-CV-June-2020.pdf

21 Miller, T. (31 March 1984). The O.M.B. writes a prescription. *The Nation*, 383–385.

Notes

22 Prager, D.J. (n.d.). Biographical information. Retrieved 13 January 2022, from Strategic Consulting Services at http://foundationimpact.com/about-denis-prager/

23 Miller, T. (31 March 1984). The O.M.B. writes a prescription. *The Nation,* 383–385.

24 ibid.

25 Conner, P. (25 August 1985). Stalling for time. *San Francisco Chronicle.*

26 Committee on Infectious Diseases, Fulginiti, V.A., Brunell, P.S., Cherry, J.D., Ector, W.L., Gershon, A.A., Gotoff, S.P., Hughes, W.T., Mortimer, E.A., Peter, G., & Plotkin S.A. (November 1982). "Red Book" Update. *Pediatrics, 70* (5), 819–822.

27 Miller, T. (31 March 1984). The O.M.B. writes a prescription. *The Nation,* 383–385.

28 Seagram, A. (29 September 2021). Email to Karen M. Starko. [Business letter from the Archivist, American Academy of Pediatrics].

29 Jennisen, M.H. (10 November 1982). Letter and attached Reye's syndrome statement from the American Academy of Pediatrics Executive Board, written on behalf of Dr James Strain to Edward N. Brandt. [Business letter from Executive Director, AAP, on behalf of the President of the AAP, to the Assistant Secretary for Health, Department of Health and Human Services].

30 deCourcy Hinds, M. (12 November 1982). Volunteer labeling plan begun on aspirin products. *New York Times* (p. 20).

31 American Academy of Pediatrics. (1982). HHS reconsiders aspirin labeling, plans new research. *News and Comment, 34,* 1–3.

32 *Public Citizen Health Research Group v. Commissioner, Food & Drug Administration,* 740 F.2d 21 (D.C. Cir. 1984).

33 Committee on the Care of Children. (16 November 1982). [Press release].

34 Heinz F. Eichenwald (Dallas, Texas), John Baum (Rochester, New York), Harvey L. Chernoff (Boston), Joseph Fitzgerald (Indianapolis, Indiana), Burton H. Harris (Boston), Robert A. Hoekelmann (Rochester, New York), David J. Lang (Baltimore, Maryland), James P. Orlowski (Cleveland, Ohio) and Consultant Sidney Gellis (Boston)

35 Miller, T. (31 March 1984). The O.M.B. writes a prescription. *The Nation,* 383–385.

36 ibid.

37 Associated Press. (19 November 1982). Aspirin-warning hinges on new studies. *Arizona Republic.*

38 *Public Citizen Health Research Group v. Commissioner, Food & Drug Administration,* 740 F.2d 21 (D.C. Cir. 1984). Refers to resignation letter of former committee chairman Dr Edward A. Mortimer, Jr, to Dr James E. Strain (17 November 1982) [JA 251]. Retrieved 24 November 2021.

39 US Department of Health and Human Services. (18 November 1982). [Press release].

40 Associated Press. (19 November 1982). Aspirin-warning hinges on new studies. *Arizona Republic.*

41 US Department of Health and Human Services. (18 November 1982). [Press release].

42 Jennisen, M.L. (19 November 1982). Letter and attached statement of the American Academy of Pediatrics, written on behalf of Dr James Strain to Richard S. Schweiker. [Business letter from Executive Director, AAP, on behalf of President of the AAP, to Secretary, Department of Health and Human Services].

43 deCourcy Hinds, M. (12 November 1982). Volunteer labeling plan begun on aspirin products. *New York Times.*

44 ibid.

45 US Food and Drug Administration. (16 November 1982). Reye's Syndrome and aspirin update. *Talk Paper,* T82–80.

46 Cobb, W.Y. (17 November 1982). Memorandum that included FDA's *Talk Paper,* Reye's syndrome and aspirin update.

47 Edlavitch, S.A. (23 November 1982). Memorandum from Chief of Epidemiology Development Branch, Division of Drug Experience, National Center for Drugs and Biologics, FDA, to Paul Fehnel. FDA.

48 Barker, E.F. (23 November 1982) Memorandum from Acting Group Leader, Neurology/Analgesics Group, FDA to Paul Fehnel, Assistant Director for Regulatory Affairs, Bureau of Drugs, FDA.

49 Judge seeks aspirin accord. (November 1982). *New York Times*.

50 Soumerai, S.B., Ross-Degnan, D.R., Kahn, J.S. (2008). The effects of professional and media warnings about the association between aspirin use in children and Reye's syndrome. In: R.S. Hornick (ed.), *Public health communication. Evidence for behavior change* (p. 275). Lawrence Erlbaru Associates. [Original published in 2002].

51 Hornick R.C. (2002). *Public health communication. Evidence for behavior change* (p. 275). Lawrence Erlbaum Associates.

52 Hurwitz, E.S. & Goodman, R.A. (December 1982). A cluster of cases of Reye syndrome associated with chickenpox. *Pediatrics, 70*(6), 901–906.

53 Starko, K.M. (7 December 1982). Note to Ted Mortimer. [Business communication Medical Epidemiologist, Bureau of Disease Control, Maricopa County Health Department, to Elisabeth Severance Prentiss Professor of Community Health and Pediatrics, School of Medicine, Case Western Reserve University].

54 Department of Health and Human Services, Food and Drug Administration. (28 December 1982). 21 CFR Part 201 (Docket No. 82N-0158): Labeling for Salicylate-Containing Drug products., *Federal Register, 47*(249), 57886–57901. [Advance notice of proposed rulemaking].

Chapter 25 – Delay, Delay, Delay, 1983–1986

1   Eichenwald, H.F. (28 February 1983). Letter to colleagues. [Business letter from Chairman, Coordinating Committee, Committee on the Care of Children, to colleagues].

2   Heckler, Margaret M. Retrieved 15 March 2022, from History, Art & Archives, US House of Representatives.

3   Shilts, R. (1987). *And the Band Played On* (p. 233). St Martin's Press.

4   Head of Consumer Affairs assesses first year on job. (30 January 1983). *New York Times* (p. 22).

5   *Public Citizen Health Research Group v. Commissioner, Food & Drug Administration*, 740 F.2d 21 (D.C. Cir. 1984).

6   The American Public Health Association. (February 1985). New data support aspirin-Reye's Link; questions on labeling delay continue. *The Nation's Health*, 1.

7   *Public Citizen Health Research Group v. Commissioner, Food & Drug Administration*, 740 F.2d 21 (D.C. Cir. 1984).

8   *Public Citizen Health Research Group v. Young*, 909 F.2d 546, 285 US App. D.C. 307 (D.C. Cir. 1990).

9   Horwitz, N. (26 January 1983). "HHS is waffling" on aspirin-Reye's. *Medical Tribune*.

10 *Emergency Reye's Syndrome Prevention Act of 1985: Hearings before the Subcommittee on Health and the Environment of the Committee on Energy and Commerce, House of Representatives*, 99th Congress. (15 March 1985). Serial No. 99-26. pp. 704–707.

11 Rensberger, B. (6 November 1984). FDA attacks pro-aspirin ad. *Washington Post*.

12 ibid.

13 Associated Press. (19 November 1982). Aspirin-warning hinges on new studies. *Arizona Republic*.

14 *Public Citizen Health Research Group v. Commissioner, Food & Drug Administration*, 740 F.2d 21 (D.C. Cir. 1984).

15 Rensberger, B. (6 November 1984). FDA attacks pro-aspirin ad. *Washington Post*.

16 ibid.

17 *Emergency Reye's Syndrome Prevention Act of 1985: Hearings before the Subcommittee on Health and the Environment of the Committee on Energy and Commerce, House of Representatives,* 99th Congress. (15 March 1985). Serial No. 99-26. pp. 644–648, Neil L. Chayet letter to Henry A. Waxman.

18 *Emergency Reye's Syndrome Prevention Act of 1985: Hearings before the US House of Representatives Subcommittee on Health and the Environment of the Committee on Energy and Commerce,* 99th Cong. (15 March 1985). Serial No. 99-26, p. 545.

19 Soumerai, S.B., Ross-Degnan, D.R., Kahn, J.S. (2008). The effects of professional and media warnings about the association between aspirin use in children and Reye's syndrome. In: R.S. Hornick (ed.), *Public health communication. Evidence for behavior change* (p. 273). Lawrence Erlbaru Associates. [Original published in 2002].

20 US Food and Drug Administration, Public Service Announcements (PSAs). (1980s). *Historical PSAs—Reye's syndrome.* [PSAs]. Retrieved 15 March 2022, from YouTube at https://www.youtube.com/results?search_query=FDA+history+and+Reye+Syndrome+PSAs

21 Soumerai, S.B., Ross-Degnan, D.R., Kahn, J.S. (2008). The effects of professional and media warnings about the association between aspirin use in children and Reye's syndrome. In: R.S. Hornick (ed.), *Public health communication. Evidence for behavior change* (p. 273). Lawrence Erlbaru Associates. [Original published in 2002].

22 ibid. p. 276.

23 Rensberger, B. (6 November 1984). FDA attacks pro-aspirin ad. *Washington Post.*

24 Soumerai, S.B., Ross-Degnan, D.R., Kahn, J.S. (2008). The effects of professional and media warnings about the association between aspirin use in children and Reye's syndrome. In: R.S. Hornick (ed.), *Public health communication. Evidence for behavior change* (p. 168). Lawrence Erlbaru Associates. [Original published in 2002].

25 Ads by aspirin group criticized. (6 November 1984). *New York Times.*

26 Rensberger, B. (6 November 1984). FDA attacks pro-aspirin ad. *Washington Post.*

27 *Emergency Reye's Syndrome Prevention Act of 1985: Hearings before the Subcommittee on Health and the Environment of the Committee on Energy and Commerce, House of Representatives,* 99th Congress. (15 March 1985). Serial No. 99-26. p. 292, written testimony.

28 Freudenburger, J. (Fall 1984). President's notes. *NRSF in the News.*

29 Starko, K.M. & Mullick, F.G. (12 February 1983). Hepatic and cerebral pathology findings in children with fatal salicylate intoxication: Further evidence for a causal relation between salicylate and Reye's syndrome. *Lancet, 321* (8320), 326–329.

30 You, K. (8 July 1983). Salicylate and mitochondrial injury in Reye's syndrome. *Science, 221* (4606), 63–65.

31 Younkin, S.W., Betts, R.F., Roth, F.K., & Douglas, R.G. (April 1983). Reduction in fever and symptoms in young adults with influenza A/Brazil/78 H1N1 infection after treatment with aspirin or amantadine. *Antimicrobial Agents and Chemotherapy, 23* (4), 577–582.

32 *Emergency Reye's Syndrome Prevention Act of 1985: Hearings before the Subcommittee on Health and the Environment of the Committee on Energy and Commerce, House of Representatives,* 99th Congress. (15 March 1985). Serial No. 99-26. p. 566, copy of *Medical Tribune* report titled "NIH, Japanese studies fail to back aspirin-Reye's tie."

33 Seabrook C. (3 February1984). CDC cites decrease in Reye's syndrome, *Atlanta Constitution.*

34 Pollack, J.D. (ed.). (1985). Reye's Syndrome IV. Proceedings of the Fourth International Conference on Reye's Syndrome. 21–22 June 1984. *Journal of the National Reye's Syndrome Foundation, 5.*

35 ibid.

36 Kannel, W.B, Sorlie, P., & McNamara, P.M. (July 1979). Prognosis after initial myocardial infarction: The Framingham study. *American Journal of Cardiology, 44*(1), 53–59.

37 Aspirin Myocardial Infarction Study Research Group. (15 February 1980). A randomised controlled trial of aspirin in persons recovered from myocardial infarction. *Journal of the American Medical Association, 243*(7), 661–669.

38 Lewis, H.D., Davis, J.W., Archibald, D.G., Steinke, W.E., Smitherman, T.C., Doherty, J.E., Schnaper, H.W., LeWinter, M.M., Linares, E., Pouget, J.M., Sabharwal, S.C., Chesler, E., & DeMots, H. (18 August 1983). Protective effects of aspirin against acute myocardial infarction and death in men with unstable angina. Results of a Veterans' Administration cooperative study. *New England Journal of Medicine, 309*(7), 396–403.

39 Mann, C.C., & Plummer, M.L. (1991). *The aspirin wars: Money, medicine, and 100 years of rampant competition* (pp. 205–309). Harvard Business School Press.

40 Hurwitz, E.S, Barrett, M.J., Bregman, D., Gunn, W.J., Schonberger, L.B., Fairweather, W.R., Drage, J.S., LaMontagne, J.R., Kaslow, R.A., Burlington, D.B., Quinnan, G.V., Parker, R.A., Phillips, K., Pinsky, P., Dayton, D. & Dowdle, W.R. (3 October 1985). Public Health Service study on Reye's syndrome and medications. Report of the pilot phase. *New England Journal of Medicine, 313*(14), 849–857.

41 Division of Viral Diseases, Center for Infectious Diseases, Centers for Disease Control, & the Reye Syndrome Task Force. (11 January 1985). Reye Syndrome—United States, 1984. *Morbidity and Mortality Weekly Report, 34*(1), 13–16.

42 Boffey, P.M. (9 January 1985). Study reported to tighten link of aspirin and Reye's syndrome. *New York Times*.

43 ibid.

44 Holtzhauer, F. (February 1985). Re: Reye's and ethical conduct [Letter to editor]. *Epidemiology Monitor, 6*, 6–7.

45 Mortimer, E.A. (19 January 1994). Letter to Donald Francis. [Elisabeth Severance Prentiss Professor Emeritus, School of Medicine, Case Western Reserve University to physician (author's husband), Genentech, Inc.].

46 Division of Viral Diseases, Center for Infectious Diseases, Centers for Disease Control, & the Reye Syndrome Task Force. (11 January 1985). Reye Syndrome—United States, 1984. *Morbidity and Mortality Weekly Report, 34*(1), 13–16.

47 Mrs. Heckler Urging syndrome warning as an aspirin label. (10 January 1983). *New York Times* (p. 14).

48 Soumerai, S.B., Ross-Degnan, D.R., Kahn, J.S. (2008). The effects of professional and media warnings about the association between aspirin use in children and Reye's syndrome. In: R.S. Hornick (ed.), *Public health communication. Evidence for behavior change* (p. 277). Lawrence Erlbaru Associates. [Original published in 2002].

49 Boffey, P.M. (9 January 1985). Study reported to tighten link of aspirin and Reye's syndrome. *New York Times*.

50 Soumerai, S.B., Ross-Degnan, D.R., Kahn, J.S. (2008). The effects of professional and media warnings about the association between aspirin use in children and Reye's syndrome. In: R.S. Hornick (ed.), *Public Health Communication. Evidence for Behavior Change* (p. 275). Lawrence Erlbaru Associates. [Original published in 2002].

51 Flu season—aspirin warnings out. (11–13 January 1985). *USA Today*.

52 United Press International. (24 January 1985). Warning to go on aspirin labels. *New York Times*.

Chapter 26 – In the Best Interest of Children, 1986

1 National Institute on Aging, US Department of Health and Human Services. (1985). What to do about flu. [Educational notice]. US Government Printing Office.

2 Emergency Reye's Syndrome Prevention Act of 1985, H.R.1381, S.538. (28 February 1985). Retrieved 15 March 2022, from GovTrack.

Notes

3   ibid.

4   *Emergency Reye's Syndrome Prevention Act of 1985: Hearings before the US House of Representatives Subcommittee on Health and the Environment of the Committee on Energy and Commerce*, 99th Cong. (15 March 1985). Serial No. 99-26, pp. 275–708.

5   ibid. p. 277.

6   ibid. pp. 283–284.

7   ibid. p. 284.

8   ibid. p. 287.

9   ibid. pp. 310–311.

10   ibid. p. 316

11   ibid. pp. 316–319.

12   ibid. pp. 326–328.

13   ibid. p. 414.

14   ibid. pp. 414–417.

15   ibid. p. 545.

16   ibid. pp. 639–640.

17   ibid. p. 518.

18   ibid. pp. 644–647.

19   ibid. p. 678.

20   ibid. p. 663.

21   ibid. p. 654.

22   Soumerai, S.B., Ross-Degnan, D., & Kahn, J.S. (2008). The effects of professional and media warnings about the association between aspirin use in children and Reye's syndrome. In R.S. Hornick (ed.), *Public health communication. Evidence for behavior change* (p. 277). Lawrence Erlbaru Associates, Publishers. (Original work published 2002).

23   FDA orders aspirin warning. (10 February 1986). *Medical World News* (p. 48).

24   *Public Citizen Health Research Group v. Young*, 909 F.2d 546, 285 US App. (D.C. Cir. 1990). Case argued February 9, 1990 and decided July 31, 1990. No. 89-5055.

25   Hurwitz, E.S., Barrett, M.J., Bregman, D., Gunn, W.J., Schonberger, L.B., Fairweather, W.R., Drage, J.S., LaMontagne, J.R., Kaslow, R.A., Burlington, D.B., Quinnan, G.V., Parker, R.A., Phillips, K. Pinsky, P., Dayton, D., & Dowdle, W.R. (3 October 1985). Public Health Service study on Reye's syndrome and medications. Report of the pilot phase. *New England Journal of Medicine, 313* (14), 849–857.

26   *Public Citizen Health Research Group v. Young*, 909 F.2d 546, 285 US App. (D.C. Cir. 1990). Case argued 9 February 1990 and decided 31 July 1990. No. 89-5055.

27   FDA orders aspirin warning. (10 February 1986). *Medical World News*.

28   US Food and Drug Administration. (17 April 2003). Labeling for oral and rectal over-the-counter drug products containing aspirin and nonaspirin salicylates; Reye's syndrome warning. *Federal Register, 68* (74), 18861–18869.

29   US Food and Drug Administration. (7 March 1986). Labeling for oral and rectal over-the-counter aspirin and aspirin-containing drug products. *Federal Register, 51* (45), 8180–8182.

30   Around the world: Britain halts the sale of children's aspirin. (11 June 1986). *New York Times*.

31   Rodger, I. (1986). Withdrawal of aspirin products for children. *Financial Times*.

32   Meikle, F. (23 October 2002). Government bans aspirin for under-16s. *Guardian*.

33   Hurwitz, E.S,. Barrett, M.J., Bregman, D., Gunn, W.J., Pinsky, P,. Schonberger, L.B., Drage, J.S., Kaslow, R.A., Burlington, D.B., Quinnan, G.V., LaMontagne, J.R., Fairweather, W.R., Dayton, D., & Dowdle, R.R. (10 April 1987). Public Health Service study of Reye's syndrome and medications. Report of the main study. *Journal of the American Medical Society, 257* (14),1905–1911.

34 Forsyth, B.W., Horwitz, R.I., Acampora, D., Shapiro, E.D., Viscoli, C.M., Feinstein, A.R., Henner, R., Holabird, N.B., Jones, B.A., Karabelas, A.D.E., Kramer, M.S., Miclette, M., & Wells, J.A. (5 May 1989). New epidemiologic evidence confirming that bias does not explain the aspirin/Reye's syndrome association. *Journal of the American Medical Association, 261* (17), 2517–2524.
35 ibid.

Afterword

1   Pinsky, P.F., Hurwitz, E.S., Schonberger, L.B., & Gunn, W. (1988). Reye's syndrome and aspirin: Evidence for dose-response effect. *Journal of the American Medical Association, 260*(5), 657–661.
2   Chu, A.B., Nerurkar, L.S., Witzel, N., Andresen, B.D., Alexander, M., Kang, E.S., Brouwers, P., Fedio, P., Lee, Y.J., & Sever, J.L. (1 October 1986). Reye's syndrome: Salicylate metabolism, viral antibody levels, and other factors in surviving patients and unaffected family members. *American Journal of the Diseases of Children, 140*(10), 1009–1012.
3   Rennebohm, R.M., Heubi, J.E., Daugherty, C.C., Daniels, S.R. (December 1985) Reye syndrome in children receiving salicylate therapy for connective tissue disease. *Journal of Pediatrics, 107*, 877–880.
4   Arrowsmith, J.B., Kennedy, D.L., Kuritsky, J.N., & Faich, G. (1987). National patterns of aspirin use and Reye syndrome reporting, United States, 1980 to 1985. *Pediatrics, 79*(6), 858–863.
5   Belay, E.D., Bresee, J.S., Holman, R.C., Khan, A.S., Shahriari, A., & Schonberger, L.B. (May 1999). Reye's syndrome in the United States from 1981 through 1997. *New England Journal of Medicine, 340*(18), 1377–1382.
6   Russell, C. (12 February 1982). Children with chickenpox, flu should not use aspirin US says. *Washington Post.*
7   Soumerai, S.B., Ross-Degnan, D., & Kahn, J.S. (2008). The effects of professional and media warnings about the association between aspirin use in children and Reye's syndrome. In R.S. Hornick (ed.), *Public health communication. Evidence for behavior change* (p. 285). Lawrence Erlbaru Associates, Publishers. (Original work published 2002).
8   Rahwan, G.L., & Rahwan, R.G. (1986). Aspirin and Reye's syndrome: The change in prescribing habits of health professionals. *Annals of Pharmacotherapy, 20*(2), 143–145.
9   Belay, E.D., Bresee, J.S., Holman, R.C., Khan, A.S., Shahriari, A., & Schonberger, L.B. (May 1999). Reye's syndrome in the United States from 1981 through 1997. *New England Journal of Medicine, 340*(18), 1377–1382.
10 Glasgow, J.F.T. (2006). Reye's syndrome. The case for a causal link. *Drug Safety, 29*(12), 1111–1121.
11 Committee on Safety of Medicines. (June 1986). CSM update: Reye's syndrome and aspirin. *British Journal of Medicine, 292*(6535), 1590.
12 Hall, S.M., Plaster, P.A., Glasgow, J.F.T., & Hancock, P. (July 1988). Preadmission antipyretics in Reye's syndrome. *Archives of Disease in Childhood, 63*(7), 857–866.
13 Glasgow, J.F.T. (2006). Reye's syndrome. The case for a causal link. *Drug Safety, 29*(12), 1111–1121.
14 Davis, D.L. & Buffler, P. (24 October 1992). Reduction of deaths after drug labelling for risk of Reye's syndrome [Letter to the editor]. *Lancet, 340*(8826), 1042
15 Doyle, L. (31 May 1987). Aspirin and deadly Reye's syndrome: warning can be missed. *LA Times.*
16 US Food and Drug Administration. (4 February 2020 4). Rulemaking history for OTC internal analgesic drug products. Retrieved 29 November 2021, from the Food and Drug Administration.

Notes

17 Swann J., & Ottes R.T. (12 November 1997) Oral history interview of J. Richard Crout. [FDA Historian interview of former, Director, Bureau of Drugs, FDA.]. Retrieved 29 November 2021, from the Food and Drug Administration.

18 US Food and Drug Administration. (23 November 2021). Over-the-Counter (OTC) drug review | OTC monograph reform in the CARES Act. Retrieved 29 November 2021, from the Food and Drug Administration.

19 Hurwitz, E.S. (2 December 1988 2). The changing epidemiology of Reye's syndrome in the United States: Further evidence for a public health success. *Journal of the American Medical Association, 260*(21), 3178–3180.

20 Rowe, P.C., Valle, D., & Brusilow, S.W. (1988). Inborn errors of metabolism in children referred with Reye's syndrome. A changing pattern. *Journal of the American Medical Association, 260*(21), 3167–3170.

21 Hurwitz, E.S. (2 December 1988). The changing epidemiology of Reye's syndrome in the United States: further evidence for a public health success. *Journal of the American Medical Association, 260*(21), 3178–3180.

22 Morgan, G. (5 May 2008 5). Copy of original handwritten line listing of data extracted from patient charts by J. Baral and G. Morgan provided to the author.

23 Baral, J. (6 June 2009). Oral presentation by Dr Jacob Baral, guest of honor and key speaker, National Reye's Syndrome Foundation's 35th Annual Meeting held in Columbus, Ohio. [Oral presentation]. Retrieved 29 September 2021, from YouTube at https://www.youtube.com/watch?v=Repw3pJyj0M

24 National Reye's Syndrome Foundation. (2011). Thanks to the FDA & NRSF "Baby Aspirin" Does Not Exist Anymore! *In the News, 37*(2).

25 Hochberg F.H., Nelson, K., & Janzen W. (24 February 1975). Influenza type B-related encephalopathy. *Journal of the American Medical Association, 231* (8), 817–821.

25 Solomons G., Markman C., & West E.J. (1953). Measles encephalitis. *Pediatrics, 11,* 473–479.

Appendix 1

1 Lucas, W.P. (1923). *Children's diseases for nurses* (p. 541). The MacMillan Company.

2 For a 6-month-old infant, one-half grain (30 mg) and for a 1-year-old, 1 grain (60 mg), to be given every 4 hours. In Marriott, W.M. (1930). *Infant nutrition*. The C.V. Mosby Company.

3 Nelson, W.E., (ed.) (1950). *Mitchell-Nelson textbook of pediatrics* (5th ed., pp. 222–224). W.B. Saunders Company.

4 Hoffman W.S. (1953). Pitfalls of acetylsalicylic acid medication. *American Journal of Diseases of Children, 85,* 58.

5 Riley, H.D., & Worley, L. (October 1956). Salicylate intoxication. *Pediatrics, 18*(4), 578–594.

6 Wehrle, P.J. (1964) Influenza. In Gellis, S.S., & Kagan, B.M. (eds) *Current pediatric therapy*. W.B. Saunders Company.

7 Shirkey, H.C. (ed.) (1964). *Pediatric therapy*. The C.V. Mosby Company p. 125 and 1059.

8 Tainter, M.L., & Ferris, A.J. (1969). *Aspirin in modern therapy. A review.* Bayer Company Division of Sterling Drug Inc.

9 Vaughan, V.C., McKay, R.J., & Nelson, W.E. (eds). (1975). *Nelson Textbook of Pediatrics* (10th edition, pp. 1445–1446). W.B. Saunders Company.

10 US Food and Drug Administration, Department of Health, Education, and Welfare. (8 July 1977). Over-the-counter drugs. Establishment of a monograph for OTC internal analgesic, antipyretic, and antirheumatic products. *Federal Register, 42* (131), 2 of 2 books, p. 35368.

11 Flower R.J., Moncad S., & Vane J.R. (1980). Analgesic-antipyretics and anti-inflammatory agents; drugs employed in the treatment of gout. In L.S. Goodman and

A. Gilman (eds). *The pharmacological basis of therapeutics* (6th ed., pp. 95–697). The Macmillan Publishing Company, Inc.

12   Dalen J.E. (2006). Aspirin to prevent heart attack and stroke: what's the right dose? *American Journal of Medicine, 119* (3), 198–202.

Appendix 2

1   Luscombe, F.A., Monto, A.S., Baublis, J.V. (1980) Mortality due to Reye's syndrome in Michigan: Distribution and longitudinal trends. *Journal of Infectious Diseases* 142, 363–371.

2   Davis, D.L., & Buffler, P. (24 October 1992). Reduction of deaths after drug labelling for risk of Reye's syndrome [Letter to the editor]. *Lancet, 340* (8826), 1042.

Appendix 3

1   Sullivan-Bolyai, J.Z. & Corey, L. (1981). Epidemiology of Reye syndrome. *Epidemiologic Reviews, 3*, 1–26.

2   Davis, D.L., & Buffler, P. (24 October 1992). Reduction of deaths after drug labelling for risk of Reye's syndrome. [Letter to the editor]. *Lancet, 340* (8826), 1042.

3   Sullivan-Bolyai, J.Z., Marks, J.S., Johnson, D., Nelson, D.B., Holtzhauer, F., Bright F., Kramer, T., & Halpin, T.J. (1980). Reye syndrome in Ohio, 1973–1977. *American Journal of Epidemiology, 112*, 629–638. (See also: Nelson, D.B., Sullivan-Bolyai, J.Z., Marks, J.S., Morens, D.M., & Schonberger, L., Ohio State Department of Health Reye's Syndrome Investigation Group. (1979). Reye syndrome: an epidemiologic assessment based on national surveillance 1977–1978 and a population-based study in Ohio, 1973–1977. In Crocker, J.S. (ed.) *Reye's Syndrome II*. Grune and Stratton, 33–49.)

4   Hurwitz, E.S., Nelson, D.B., Davis, C., Morens, D., & Schonberger, L.B. (1982). National surveillance for Reye's syndrome: a five-year review. *Pediatrics, 70*, 895–900.

5   Hurwitz, E.S, Barrett, M., Rogers, M., & Schonberger, L.B. (1984). Grade I Reye's syndrome. [Letter to editor]. *New England Journal of Medicine, 310*,128–129.

6   Sullivan-Bolyai, J.Z., Marks, J.S., Johnson, D., Nelson, D.B., Holtzhauer, F., Bright, F., Kramer, T., & Halpin, T.J. (1980). Reye syndrome in Ohio, 1973–1977. *American Journal of Epidemiology, 112*, 629–638.

7   Hurwitz, E.S., Nelson, D.B., Davis, C., Morens, D., & Schonberger, L.B. (1982). National surveillance for Reye's syndrome: a five-year review. *Pediatrics, 70*, 895–900.

8   Luscombe, F.A., Monto, A.S., & Baublis, J.V. (1980). Mortality due to Reye's syndrome in Michigan: Distribution and longitudinal trends. *Journal of Infectious Diseases, 142*, 363–371.

9   Lichtenstein, P.K., Heubi, J.E., Daugherty, C.C., Farrell, M.K., Sokol, R.J., Rothbaum, R.J., Suchy, F.J., & Balistreri, W.F. (1983). A frequent cause of vomiting and liver dysfunction after varicella and upper-respiratory-tract infection. *New England Journal of Medicine, 309,* 133–139.

Appendix 4

1   Danks, D.M. (10 October 1987). Reye's syndrome and aspirin. [Letter to editor.]. *Lancet, 330* (8563), 864.

2   Newgreen, D.B. (February 1998). *Review of non-prescription analgesics.* Report prepared for the Therapeutic Goods Administration.

3   Orlowski, J.P., Gillis, J., & Kilham, H.A. (November 1987). A catch in the Reye. *Pediatrics, 80* (5), 638–642.

4   ibid.

5   Cullity, G.J., & Kalulas, B.A. (1970). Encephalopathy and fatty degeneration of the viscera: An evaluation. *Brain, 93* (1), 77–88.

6   Largent, M. (2015). *Keep out of reach of children. Reye's syndrome, aspirin, and the politics of public health* (pp. 186–200). Bellevue Literary Press.

Notes

7   James, S. (April 2004). *Review of aspirin/Reye's syndrome warning statement.* Report prepared for the Medicines Evaluation Committee, Department of Health and Aging, Therapeutic Goods Administration.

8   Orlowski, J.P. Gillis, J., & Kilham, H.A. (November 1987). A catch in the Reye. *Pediatrics, 80* (5), 638–642.

9   James, S. (April 2004). *Review of aspirin/Reye's syndrome warning statement.* Report prepared for the Medicines Evaluation Committee, Department of Health and Aging, Therapeutic Goods Administration.

10 Jeffreys, D. (2005). *Aspirin: The remarkable story of a wonder drug aspirin* (p. 207–209). Bloomsbury.

11 The acetaminophen molecule—Tylenol. (n.d.). Retrieved 13 January 2022, from World of Molecules.

12 Jeffreys, D. (2005). *Aspirin: The remarkable story of a wonder drug aspirin* (p. 209). Bloomsbury.

13 Glasgow, J.F.T. (2006). Reye's syndrome: A case for a causal link with aspirin. *Drug Safety, 29* (12), 1111–1121.

14 History of Tylenol. (n.d.). McNeil Consumer Healthcare Company Worldwide Consumer Pharmaceutical Intranet Site Content. Retrieved 4 November 2021, from http://www.nancywest.net/pdfs/McNeilConsumerHealthcareCompany.pdf

15 Arrowsmith, J.B., Kennedy, D.L., Kuritsky, J.N., & Faich, G.A. (June 1987). National patterns of aspirin use and Reye syndrome reporting, United States, 1980 to 1985. *Pediatrics, 79* (6), 858–863.

Appendix 5

1   Starko, K.M., Ray, C.G., Dominguez, L.B., Stromberg, W.L., & Woodall, D.F. (1980). Reye's syndrome and salicylate use. *Pediatrics, 66* (6), 859–864.

2   Waldman, R.J., Hall, W.N., McGee, H., & Van Amburg, G. (11 June 1982). Aspirin as a risk factor in Reye's syndrome. *Journal of the American Medical Association, 247* (22), 3089–3094.

3   Halpin, T.J., Holtzhauer, F.J., Campbell, R.J., Hall, L.J., Correa-Villaseñor A., Lanese, R., Rice, J., & Hurwitz, E.S. (13 August 1982). Reye's syndrome and medication use. *Journal of the American Medical Association, 248* (8), 687–691.

4   Waldman, R.J., Hall, W.N., McGee, H., & Van Amburg, G. (11 June 1982). Aspirin as a risk factor in Reye's syndrome. *Journal of the American Medical Association, 247* (22), 3089–3094.

5   Partin, J.S., Partin, J.C., Schubert, W.K., & Hammond, J.G. (23 January 1982). Serum salicylate concentrations in Reye's disease. A study of 130 biopsy-proven cases. *Lancet, 319* (8265), 191–194.

6   Hurwitz, E.S., Barrett, M.J., Bregman, D., Gunn, W.J., Schonberger, L.B., Fairweather, W.R., Drage, J.S., LaMontagne, J.R., Kaslow, R.A., Burlington, D.B., Quinnan, G.V., Parker, R.A., Phillips, K., Pinsky, P., Dayton, D. & Dowdle, W.R. (3 October 1985). Public Health Service study on Reye's syndrome and medications. Report of the pilot phase. *New England Journal of Medicine, 313* (14), 849–857.

7   Hurwitz, E.S., Barrett, M.J., Bregman, D., Gunn, W.J., Pinsky, P., Schonberger, L.B., Drage, J.S., Kaslow, R.A., Burlington, D.B., Quinnan, G.V., LaMontagne, J.R., Fairweather, W.R., Dayton, D., & Dowdle, R.R. (10 April 1987). Public Health Service study of Reye's syndrome and medications. Report of the main study. *Journal of the American Medical Association, 257* (14),1905–1911.

8   Forsyth, B.W., Horwitz, R.I., Acampora, D., Shapiro, E.D., Viscoli, C.M., Feinstein, A.R., Henner, R., Holabird, N.B., Jones, B.A., Karabelas, A.D.E., Kramer, M.S., Miclette, M., & Wells, J.A. (5 May 1989). New epidemiologic evidence confirming that bias does not explain the aspirin/Reye's syndrome association. *Journal of the American Medical Association, 261* (17), 2517–2524.

Index

Index

Index

Index

Index